Praise for *It's Not Mental*

"I was starved for a book from another parent who really gets what we are going through. Ms. Wolfson's research on seemingly unconnected symptoms and solutions has helped put her daughter's life back together. This is a story that raises expectations and validates persistence." *Darryl Kilsdonk, CABF (Child and Adolescent Bipolar Foundation) volunteer and board moderator*

"My husband and I have been riding the same roller coaster for many years, and it has definitely taken its toll. Only someone who has been through this hell can relate to the visual of 'blowing one's brains out.' This book gives me hope for a better tomorrow." *Gloria Burd, mother of two young adult children with biological brain disorders*

"Psychiatrists, psychiatric nurses, therapists, and ancillary staff working in direct patient care of the 'mentally ill' should be required to read this book as a precondition of employment." *K. P. Gail, R.N., psychiatric nurse*

"It's Not *Mental* depicts the true horrors parents go through in attempting to get medical treatment for their children. I relived my own struggles as a parent of a child with a disability. It should be required reading for every first-year medical student. It's time to change mental health care in our country and simply call it 'health care'—period!" *gg Burns, advocate and instructor of NAMI's Family-to-Family programs*

"Every doctor needs to read this book. They need to move beyond looking at one symptom or one test. Patients need collaborative care." *Kay Davis, medical technologist*

"The story is very interesting, moving, and gripping; combining observations, emotions, and references to research when appropriate. I love the sidebars, especially the comments from a psychiatric nurse." *Martha Hellander, Co-Founder of CABF (Child and Adolescent Bipolar Foundation)*

It's Not *Mental*

Finding innovative support and medical treatment for a
child diagnosed with a severe mental illness

◊

Jeanie Wolfson

◊

Foreword by
Robert Fredericks, M.D.

Cerebella Publishing
2010

It's Not Mental—Finding innovative support and medical treatment for a child diagnosed with a severe mental illness

Copyright © 2010 by Jeanie Wolfson

This book was written purely to convey one family's journey of discovery and learning that led to the road of recovery for one child. No information in this book is meant to offer medical advice to any other family. The publication of this book does not constitute the practice of medicine, nor is it to be used as a replacement for a physician, pharmacist, or other health care professional. You are advised to consult with the appropriate health care practitioner about any and all health care decisions regarding prescription and non-prescription medications, vitamins, food supplements, exercise, diet, and other forms of therapy.

All rights reserved. Printed in the United States of America. No part of this book may be used or reproduced in any manner whatsoever without written permission except in the case of brief quotations embodied in critical articles and reviews. For more information, contact:

Cerebella Publishing
http://www.cerebellapublishing.com

Publisher's Cataloging-in-Publication Data

It's not mental: finding innovative support and medical treatment for a child diagnosed with a severe mental illness / Wolfson, Jeanie.

Includes biographical references and index.

ISBN 978-0-9828052-0-6

Library of Congress Control Number: 2010938258

1. subject- medical / psychiatry / child & adolescent
2. subject- biography / medical
3. subject- parenting

Acknowledgments

I thank my editor, Susan Owens, and my mentor, Neil Chethik, for helping turn my initial ramblings into a real manuscript fit for publishing. All errors are mine alone.

This book would never have been written without the encouragement and support from an army of friends and family, including those from my NAMI and CABF families. You know who you are—Angelina, Beth, Bob, Cat, Darryl, David, Gail, Gina, Gloria, Janice, Jenny, Joan, Kay, Kelly, Madonna, Mama Faye, Martha, Michele, Phill, Preeti, Rachel, Roberta, Sheyna, Valerie . . . the list goes on.

I especially want to thank my brothers, Sam, Mark, and John, and my parents, Herb and Sylvia, for giving me a shoulder to cry on during the early years and for putting up with my tirades in the later years.

I thank my daughters for their trust and confidence in me, even when I lacked it in myself. And to my son-in-law, Philip—your technical expertise and support have been invaluable.

K.P. Gail . . . I will be ever grateful for your patient reading, encouragement, and reading some more . . . and for making me stop for our long walks.

As for my husband, Greg, thank you for bringing my coffee every morning, putting together dinners when I didn't want to stop working, and finally dragging me out of my chair when enough was enough. I'd be remiss not to mention my furred and feathered friends who kept me company and also made sure I got up and out whether I wanted to or not—Mugsy, Chieena, Bumper, and Chloe.

And not a day goes by that I do not think of those who rooted for me in life: my vivacious aunt, Maggie, and my loving mother, Doris.

Cover Design, Brittany Thompson and Chris Walls.

Back Cover Art, Original photo by Ele Peavy. Painting by Angelles LaVeau, Angelles Art International, LLC. Used with permission.

This book is dedicated to my two mothers,
Sylvia and Doris

and to my two daughters,
Candace and Kerachel

Dor L' Dor

Table of Contents

Foreword 13

Introduction 17

In the Beginning Birth through Age Two 23

    CHAPTER 1 − DIFFERENT FROM BIRTH 25
    CHAPTER 2 − BABYSITTER SATISFACTION AND AWFUL ALLERGIES 41
    CHAPTER 3 − DAY CARE DILEMMA 51

The Calm Ages Three to Nine 61

    CHAPTER 4 − MUSIC AND MONTESSORI MANIA 63
    CHAPTER 5 − MONTESSORI MADNESS AND SCALPEL SUCCESS 75
    CHAPTER 6 − THE LITTLE SCHOOLHOUSE ON THE PRAIRIE 81
    CHAPTER 7 − WRITING WOES AND DEALING WITH DEATH 89

Before Ages Nine to Ten and a Half 95

    CHAPTER 8 − SCHOOL SCRUTINY 97
    CHAPTER 9 − TIC ... TIC ... TIC 103
    CHAPTER 10 − DEPRESSION 107
    CHAPTER 11 − GETTING ON THE ROLLER COASTER 111
    CHAPTER 12 − SOCIALLY SECURE AND SPREADING HER WINGS 117
    CHAPTER 13 − A NEW PSYCHIATRIST, A FRESH LOOK 121
    CHAPTER 14 − RITUALS AND ROUTINES 129

The Brewing Storm Ages Ten and a Half to Twelve 137

    CHAPTER 15 − ALL SEEMS WELL 139
    CHAPTER 16 − MAYBE NOT SO WELL 149
    CHAPTER 17 − WHAT THE . . . ??? 155

Hell Age Twelve 171

    CHAPTER 18 − BLINDSIDED 173
    CHAPTER 19 − AT THE HOSPITAL 177
    CHAPTER 20 − AT HOME 183
    CHAPTER 21 − MONSTERS 189
    CHAPTER 22 − OF SISTERS AND SPIDERS 197

Darkness Ages Twelve to Thirteen 201
 CHAPTER 23 – ON THE FAR SHORES 203
 CHAPTER 24 – THE ROLLER COASTER THROUGH DARKNESS 209
 CHAPTER 25 – OUR MARRIAGE, OUR DEPRESSION 215

The Long Tunnel Ages Thirteen to Sixteen 227
 CHAPTER 26 – DETERMINATION 229
 CHAPTER 27 – THE BOO-BOO MOBILE 235
 CHAPTER 28 – MEDICATIONS AND FOOD SUPPLEMENTS 239
 CHAPTER 29 – HIGH SCHOOL 243
 CHAPTER 30 – DASHED DREAMS 255
 CHAPTER 31 – THE ENDOCRINOLOGIST WHO COULD HAVE (BUT DIDN'T) 259
 CHAPTER 32 – SURVIVING SCHOOL 263

Light at Tunnel's End Ages Sixteen to Nineteen and a Half 267
 CHAPTER 33 – LOOKING TO THE FUTURE 269
 CHAPTER 34 – A SERVICE DOG FOR KERI 275
 CHAPTER 35 – FINDING ANSWERS 283
 CHAPTER 36 – COLLEGE 293

Sunshine Ages Nineteen to Twenty-one 301
 CHAPTER 37 – ENDOCRINE TREATMENTS 303
 CHAPTER 38 – INTEGRATED TREATMENT 317
 CHAPTER 39 – SLEEP 327
 CHAPTER 40 – A LIFE RESTORED 333

Epilogue 343

Appendix A: The Thyroid Connection 359
Appendix B: Medical Tests 365
Appendix C: Charting Symptoms 377
Appendix D: Preparing for Doctor Visits 379

Photos 385

References 391
 BOOKS 391
 MUSIC, POEMS 397

Index 399

A Note from Keri 405

List of Tables

Table 1: Useful Lessons from Year One 38
Table 2: Characteristics: Prenatally, at Birth, and During the First Year ...39
Table 3: Characteristics: Ages 12 to 24 Months 49
Table 4: Useful Lessons from the Toddler Years 59
Table 5: Characteristics: Age 2 60
Table 6: Characteristics: Ages 3 to 6 80
Table 7: Additional Characteristics: Age 7 88
Table 8: Characteristics: Age 8 94
Table 9: Characteristics: Age 9 110
Table 10: Glitches in the Hypothalamic-Pituitary-Adrenal Axis 127
Table 11: Diagnoses: Age 10 134
Table 12: Characteristics: Age 10 135
Table 13: A Non-Medical Explanation of the Differences between Bipolar Disorder with Psychotic Features, Schizophrenia, and Schizoaffective Disorder 167
Table 14: Characteristics: Age 11 169
Table 15: Comparison of Seventh- and Eighth-Grade CTBS Scores 208
Table 16: Diagnoses: Ages 12 to 12½ 223
Table 17: Chronology of Symptoms and Drug Regimen: Ages 12 to 12½ 224
Table 18: Medication History Chart: Ages 12 to 12½ 225
Table 19: Diagnoses: Ages 12½ to 16 265
Table 20: Characteristics, Problems, and Chronology: Ages 12½ to 16..266
Table 21: How a Well-Trained Dog Can Help at Home 282
Table 22: Possible Signs of Hypothyroidism 284
Table 23: Some of the Puzzle Pieces at Age 16½ 288
Table 24: Summary of Medical Issues (for college) 295
Table 25: Summary of Service Dog's Public Tasks (for college) 296
Table 26: Diagnoses: Ages 16 to 20 300
Table 27: Tests: Diagnoses with Neuropsychiatric Symptoms 366
Table 28: Tests for an Endocrine Workup 370
Table 29: Tests: Adrenal Function 371
Table 30: Tests: Bone Metabolism 372
Table 31: Tests for Medication Side Effects: Glucose 373
Table 32: Tests of Metabolic & Mitochondrial Health 375
Table 33: Charting Key Symptoms 378
Table 34: Symptom History Chart 380

List of Figures

Figure 1: Pituitary—The Master Gland 125
Figure 2: Good Day Math Sample 204
Figure 3: Bad Day Math Sample...204
Figure 4: Sample of a Daily Journal..211
Figure 5: Typed Summary for Doctor 212
Figure 6: Plan from Doctor 213
Figure 7: Hypothalamic-Pituitary-Thyroid Axis......................................312

Foreword

When Jeanie Wolfson contacted me regarding her daughter, Keri, then age 16, she was searching for answers. Like many of my patients, Keri was beset by a diverse array of health issues. Several of her symptoms suggested a physical cause, but based on her behaviors, emotional lability, and hallucinations, her illness had been diagnosed as mental. Treatment, for the most part, was constrained by the procedures and assumptions of America's health care system for patients termed mentally ill. However, Keri's family was unwilling to ignore the possibility that underlying medical issues, including endocrine factors, could be causing at least some of their daughter's symptoms.

The fact that Keri's parents found it so difficult to obtain effective medical care for her—a fresh look at her case with in-depth testing—in my opinion reveals a malaise in our technologically based system of health care. Instead of broadening possibilities for understanding and treatment of the individual, the manner in which technology is applied today often limits such possibilities. The answers many people receive as to "what ails them" forces them into one or more standardized boxes, often with the poor fit that comes from a one-size-fits-all approach.

The question of the moment for the health insurance industry seems to be: How can we most appropriately use advances in technology to resolve the problems in our lives? There's nothing wrong with this question; after all, technology has made possible medical advances undreamed of even a generation ago. However, before computers can be given the authority to make decisions regarding our needs and wants, we must be certain they are capable of understanding who we are—not as targets for the marketing of treatments, no matter how revolutionary, but as complex individuals with unique medical profiles.

Without this recognition of the differences between people, the application of digital technology to our social systems leaves us feeling like the enemy in a war directed against the sense of self. Instead of being understood, we are fragmented and standardized. Falling by the wayside may be the ethical obligation to treat the patient as an individual case.

Writing from a physician's point of view, we encounter difficulty when the application of our efforts is inconsistent with our expectations. The ensuing discord is experienced as stress, and we search for a means to explain the events that challenge our sense of security. A common strategy is to dismiss the situation as an unimportant aberration, taking solace in the exception proving the rule. It is better, perhaps, to state that the exception *frames* the rule, seeing the exception as contrasting with the expectation. Albert Einstein is often quoted as having said, "What does a fish know of water?" Only in leaving the water to explore the terrestrial environment does it becomes evident that the sea is a special case, with the challenges of leaving it in need of clarification.

Practicing medicine applies our experience from a multitude of cases while developing the understanding needed to explain our observations. We feel secure when the outcomes confirm our expectations. We then attempt to engage the principles learned to make predictions on which to base future actions. This process serves to continually refine the assumptions and applications of our ideology.

Cases that do not conform to expectations are considered difficult. In cases such as Keri's, in which diagnostic labels are applied using subjective symptoms according to a manual—a task that can be accomplished without consideration of complexity while selecting from the plethora of data available relating to individual physiology—doctors may become so enmeshed in a failing ideology they fail to recognize that "difficult cases" are the source of the insights required to rectify the system. Ideology must be consistent with reality; otherwise, it gets in the way of solving the problem. Difficult cases force the recognition of the inadequacies of a strategy. As such, they are often resented by the defenders of flawed ideologies.

Managing human health requires us to adjust our approach consistent with the observations of human variance. Refining our understanding of complexity as the foundation of addressing variance is fostered by paying attention to those cases that expose our ignorance. Our ideologies are always simplified when compared to reality; thus, we need new ways of thinking that capture the complexity of disruptions in adaptation to environment that compromise health. When it becomes possible to engage the seemingly ambiguous and conflicting data derived from pragmatic experience with difficult cases, we sense progress has been made, and we are rewarded for engaging the curiosity and compassion so necessary for comprehensive, effective health care for all.

Success in this venture should lead to resolution of cases considered difficult while acquiring the knowledge necessary to avoid perpetuating the mistakes unrecognized in those patients enjoying the innate complexity to compensate for them. If difficult cases are considered to be on the fringe, then as in textiles, careful study of that fringe permits a more detailed and appropriate understanding of the cloth as a whole. Attention to difficult cases promises to benefit all.

Robert Fredericks, M.D.

Dr. Robert Fredericks is a practicing endocrinologist and Medical Director of the Center for the Advancement of Structural Ecology.

Introduction

One night, my daughter Keri was whipped. Over and over, the lash struck her back, arms, and legs. As she felt her skin shredding, she screamed in agony.

The whipping was a hallucination; there were no visible scars. Yet my preteen daughter felt the same pain and was as wrecked emotionally as one might expect a lashed child to be.

~~~~~~~~~~~

Scientists do not know what caused the mix of clinical symptoms that unfolded in my daughter's life, some of them manifesting themselves as early as her birth, but when my husband, Greg, and I first held our beautiful baby girl, there was no clue as to how complex her care was going to be.

As an infant, Keri slept only in small bursts and sometimes screamed as if in pain. She also was excessively startled by sounds, and she didn't want strangers to look at her. The pediatrician told us not to worry; Keri's behavior was within the normal spectrum of infancy. After turning a year old, however, her symptoms escalated, leading us to our first visits with medical specialists and later into the mental health care system.

Doctors tossed around many labels for Keri's increasingly bizarre symptoms in the years to follow: colic, migraines, allergies, night terrors, highly gifted, learning disabled (LD), gifted-LD, major depressive disorder (MDD), obsessive-compulsive disorder (OCD), Tourette syndrome (TS), attention deficit hyperactivity disorder (ADHD), sensory integration (processing) dysfunction (SID/SPD), bipolar disorder, psychosis-NOS (not otherwise specified), schizoaffective disorder, constitutional delay, delayed menarche, fibromyalgia, chronic fatigue syndrome, Kleine-Levin syndrome, narcolepsy, and more. Still, some of her problems went undiagnosed for far too long, with devastating repercussions.

The medical and psychiatric professionals who knew Keri best—her pediatricians, psychiatrists, psychologists, and therapist—said her symptoms of depression, and later, mood swings and hallucinations, were of a physiological (biological/physical) nature and not due to a psychological problem. She did not have disciplinary or emotional issues causing out-of-control or attention-seeking behavior. Neither were her severe symptoms manifestations of maladaptive coping strategies adopted as a result of some traumatic life event.

In the meantime, our beautiful young daughter was struggling with a complex medical mystery affecting both body and brain. As this mystery grew, she was given escalating diagnoses of what we refer to collectively as "mental illness."

Being labeled with a mental illness shut doors for Keri. It was a stigma that caused misunderstanding in all areas of her life—especially in doctors' offices. *Mental* meant her problems were emotional, or behavioral, or both. *Mental* meant she needed better parenting. *Mental* meant she was not really sick. Even worse, *mental* meant she had already been given a diagnosis. And once a diagnosis existed, why should anyone look past it to discover and treat what truly ailed her?

As parents, we accepted Keri's various mental-illness diagnoses and tried to help her live a full life in spite of them. We still made occasional forays into the medical health field, but our requests for tests were rebuffed and our concerns, as well as those of our daughter, her pediatrician, and her psychiatrist, were cavalierly dismissed. Confused by the rift between the *mental* and the *medical,* we found ourselves at an impasse. For nearly a decade we made no progress in understanding or treating our daughter's slowly escalating physical malaise.

When Keri was very young, she was a bright child who was kind, caring, responsible, and creative, but she also was a child who spent countless hours either screaming and crying, or immobilized with pain or fear. As a result, her life was limited, her body was deteriorating, and her illness, whatever it was, was progressing largely untreated. Just as she turned 12, it stripped her of her sanity, and almost of her life, as she plunged into psychosis. But as Keri herself pointed out, psychosis is a symptom, not a cause. *What was the cause?*

The cause, we were told, was called schizoaffective disorder, a diagnosis that falls somewhere in severity between bipolar disorder and schizophrenia, with symptoms of both. Childhood-onset schizophrenia (COS), I discovered when I began to read about it, is a very serious disease from which we could anticipate difficult-to-treat symptoms, cognitive deterioration, extensive hospitalizations, and disruptions to normal childhood development.

Though psychoactive drugs could not restore Keri to her previous level of functioning, they did help to control the worst of the psychosis and mood swings. With a semblance of stability, she was considered in the recovery stage of mental illness. Keri accepted her new physical and mental limitations, but she was also a fighter. She was determined to accomplish much, to improve her lot in life, and to retain hope for a better future. Greg and I put in a support system to assist her.

Psychological therapies and a loving, supportive home helped her adapt to her physiology and to overcome the inevitable psychological trauma resulting from her illness. A psychiatric/medical-assist service dog increased her confidence and independence. But the fact remained that the manifestations of her illness were no more mental than those of a person suffering from thyroid hormone imbalance, narcolepsy, or multiple sclerosis.

Then, when Keri was 16, word-of-mouth led us to two medical doctors who changed our lives. They did what the other medical specialists had been loath to do: They ran extensive batteries of tests, and they ordered a sleep study. The test results showed very real physical problems that were affecting Keri's body and brain, and which, in turn, were influencing her thoughts, emotions, perceptions, and behavior.

Ultimately, my daughter's fate was not determined by a specific set of diagnoses or prognoses, nor by the esoteric debates of schizophrenia researchers far removed from the case of this one particular child. Rather, Keri benefited most from an understanding of the underlying physiology of *her* particular set of symptoms. Only then were we able to determine how best to assist her individual biology in an integrative, functional, biomedical manner—emotionally, nutritionally, dietetically, hormonally, immunologically, supportively, therapeutically, and pharmacologically.

Keri's case truly blurs the line between what we call a mental illness and what we term a medical condition. Some doctors argue that if a patient's symptoms are ameliorated through a non-psychiatric approach, i.e., by improving physical health via medical, biomedical, functional, and/or nutritional means, then a psychiatric diagnosis is inappropriate. Others insist that alleviation of symptoms with a medical approach simply means the patient's medical, nutritional, and/or hormonal needs, etc., *are*, collectively, their mental illness.

Regardless of how an individual's symptoms are ameliorated, or whether we call those symptoms a mental illness or a neurobiological disorder (a biological/medical problem affecting the brain), treatment must be designed to meet each person's unique needs.

Keri had a good home life. She was psychologically healthy. These facts neither prevented nor treated her mental illness. Later, we put in place psychiatric treatments to stabilize her and help her to recover. These treatments neither prevented nor treated the deterioration of her body. Missing was a program of sane, medically oriented treatments designed to prevent further deterioration of, and to help heal, both mind and body.

My now adult daughter is a successful college student with a bright future. With two college degrees already under her belt, she is going for another in dietetics, a medical-related field near and dear to her heart. After all, she has a personal connection with the prerequisites in biology, physiology, and nutrition.

This book is a story of the impact Keri's illness has had on her and on our family. Greg and I learned the hard way that parents need to take control of their children's medical/psychiatric care in a way we did not, until it was almost too late. Inasmuch as the lessons we learned may be applicable to the circumstances of another, I have attempted to offer insights into coping with the problems of a severely ill child and of ultimately becoming the child's advocate, including a review of lessons learned about navigating the convoluted maze of the medical/mental health care system. But ultimately, this is a story of concern, fear, denial, and mourning that led to a story of acceptance, hope, and wonder.

It is my sincere wish that others traveling similar paths may gain insight, ideas, inspiration, solace, and hope from reading this book. Most of the story is told from my perspective as a mother, but I've also included other viewpoints, such as words of wisdom from "Psych Nurse," a registered nurse (R.N.) with 13 years of experience at the local state psychiatric hospital, as well as thoughts from Keri herself. Keri is a bright, articulate young woman with deep insight into her own neurobiology. She is also the heroine of this tale.

In the Beginning

Birth through Age Two

I love your body
    As I love my own.

Not just your curly hair,
    Nor chubby hand within my own,

But in that I want your body
    To have no pain,
        Feel no hurt,
            Be relaxed and loved,

And I want the person within,
    To feel the same.

— Jeanie

Chapter 1
Different from Birth

I stood in the doorway to my baby daughter's room, listening to her screams, determined to compose myself. I loved my daughter fiercely, yet I had visions of picking her up and throwing her across the room. The image was simultaneously horrifying and cathartic. If I added my screams to hers, would they intertwine and rise to the heavens like a prayer for relief? With love overpowering everything, I knew I needed to compose myself before I entered the room.

I took a long, deep breath through my nose, expanding my abdomen and using my diaphragm to fill my lungs. Then, holding the tip of my tongue to the roof of my mouth directly behind my front teeth, I exhaled slowly, completely. I repeated this favorite relaxation technique over and over, releasing more tension with each cycle until I felt calm. Images of serenity entered my mind. Fully relaxed, I could now give my full attention, love, and care to the wailing infant who was merely responding instinctively to some need only she could feel.

I would never act on the horrifying thoughts that went through my mind on this occasion and many others. I felt profound shame for even having them. In contrast, I basked in the glow of good fortune. I had a supportive, caring husband who adored me. I had a job that had allowed me to pay off my car loan and save money before the birth of this beautiful, deeply wanted baby girl. Candace, our older daughter, was smart, fun-loving, and compassionate—I called her our sunshine daughter. She was so happy to be a big sister. My life was good, or so it seemed.

~~~~~~~~~~~

My pregnancy had been a joyful time. I was 30 years old and ready to be a mother to a second child.

One of my best friends, Sophie, married to my brother John, was pregnant at the same time. Sophie and John lived just minutes away. My father, Herb, and my stepmom, Sylvia, lived in another city, but they also leant their support. To help Sophie and me prepare, they had each of us pick out a plush, La-Z-Boy rocker-recliner as a comfortable nursing chair.

At the end of my first trimester, I contracted chicken pox. (It was still some years before a chicken pox vaccine would be available.) I had a low-grade fever, but I never got very sick. Instead, my pampered two weeks away from work felt like a vacation. My obstetrician and pediatrician, however, were both concerned about the baby's well-being. The chicken pox virus resides in nerves and can later cause a painful condition called shingles. The doctors prepared us for the possibility our baby might be born with this condition. They weren't really sure what to expect.

To further complicate matters, I was suffering from severe allergic rhinitis, which caused back-to-back respiratory infections. Normally I took antihistamines and decongestants to control my allergies, but I'd stopped taking these medications for the first two trimesters of my pregnancy. Despite wearing a pollen/dust mask religiously when I was out of doors, I was chronically sick, necessitating repeated doses of antibiotics. Finally, during the last trimester of pregnancy, I resumed the antihistamines. My obstetrician, allergist, and pediatrician, after a three-way consultation, concluded this was a safer course of action—for baby and mother alike.

At the end of my pregnancy there was another complication. The baby was in breech position and her head was quite large. She was not dropping. Delivery by Cesarean section was medically necessary. Sylvia flew in to support me.

Our baby girl was born full-term on a sunny autumn day in 1987, weighing in at a perfect 8 pounds, 2 ounces (3.7 kg). We named her Keri. My brain, awash with maternal hormones, declared her to be the most beautiful, perfect baby in the world. Her feel, her smell, even her cry evoked my love. I had no problem supplying breast milk, and she nursed heartily from the start. She was alert, gazing up into our faces. Candace, the proud big sister, loved cradling the baby tenderly in her arms.

Greg and I, stepmom Sylvia, and even the doctors breathed a collective sigh of relief. In spite of being exposed to chicken pox, repeated infections, antibiotics, and antihistamines; having a large head; being in breech position; and being born via C-section, Keri appeared to be just fine. My father, however, remained concerned, though at the time he kept those concerns to himself. Dad is an intelligent person, an astute observer, and a lover of science. He'd done extensive reading on how perinatal complications and disorders, including viral infections, can affect the brain of a fetus, increasing the risk of psychiatric problems later in life. Today, scientists think the mother's own immune response might affect the baby's brain development.[1]

> The hormone oxytocin, released by the mother during normal labor, may help protect the baby's brain from hypoxic or hypoglycemic insult (low oxygen or glucose, respectively) and act as a "switch" to change the way an important neurohormone, gamma-aminobutyric acid (GABA) functions. C-section babies may not get that infusion of oxytocin that switches GABA function.
>
> An impaired GABA transmitter system is implicated in a range of disorders affecting the brain, including epilepsy, bipolar disorder, schizophrenia, Alzheimer's disease, anxiety, depression, and Down syndrome.
>
> Brown, et al., 2007; Busko, 2007; Lee, et al., 2007; Obreitan, et al., 2002; Tyzio, et al., 2006.

Dad learned that C-sections can slightly increase the odds of the baby's still-developing brain being affected on a molecular level. And then there was the genetic factor: Both of Keri's biological grandmothers had been afflicted by schizophrenia-like brain disorders.

---

[1] Smith, et al., 2007.

Had my father voiced his concerns to me at the time of Keri's birth, I would have scoffed, yet much of what he'd learned turned out to be relevant. Furthermore, what we didn't know then was that *the mother's* extensive use of antibiotics during pregnancy, which—without the countering effect of probiotics—depletes the normal flora (bacteria) in the gut, would someday be theorized as contributing to inflammation, immune dysfunction, malabsorption issues, and brain disorders in the baby.

To care for our growing family, I was able to take a three-year leave of absence from my job as a computer software developer with IBM, retain our family's health insurance, and still maintain my position with the company. I also had the option to resume my job part-time while on leave, or to end my leave early and return to work full time. I was not at all stressed by finances, a rocky marriage, a lack of emotional support, anxiety, or depression. When my baby was alert and happy, I was in heaven. But because she soon proved to be such a high-needs, extremely sensitive baby and cried so much, I often felt like a prisoner being subjected to some perverse form of torture.

Greg worked hard as an engineer, fixing high-tech scientific equipment. Although most of his work was local, he was sometimes on the road for several days, traveling to various medical, research, and commercial facilities. When he was home, he helped at night by changing Keri's diaper and bringing her to me to nurse so I could rest as much as possible. He did projects with Candace and took her to the park. He played with Keri and gave her baths. In other words, he was a great dad when the kids felt well, but he did not understand how to comfort sick children. He lacked patience when they were sick or crying.

Our pediatrician was a jolly, diminutive woman who'd been in practice for decades. I first admitted my shame to her when Keri was just a few weeks old. "Sometimes I feel overwhelmed by the crying and my inability to comfort her," I confessed.

The pediatrician gave me comforting reassurance. "Some babies are just like this," she said. "They have colic. You can give her some drops to help relieve her discomfort. Don't worry; the crying and colic episodes will soon pass."

A visit with Sylvia and my father when Keri was five months old gave them an opportunity to witness how their little granddaughter woke from a sound sleep shrieking, as if she were being tortured. Surely something must be causing Keri's acute distress, they thought. They stripped her to see if something was sticking her. Nothing was. We tried holding and rocking her. No success. I offered her my breast. She refused it. Drops for colic did nothing. Eventually, the wailing abated, apparently completely unrelated to anything we had done.

Years later, Sylvia told me it was then my dad first expressed fear that the same biological problems which underlie some types of schizophrenia might be causing his granddaughter's severe distress. At the time, however, he couched his concerns to me in the form of a serious discussion about Keri's hysterical, inexplicable screaming-crying-wailing. "This," cautioned both Dad and Sylvia, "is *not* normal." They did not think she had colic.

Years later I discovered that other gastrointestinal problems—more severe than colic—can cause such distress. One common condition commonly misdiagnosed as colic is a type of reflux other mothers referred to as "silent reflux." After Keri was diagnosed with migraines at age two, I read that babies with migraines are often thought to have colic.

> Migraines in infancy are usually diagnosed in retrospect, after the child is diagnosed with migraines as a toddler. Often, the child was colicky as an infant.
> In toddlers, the migraines are often accompanied by vomiting, head pain, falling down, and sensitivity to sound and light.

Keri usually interacted joyfully with her family and played like any normal baby, but she did have her quirks. At just three months old, she was already guarded around strangers. When a friend came to visit and their eyes met, Keri started screaming. In public, people naturally wanted to look at this adorable baby, but if they looked directly at her, Keri had a fit. At home, I learned to warn visitors not to make eye contact. "Give her a chance to get used to you," I told them. I also discovered that hugging my visiting friends enthusiastically while Keri was watching greatly reduced the time it took for her to accept them. After she felt comfortable, the visitor could look her in the eye and interact with her directly. As Keri got older, we called this "just being cautious."

Was such behavior normal for a three-month-old? "Yes," the pediatrician replied. "Usually, stranger anxiety kicks in at about eight months of age. Keri seems to be quite precocious to be at this stage already, but it is a normal stage of development."

The doctor may be right, I thought, but "normal" was the last word I'd have used to describe my daily existence.

~~~~~~~~~~~~

For the first year of Keri's life, I lived in a blur of exhaustion and sleep deprivation. Her overall *lack* of solid sleep had me desperate. I took Keri back to the pediatrician. "She doesn't sleep!" I complained.

"Of course she does," chuckled the pediatrician. "It just *seems* like she isn't sleeping enough. Her sleep might be in bits and pieces, but babies get the rest they need."

Was she right? I started logging her sleep time both during the day and at night. She slept in short intervals, ranging from 5 to 90 minutes. Her total sleep time in a 24-hour period was 8 hours. I thought infants were supposed to sleep more than that. I took the sleep log with me to Keri's next appointment. With a compassionate air of patience, the pediatrician again reassured me, "Your baby is fine. You're not the only mother who is exhausted and sleep-deprived."

One evening, as I sat in my wonderful La-Z-Boy chair, quietly nursing, I relished the fact that Keri seemed content. As I changed her diaper and put her in her crib, the room had just enough of a soft glow to see by. I tiptoed out and joined the rest of the family in Candace's room. Candace was already tucked in bed, and Greg was reading her a book about horses, one of her favorite animals. This was Candace's time. When the book was finished, we kissed her good night, and went into the kitchen to finish cleaning up and getting ready for the next day.

Suddenly, Keri was wailing. She'd slept only 45 minutes. We looked at each other, sighed, and almost laughed. We knew from experience that just going in and putting a hand on Keri, trying to soothe her but keep her drowsy, was not going to work. I went into her room and took her out of the crib. She was wide-awake. As I sat with her in the La-Z Boy, she relaxed in my arms and touched my face gently. *This is good*, I thought. *It sure beats a screaming fit*. Within half an hour, she was dosing off, and I put her back in the crib. *Ahhhh. Now I can now get ready for bed.*

I was asleep the moment my head hit the pillow. A half-hour later we were awakened by a blood-curdling scream from Keri's room. I was at her side in seconds. *Oh*, I thought, once I made sure she was safe in her crib, *it's that colic again*. Fortunately, Candace could sleep through a tornado. But Greg couldn't. He rolled over and covered his ears with a pillow, wanting desperately to sleep. I gave Keri the drops the doctor had recommended for colic. I walked, rocked, and comforted her while the screams went on and on. My ears were ringing. My tired brain wondered if I was going to suffer permanent damage to my hearing.

An hour later, Keri abruptly stopped crying and went back to asleep. *Is she as exhausted as I am?* I wondered as I stumbled into bed. Ninety minutes later she was crying her usual "I'm hungry and soiled" cry. I moaned. Greg unhappily got out of bed, changed her diaper, and brought her to me to nurse. In a fog, I fed her. When she finished, I just wanted to fall back asleep. Let her just stay where she was. But Greg didn't think kids should sleep in bed with their parents. The prominent parenting professionals were saying that for good sleep habits, babies should sleep in their own cribs. I sighed, got up, put Keri in her crib, and staggered back to bed.

I dozed off, only to be awakened at 2:30 a.m. by the telephone. An out-of-state friend desperately needed emotional support and my shoulder to cry on. She and her husband were splitting up. She felt wildly grieved. But I had no shoulder to offer. I was so exhausted I had nothing left to give, not even five minutes of sympathy. All I wanted was to be asleep for the few minutes before Keri started crying again. My friend never forgave me.

Twenty minutes later Keri was crying again. This time she had the hiccups. She often had the hiccups. She'd had them in utero as well. The thump, thump, thump of her hiccups had been amusing when I was pregnant. It wasn't funny anymore. The pediatrician referred to them as simply a product of the baby's immature nervous system. Maybe, but immature or not, they were one more thing disturbing Keri's sleep, and, by extension, mine and Greg's.

It took a while for Keri to fall back to sleep. But just 10 minutes later she was making whimpering sounds. These were loud enough to disturb us, but we also knew they were sounds we could ignore. Forty minutes later, she started back with full-blown wails. Once again I got up for a few minutes to tend her.

When the alarm went off, Greg and I lurched out of bed, wondering how we were going to make it through another sleep-deprived day. Keri was still asleep but woke soon after. Seated in her high chair across the breakfast table from Candace, she grinned widely. Candace made a funny face. Keri howled with delight, which launched Candace into peals of laughter. Keri chortled even more. Except for the dark circles under my eyes, there was no evidence of the night before.

> White noise (sound-masking/screening/conditioning devices) helps *some* hypersensitive babies who easily startle from sleep.

Keri's daytime sleep was no better.

Keri dozed off, making delicate sucking movements with her lips. Moments later our little dog, Napkin, who was lying on the floor nearby, let pass a small burst of flatulence. Immediately, Keri was wide awake and screaming. Some sounds, especially when unexpected (and she reacted to many sounds as if they were unexpected), provoked an intense reaction, as if these sounds foretold the end of her world.

> Prepulse inhibition (PPI) describes the ability most people have to filter out expected stimuli and not get overly startled by it. Some people with schizophrenia show excessive startle response to auditory stimuli.
>
> Some birth circumstances, such as C-section births and those with oxygen deprivation, can cause long-term changes in dopamine-mediated behavior, disrupting this acoustic startle response.
>
> Swerdlow, et al., 2006; Vaillancourt, et al., 2000.

Because Keri loved riding in the back carrier, I was wearing her as I did chores around the house. She dozed off for about 15 minutes, after which she got squirmy and fussy. She wasn't hungry. She wailed when I put her in her crib, but calmed when I placed her on a play mat in the living room. She started screaming when I turned on the radio.

I began switching radio stations, pausing briefly at each one. To my surprise, she quieted when I came to classical music. Was the classical music calming to her, or was it that the other music caused her distress? I experimented, determining that any music other than classical, jazz, or certain vocal folk music caused instant screaming. I later played music she liked during one of her wailing fits, hoping it would soothe her, but it did not.

I enjoyed nursing time, partly because it allowed me to indulge in one of my own favorite pastimes—reading. I read out loud, softly, in a monotonous tone. While suckling, Keri often watched me intently, occasionally reaching up to pat my face.

Shortly after Keri was born, John and Sophie had a baby girl whom they named Roberta. Candace loved playing with their older daughter,

Maria. Now Keri had her cousin Roberta. Keri and Roberta loved each other even as infants, though the differences in their personalities were startling.

Roberta rarely cried. She had a more mischievous and playful attitude than Keri. She was also more physically adept. Nevertheless, they loved playing together and complemented each other well.

One clear, chilly day after school, Sophie came over with her children. While walking in the neighborhood, Roberta slept peacefully in her stroller; Keri fussed and squirmed. We cut the walk short and went home. While Candace and Maria played, Sophie and I nursed our babies and talked quietly. We discussed joining a mother-baby swim class (no actual swimming was involved) at the YWCA for babies six to ten months old. I thought Keri might like it because she enjoyed water so much.

After Keri turned six months old, I enrolled us in the class and, as expected, she loved it. But each time we put our babies on their backs to float, Keri instantaneously fell into a deep sleep! Teasingly, other parents started calling her the narcoleptic baby.

Sometimes John and Sophie left Roberta with us so they could go out in the evening. I would have loved to leave Keri with them so Greg and I could have a night out, but Keri did not stop crying when we left her with someone else, not even with her beloved Aunt Sophie.

Around the time Keri was about five months old, I had to leave her with Sophie on two different occasions while I underwent minor surgery. (One of these surgeries was for a tendon I damaged by carrying Keri so much.) When I returned, I found my daughter screaming and my sister-in-law ragged with fatigue. Keri had taken no nourishment and no fluids during the eight hours I was gone, crying almost constantly, and stopping only for occasional short dozes when she was just too exhausted to continue.

Despite the many incidents of Keri's distress, however, our life was not pure hell. She enjoyed being talked to, getting bathed, and playing with the dog and her toys. She also loved being with her big sister, being held by her daddy, and sleeping on Greg's father's chest when Grandpa Larry came to visit.

Still, when I decided to go back to work part-time, it was with a sense of relief. My job offered the sanctuary of a private office along with the opportunity for lots of interaction with co-workers. I loved the challenges, creativity, and satisfaction of writing computer software, solving the puzzles behind software glitches, and collaborating on projects with colleagues. I felt exhilarated by the ongoing learning that was an intrinsic part of the job. After months of non-stop care for an extremely high-needs baby, the hours away each day would feel like mini-vacations, a series of opportunities to recharge my batteries.

It took a lot of investigating before I found a wonderful caregiver. Sally was a grandmother who took only infants up to a year old. She'd been taking care of babies, including foster babies, for 28 years. Secure in the knowledge that my now eight-month-old baby girl would be well taken care of, I made plans to leave her for a few hours each day.

I knew how important it was for Keri to trust anybody with whom she interacted, so we did some advance preparation. Wanting to give Keri plenty of time to become accustomed to Sally, I took her there many times before I returned to work. At first, I let Keri interact and play while I just sat and chatted. Then I started leaving her for short periods. While I was gone, Keri cried. Sally assured me most babies cry at first, but they quickly adjust.

I returned to work.

Each day when I picked up my daughter, Sally asserted that something was wrong. All Keri *did* was cry, and her constant crying was distressing the other babies. In all her years of caring for infants, Sally had never known a baby to cry so much. She didn't want Keri there anymore. Each day, I sat and listened sympathetically while Sally vented her distress and frustration. Each day, she relented and agreed to try again. This went on for 10 weeks.

At some point in the 11th week, Keri stopped crying and reached for a toy. Sally was so excited she took a picture. From then on, Sally had much to tell me each day. She found Keri loved to feed herself fruits and was curious and playful. She was surprised to discover how much

Keri could already talk. In fact, it was during this time Keri created her first joke—a play on words. Making the connection between Napkin the dog and the napkins used at meals, Keri lifted a paper napkin from the table and chortled "Doggie." She then proceeded to giggle gleefully at her own wit.

Just as Keri turned a year old, she began talking in complete sentences. Expressing her feelings to me with her first full sentence, she angrily stated, "You fwustwate [frustrate] me!"

Physically, she had less-than-average flexibility, but her skills were still considered on target. She began walking at 10 months. By 12 months she was toddling around without assistance. She had good manual dexterity, but her hand-eye coordination and gross motor skills (such as climbing stairs, hopping, and skipping) lagged behind, though not enough to raise any concern.

Later, Keri created a touching tribute to Sally's loving nature and to the affection that developed between them. Eight months after Keri last saw Sally and no longer actively remembered her, she still must have associated Sally's name with something good in her life. When she was given a new doll, she named it Sally.

I knew all babies needed a period of adjustment when starting with a day care center or a babysitter. Ten weeks of non-stop crying was extreme, I admit, but at the time I reasoned it must be normal because *my* baby did it, and *my* baby was normal. Some years later, Sally told me she'd recently cared for another baby who cried as much as Keri. "Really?" I queried.

"Yes," Sally continued, "a crack baby."[2]

I didn't know what to say.

Yes, I'd suffered from allergies, chicken pox, and sinus infections while I was pregnant. I'd also taken numerous antibiotics, used antihistamines, and delivered via C-section. But I hadn't taken even a sip of alcohol or caffeine, and I don't smoke. I'd also been quite diligent during pregnancy about avoiding known sources of toxins, such as

---

[2] A crack baby is born affected by, and addicted to, a highly destructive form of cocaine used by the mother during pregnancy.

paints, cleaning supplies, and pesticides, although I'd been exposed to them throughout my life, as have most of us.

Greg and I never considered there might be a genetic basis for any of Keri's issues, even though both our mothers had been diagnosed with a bipolar-schizophrenia spectrum disorder. After all, our mothers' problems didn't really flare up until they were adults with children of their own. And in each case, we were led to believe the electroconvulsive therapy (ECT)—also known as shock treatments—they'd received in the late 1950s and early 1960s, for what might actually have been postpartum depression, had resulted in their psychotic mood disorders. Before their ECT, our memories were of bright, loving mothers.

Eventually, my mother responded favorably to an old-fashioned, typical neuroleptic (antipsychotic) medication, but she died of heart failure shortly thereafter. I thought I was quite familiar with mental illness, but in retrospect, I hadn't really thought beyond the label itself.

> The interchangeable terms neuroleptics and antipsychotics describe medications that manage symptoms of disrupted brain neurochemistry. They are used to treat the tics of Tourette syndrome, severe depression, mania, mood swings, sleep disturbances, aggression, and agitation caused by brain injuries, severe obsessions and compulsions, paranoia, hallucinations, and anxiety.
>
> The term neuroleptic may carry less stigma simply because, being less familiar with it, people do not immediately associate the medication with preconceived ideas about the person taking it.

I knew our mothers had developed mental illness even though they were raised in loving, stable homes, had cheerful dispositions, and suffered no major traumatic events. Still, the term *mental* did not conjure up images of genetics, inflammation, environmental toxins, diet, hormones, viruses, or biology. We had no reason to worry about our baby.

What I didn't know was that one day, through loving my daughter, I would better understand my mother, and from loving my mother, I would better understand my daughter.

Table 1: Useful Lessons from Year One

- A baby's special needs and sensitivities must be respected regardless of social dictates about how babies should be cared for.
- A soothing sound (white noise) helps some highly sensitive babies to sleep.
- It's important to be very sensitive to the type of music (and sounds in general) that babies like and dislike.
- Pediatricians don't always understand the severity of a problem. A baby who cries or does not sleep well is normal in the eyes of most physicians. Keeping a log of your baby's sleep and crying patterns, and then summarizing that log into simple numbers, may factually convey the true picture of what's going on.
- Avoid television and videos in favor of letting babies participate with family and nature.
- Wear the baby on your person if he/she likes it.
- In response to crying, use earplugs to help protect your hearing and reduce your own stress.
- Learn to breathe!

Table 2: Characteristics: Prenatally, at Birth, and During the First Year

Prenatal
- Genetic predisposition: family history of depression, psychosis, ADHD, movement disorders (essential tremors), tics, and learning disorders (LDs).
- Parental age at conception: mother, 30; father, 38.
- Viral exposure *in utero* to chicken pox (varicella-zoster virus).
- Medications (under the care of a conferencing team of three doctors— allergist, ob-gyn, and pediatrician):
    - Promptly after conception—mother stopped taking antihistamines and decongestants for allergies.
    - First two trimesters—took antibiotics and Sudafed® for sinus and tonsil infections due to allergies.
    - Third trimester—resumed taking antihistamines/decongestants but stopped taking antibiotics.
- Fetus had lots of hiccups.

Birth
- Breech. Delivered by Cesarean section, face up; needed suctioning.
- Average weight and size (50th percentile).
- Large head size (> 95th percentile).
- Less-than-average flexibility.

First Year
- Breastfed, normal physical development, and above-average language development.
- Hypersensitive to sounds and disliked popular music.
- Displayed excessive startle reaction.
- Poor sleeper, often disturbed by hiccups, sounds, smells, pain, and for other unknown reasons.
    - Slept 5-90 minutes at a time and averaged a combined total of 8 hours of sleep per day.
- Extremely attached to mother; fear of separation and fear of strangers by 3 months of age.
- Intolerant of strangers meeting her eyes.
- Sometimes screamed as if in severe pain.

Chapter 2
Babysitter Satisfaction
and
Awful Allergies

Bam! Keri pitched nose-first onto the concrete driveway. She'd been standing next to me and was neither bumped nor jostled. She had just celebrated her first birthday. She'd been feverish on that special day, so we all ate just a little cake and gave her a few gifts. By the following week, she'd recovered from her illness and seemed to be doing fine, at least, that is, until she stopped her fall with her nose.

The fact that she fell spontaneously, with no apparent provocation, puzzled me enough to take her to the pediatrician. I felt relieved at the diagnosis: an ear infection. She didn't display any common signs of an ear infection, such as crying or tugging on her ear, but it must have caused her to experience an episode of vertigo. Armed with antibiotics, we returned home. The antibiotics seemed to work. She didn't fall again, and by Halloween, some weeks later, she seemed fine. Dressed as a pumpkin, with her chubby pumpkin belly and her poor scraped nose, she looked adorable. For years after, I called her my little pumpkin.

I shouldn't have been so complacent. As it turned out, Keri's first birthday ushered in a world of health issues, though none of them, alone, seemed critical. She had recurring allergies and ear infections, often accompanied by gunky eyes. In fact, we got to the point where we could diagnose an ear infection merely by observing Keri's eyes. We sometimes laughed about the fact she seemed the most normal—not screaming, but calm and contentedly playing—when she was no longer in pain yet running a slight fever. Oddly, at other times when she seemed quite sick, her temperature dropped several degrees *below* normal, which caused her to feel cold and sleep a lot. This led to a family joke that Keri hibernated when she was sick. Her fluctuations in temperature (up *or* down) didn't seem to do her any harm, however, and she recovered from illnesses quickly. As she got older, her temperature over the course of a day often ranged from 95.5°F to 101°F (35.3°C to 38.3°C) when she was sick. Although 101°F wasn't high enough to cause a doctor's concern, this bouncing temperature spread made Keri miserable, as she alternated between feeling extremely cold and burning up.

Then she stopped growing—completely. By the age of 18 months, she'd dropped from the fiftieth percentile on the growth chart to below the fifth percentile. Fortunately, her weight remained within normal range. The normally reassuring pediatrician now expressed alarm. She thought Keri might have a genetic or endocrine problem. Keri's lack of growth, plus other physical attributes such as the large size of her head, her body structure, and her lack of flexibility, caused the doctor to suspect dwarfism.

> Slower growth in early life correlates with an increased risk of later developing bipolar and schizophrenia-spectrum disorders. Slower growth in infancy is indicative of early disruption in a growth factor (IGF-1) that plays a major part in the regulation of growth. Some researchers speculate that a disruption in IGF-1 might be a cause of abnormalities in neurodevelopment.
>
> Perrin, et al., 2007.

By the time Keri was able to see a pediatric endocrinologist a few months later, she was growing again, albeit slowly. Blood test results appeared normal. Coupled with her recent growth, she earned a clean bill of health. Again, on the surface all seemed well. I didn't know that more than a simple blood test was necessary to determine whether a child had a medical problem affecting growth.

During the ensuing years, Keri stopped growing several more times. When it happened next for a period of several months just before she was three, the endocrinologist opined Keri's growth pattern indicated either a growth-hormone deficiency or a genetic condition called Turner syndrome or Turner mosaic. However, the pediatrician decided that having Keri undergo another blood test to confirm either of these possibilities, especially since her last test had been normal, would be cruel.

My friend Cat, who suffers from an endocrinological disorder, later explained that imbalances come and go, and that a blood test won't reveal the problem unless it is taken during a time of imbalance. That's what had happened to Cat, whose body had been deteriorating for six years before her doctor happened to draw blood during one of her bad times and discovered something wrong.

It was just such elusiveness that led Keri's pediatrician to decide that her stop-go growing must be normal. Keri was just growing *at her own pace*.

~~~~~~~~~~~~

Shortly after Keri turned a year old, we'd had to bid her babysitter goodbye. Sally only cared for infants up to the age of one. Keri's new sitter, Valerie, had two children of her own—a three-year-old named Elizabeth and an infant named David. Valerie was cheerful, a kind and loving person. Keri was the only child she was caring for besides her two. I was relieved my daughter enjoyed her new environment immediately. She grew attached to Valerie's children. She loved to play with dolls, talk to Elizabeth, play with David, and go on excursions to the park.

And even if Keri was not growing in height, she was growing intellectually. "No, no," I exclaimed once when she brought some non-food item to her lips. "We only put edible things into our mouth." Afterward, the tiny tot went through a phase of picking up an object and asking, "Is it edible?" She'd then pause waiting for a "Yes" before eating the questionable item.

Contrary to statistics that indicate most children later diagnosed with psychotic disorders have poor verbal development and lower IQs, especially verbal IQs, Keri's vocabulary developed rapidly into the gifted range. When she was 14 months old, we visited Greg's sister, Connie. When Connie picked her up, Keri stiffened and said sternly, "Please put me down. I did not *want* to be picked up!" Keri's aunt almost dropped her in shock. "What *is* she?" she asked, as if Keri were some alien being. "I thought I was picking up a *baby!*"

When Keri was 19 months old, she watched Valerie potty training Elizabeth. She then proceeded to potty train *herself* the same way at home. She took books to read while sitting on the potty, just as Elizabeth did. Then she *did* it—she peed! She was bursting with pride. Shortly thereafter, she also quit crying when we put her to bed. It was just like the potty training—as if a switch had been flipped between one day and the next. "Cover me up, Mom," she now said, and asked for her doll.

Because Keri lagged behind most 18-month-olds in gross motor ability, we tried to get her to play more actively. She, however, preferred verbal interaction with older children and pretend-play to more physically active pursuits. Even her expressions of curiosity were more verbal than physical. "Do dogs have belly buttons?" she would ask. Then, after hearing the explanation about mammals and umbilical cords, she wondered whether animals that hatch from eggs, such as birds, have belly buttons.

During a visit to the National Museum of the U.S. Air Force, Keri decided to be a pilot when she grew up. She thought for a moment and then asked if she could be *both* a mother and a pilot because, first and foremost, she wanted to be a mommy.

Meanwhile, I continued to work part-time. I was happy to be home when Candace returned from school. I loved taking both children to the park, to the pool, on walks, and to visits with their cousins. Keri adored her big sister. They entered fairy worlds accessible only to children, dressed up the dog as a horse, reindeer, or whatever they wanted him to be at the moment, and used dolls to populate imaginary stores, cities, and forests.

Candace, then nine, was in fourth grade and busy with school, piano, gymnastics, and Girl Scouts. While she was involved with her activities, Keri and I made happy use of the time. We went on nature walks, shopped for groceries, or, if it was pouring rain, remained in the car to read and play.

Though most of the time Keri seemed happy, there were still problems. She went to bed without a fuss, but she slept restlessly, thrashing and crying out in her sleep for hours. She had nightmares and night terrors. She woke several times each night, needing comforting. She dozed off frequently during the day yet was unable to maintain extended sleep during nap time. For me, a good night's sleep was a distant memory.

As she approached her second birthday, Keri started having strange tantrums—screaming, crying, wailing episodes—that escalated tremendously over the next few years. I knew what normal tantrums were like, and of course, Keri had her moments of acting like a normal toddler, throwing herself down on the ground and yelling "No!" This behavior was short-lived and quickly outgrown. The other episodes seemed to occur at random—not provoked by a disappointment such as not getting something she wanted or for any other apparent reason. We started calling them her "fits."

> Healthy children tend to have less-frequent, less-aggressive, and shorter tantrums. They also tend to be able to calm themselves.
>
> Severe tantrums may indicate depression, allergies, or some other medical problem.

The only thing we knew to do for Keri during a fit was to leave her alone. Because her behavior was so upsetting to the family, and since what she wanted at such times was solitude, by the time she was two and a half she learned to run into the playroom or her bedroom to have her fit. Usually she made it. Sometimes she didn't, leaving us with no choice but to disperse for our own sanity. Trying to calm her, as opposed to leaving her alone, only increased her agitation. Once, she flat out told us, "I *need* to cry!" On really bad days, the fits lasted up to four hours. When she was done crying, Keri either fell asleep or came smiling back to us for hugs.

Keri often peed during these fits, even when she was older. One day, Greg said in front of her, "I think she does it [pees] on purpose."

"I do *not* do it on purpose," Keri yelled, heartbroken, and began to sob. Too upset to say anything else, she gasped out "Mommy! I am having trouble talking!" Abashed, Greg apologized. Later, I told him there was no way Keri was peeing on purpose. Even five-year-olds can cry so hard they pee. Greg said he sometimes forgot how young Keri actually was.

Keri underwent extensive (for the time) immunoglobulin E (IgE) skin scratch allergy testing when she was 18 months old. This test of immediate immune response showed she had allergies to dust and numerous types of pollen. She also had mild reactions to *many* foods, but a food-elimination trial did not help to alleviate any of her symptoms. Perhaps this was due to eliminating too few foods or to conducting the trial for too short a time. Also, we did not take into consideration the possibility of delayed food allergies caused by immunoglobulin G (IgG) immune response (an inflammatory immune reaction hours or days after consuming a food), or even the response of immunoglobulin A (IgA), useful in detecting celiac disease because it's made in the small intestine, causing inflammation in people sensitive to gluten. Also, I was still breastfeeding, but I was not told to eliminate the corresponding foods from my diet. Eighteen years later, another round of allergy testing revealed that some of the foods initially identified were still an issue, some were not, and others for which she had tested negative as a toddler were now causing havoc in her gut.

When Keri's pollen allergies worsened each spring and autumn, her fits became more severe and frequent, and she became cranky and very irritable. With antihistamines, the fits lessened. Even her already disturbed sleep became more fitful when her allergies were aggravated by outdoor allergens. The pediatrician suspected Keri's allergies were causing her frequent stomachaches, either directly from the food she ate or from excessive sinus drainage.

At age two, Keri began to have episodes in which she simply dropped to the ground and could not get up or walk. The pediatrician called this condition ataxia, although the term more commonly describes an uncoordinated, stumbling walk, frequently resulting in falls. Severe head pain quickly followed. Keri lay in bed with the shades drawn, wanting complete quiet. Silently, tears squeezed between closed eyelids. She could not even endure the sound of her own sobs, so she just lay there inertly. Back at the pediatrician's office, the diagnosis seemed benign. "These are migraines," we were calmly reassured. "Pediatric migraines are not the same as adult ones. Children can sleep them off." I didn't even know a child could get a migraine! The pediatrician continued, "The migraines might be because of her allergies." She prescribed pediatric liquid Advil.[3]

> A pediatric neurologist should be consulted about migraines in children.

Keri did not outgrow her allergies and sensitivities. Rather, they continued to fester, stressing her body and her brain. She also became allergic to many metals, including silver, nickel, copper, and steel.

> Giving probiotics to children under the age of five who were delivered by C-section may reduce their risk of developing allergies.
>
> Kuitunen, M., M.D., et al., 2009.

When she was five, we learned she was also unusually sensitive to the chemicals in plastics considered "endocrine disruptors." At the time, she developed a strange estrogen-related endocrine problem. The endocrinologist was at a loss. It was the pediatrician—a full decade before the information about the potential dangers of plastics became more widely published—who put two and two together. "This

---

[3] The main ingredient in Advil is ibuprofen. At the time, pediatric liquid Advil was a prescription medication.

is off the record, but I feel strongly you should know this," the doctor explained. "Chemicals in plastics called phthalates can mimic estrogen. I suspect Keri may be extremely sensitive to them. Get rid of them. Stop using any plastics in the microwave or in conjunction with warm food. They mimic our own hormones and can scramble signals during development."

Phthalates and another potential endocrine disruptor, bisphenol-A (BPA), were common in plasticware used for food and drinks, plastics lining the inside of food cans, and plastics widely used for cooking. ("Cook the roast in the bag to retain moisture and make cleanup easy!" and "Just throw the bag of food into a pot of boiling water" were the cheerful refrains from food companies.) Greg and I meticulously eliminated plastic plates, plastic containers, plastic wraps, and Styrofoam from use with warm or hot food and beverages. Keri's symptoms disappeared.

I thought Keri must be unique in this sensitivity, but one day at the cafeteria in the building where I worked, Keri wanted a hot beverage. All the stirrers and spoons were plastic, so I asked if there was anything else available. I was surprised by the answer. Wooden stirrers were kept for those sensitive to plastics. Until then, I had never heard of anyone other than Keri who had this problem.

In the coming years, more research on chemicals that leach from plastics would link them to problems ranging from obesity and allergic asthma to mood problems and a decrease in reproductive health. Studies on normal exposure levels of BPA would verify the potential of this chemical to interfere with hormonal function, causing problems in the brains of infants and children[4] and thus supporting the possibility that exposure to certain plastics may contribute to the development of symptoms of neurological illnesses which are sensitive to sex hormone levels—such as schizophrenia.[5]

---

[4] Layton, Lyndsey, 2008.
[5] University of Guelph news release, 2008.

There were many things Keri's pediatrician missed or misdiagnosed, but we are eternally grateful she caught this one.

Table 3: Characteristics: Ages 12 to 24 Months

- Developed allergies and ear infections.
- Body temperature sometimes dropped when sick.
- Had screaming-crying fits, unlike normal temper tantrums.
- Stopped growing. Intermittent growth pattern caused height to fall from the 50th percentile to below the 5th percentile; weight remained average.
- Had less-than-average flexibility but was still considered normal.
- Displayed well-developed fine motor skills but poor gross motor skills. Gross motor development considered less than average but not abnormal.
- Displayed advanced verbal skills. Spoke in complete sentences with proper use of pronouns. *Large* vocabulary.
- Toilet trained voluntarily at 19 months. Continued to need diaper-like training pants because of numerous urine accidents when sleeping and when having screaming-crying fits.
- Became hypersensitive to sounds, touch, and cold. Displayed a minor sensitivity to heat.

Chapter 3
Day Care Dilemma

Greg and I continued to be challenged as we tried to meet the emotional needs of a precocious, sensitive two-year-old.

I sometimes sang a song to Keri from a book titled *Love You Forever*,[6] except I changed a few words. The song had a line that went "as long as I'm living," which I always sang as "forever and ever." After all, "as long as I'm living" might conjure up thoughts of death. I didn't want Keri, a precocious toddler, to have those thoughts to ponder. My attempt at protectiveness didn't work.

One night after lovingly singing that I'd love her forever, Keri told me sorrowfully, "No, Mommy. You are wrong."

"Huh?"

"You can't love me forever."

"Keri! *Of course* I will love you forever!"

As if talking to a young child, Keri explained to me somberly and with compassion, as if she were telling me something shocking I might not have thought of, "You cannot love me forever, Mommy. We do not live forever. Someday you will die. After you die, you will not be able to love me. Therefore, you cannot love me *forever*."

Oh, God! I scooped her up in my arms and had a long talk with her about God and souls and how I *will* love her forever and ever.

~~~~~~~~~~~

It was time to put Keri into day care while I continued to work part-time. I spent several mornings at various centers before carefully choosing one. Then I slowly transitioned her into this new setting.

---

[6] Munsch and McGraw, 1995.

Naturally, Keri was assigned to the two-year-olds' room with children her age. However, the other children, for the most part, could not yet converse with her, and rather than ask for items she was playing with, they just grabbed them. This change was a shock to Keri, who was used to politeness, sharing, taking turns, and pretend-play. She talked to me about the other children, trying to understand their actions. I explained they were very young but would soon learn politeness. So when something was yanked away from her, she told the teachers that so-and-so had not yet learned to be polite. Finding this resolved nothing, she simply learned to go play with something else, but she still found this new world disturbing. On the plus side, she was exposed to a lot more physical activity, hands-on play, group singing sessions, the alphabet, and general information about life and the world around her. Keri would spend 10 months in this day care center prior to starting at a Montessori preschool.

> In general, group settings such as day care are more stressful to young children than smaller, quieter settings such as family homes.
>
> Some children may be better off staying at home or in a small family setting.
>
> Geoffroy, et al., 2006.

She picked up new rules at day care. One day I offered her some of my juice, and she informed me, "No, Mommy, we are not supposed to share germs."

I countered with another rule: "It's okay for family to share germs." The next day Napkin had a little ball in his mouth. I could not believe it when Keri took the ball from the dog's mouth and popped it into her own. "Spit it out," I gasped. "It's dirty." She took out the ball and patted me on the arm.

"It's okay, Mommy," she said, reassuringly. "Napkin is family, and family shares germs."

When we got her a tricycle to try riding in our kitchen, Keri refused to get on it until we bought her a helmet. She had learned at day care she should wear a helmet when riding a bicycle.

Her innate love of gentleness, order, and rules made life easier for us as parents. We evoked easy compliance from Keri just by telling her something was a rule. She kept her room neat, and when she was older, she loved to organize the house. On the other hand, she did not do well in situations that were not planned in advance, nor could she cope with children and adults who did not follow rules. Why did people litter when the rule was to throw trash in the trash can? Why do the children not share when the rule is to take turns and share?

Teachers at the day care center informed me Keri was reading books with inflection and feeling. Keri pretended to be the teacher, placing dolls as if they were a group of day care children. "Now you must sit, S-I-T," she told them, and then proceeded to read simple books to them, being sure to turn the books so the dolls could see the pictures.

Skeptical, I suggested Keri probably memorized books the teachers had read aloud. "No," they insisted, "We've never read these books to the children."

Keri also became a classical music fanatic, enthusiastically listening to violin music at night and declaring she wanted to "dance to Mozart." Becky, one of my co-workers, taught me a little about symphonies and gave me a recording of Beethoven's Sixth. I played it for Keri in the car on the way to pick up Candace from piano class. When we stopped, Keri pleaded, "Mommy, don't turn off the music. I will stay here and listen to the music. Don't turn it off!"

When we got home, Keri was ill, so she lay on the living room carpet listening to the entire symphony while watching the fish in the aquarium. Fortunately, Becky had told me about movements, because Keri recognized a change and asked me what the new music was called. Not understanding at first, I said, "Beethoven's Sixth Symphony."

She said, "No, it changed." Oh! So I explained there were different parts called movements that together composed the symphony. Of course, she then wanted to know what the movement was called, but I had no idea which one was playing. It all sounded the same to me. Keri *listened* to the music; I merely *heard* it.

Keri's reactions to classical music differed, depending on the piece. After just a few moments of Beethoven's Fifth, she covered her ears. Eyes welling with tears, she told us, reproachfully, she was too young for something that scary; it made her think of dangerous bears. Other music made her laugh. Puzzled by such an odd reaction, I took the music to Becky and asked why my daughter always laughed at a certain part. Becky said it was meant to be funny. It was a musical jest called a scherzo.

At times, Keri's vocabulary, deep thoughts, and self-discipline astounded us. When she was not yet 18 months old, a hive of honey bees decided the eaves of our house would make a good home. We felt protective of the non-aggressive little bees. It was a great opportunity to learn about this wonder of nature. However, when they sometimes landed on us, it was scary. I explained that when a bee got on us we needed to be very still so it wouldn't get scared and sting. One day, I realized Keri was not moving. I went to her and saw tears rolling slowly down her cheeks. A bee was crawling on her face. She never flinched, and the bee didn't sting her. Afterward, she was calm and talkative. "I was scared," she said. Then she wondered, "Why did the bee want to be on my face?"

One day Keri was meticulously putting together a complicated, 47-piece picture of a Jeep composed of sticker shapes from an activity book. Getting tired toward the end, she allowed me to help. She politely requested stickers saying "I need a long thin rectangle" and "A small half-circle, please."

Another evening, we were at the dinner table discussing a notice Candace had brought from school about a new public Montessori magnet school. Keri was due to start at a private Montessori preschool, called Providence Montessori, in the fall, just as she was turning three. The public Montessori school would start at the kindergarten level. However, because her birthday was several days past the cutoff date, she would not be able to start kindergarten at the public Montessori until she was turning *six*. We continued talking while Keri sat in her high chair, mumbling and looking at her fingers. She then held up four fingers and asked, "So, first I will go to a school called Providence Montessori; then, in *four years*, I will go to a school named Public?"

At this point Candace started to freak out. Her chair fell over backward as she jumped up, saying, "My sister is a genius!"

I laughed. "No," I told Candace and calmly asked Keri how she figured out it would take four years for her to be six.

Keri explained. "Well, I'm two now. I'll be six in Public. So three—she held up one finger, four—she held up a second finger, five—she held up a third finger, six—and she held up the fourth finger. See . . . four!"

Candace kept muttering about her sister being a genius until I assured her Keri was not a genius, just a little advanced. I knew Keri could not do addition and subtraction as we know it. She just got inspired and worked her young brain to figure out the difference between two and six. I was content to let it drop and enjoy our happy home and our cute toddler.

As the finger-counting incident showed, Keri was fascinated by the concept of time. She put up a calendar in her bedroom and kept track of the months and the days of the week. She once voiced concern about her perception of the passage of time. The idea that time seems to pass faster when a person gets older was worrisome to her. At two and a half, she said, she felt time passing faster than when she was two, and even faster than when she was less than two. "If time already passes so fast for me, I'm scared for it to feel like it is going any faster."

~~~~~~~~~~~~

Since Keri was unable to fit in with children her own age, day care posed a dilemma. So did the religious education room for two-year-olds at our Unitarian Universalist (UU) church. She didn't like the aggression and impoliteness of non-verbal children her age. The noise level was painful to her.

Both places, independently, resolved the issue in similar ways.

Some inspiration came when the two- to five-year-olds practiced together for a winter holiday show at the church. Though Keri was the only child under four to participate in the actual performance, she did everything perfectly. She was happy.

Afterward, the church educators simply moved two-year-old Keri into the kindergarten/first-grade room. She had the manual dexterity to cut, paste, and color at least as well as the average kindergartener. She had the added benefit of being able to read, concentrate, and follow directions like an even-older child.

When Keri was three and a half, she was moved into the Sunday school class for second- and third-graders. The other children and the teachers treated her no differently than any other child. The kids accepted her even though she was so tiny. The only area where Keri lagged was in her ability to write, which was not an issue in this Sunday school. And as we found out later, an extra couple of years wouldn't have fixed her lag in writing, anyway.

Meanwhile, she complained about the other children at day care not understanding things. "Do you understand?" she'd keep saying after telling us something. Puzzled, I asked her if the teachers at day care said this to the children. She replied, "No, *I* say it to the children." I could see why. Even I had difficulty keeping up with her vocabulary. For example, Keri would speak of colors such as chartreuse, magenta, and vermillion, but I kept forgetting which was which. Where did she learn these things?

Yet in spite of this stunning vocabulary, she still sometimes grew frustrated trying to communicate with us. Her winter shirts did not easily go over her large head. For days she kept saying, "This shirt needs help!" I did not understand. Then one morning her face twisted as she searched for words. She carefully explained. "This shirt must be properly situated on my head before you pull down, or else it bends my neck." We worked together to develop a way to get her shirts on in a more comfortable way.

I also was puzzled by another of Keri's comments about day care. "The other children don't understand things that are funny because they are too young."

I asked the teacher about it. "We [the teachers] sometimes act out things that are funny, but Keri is the only child who understands and laughs her head off. She is so aware of everything. She overhears us talking with each other and responds like another adult in the room. She really doesn't belong in this room with other two-year-olds. She really needs to be moved up." She paused, expecting a response.

"So, are you saying she should be with the three-year-olds?"

"Actually, no. I don't think she would be any happier there. In fact, she might be even worse off because the children are bigger, rowdier, and still not mature enough."

I didn't get it. "What are you suggesting?" I queried.

"I don't actually have a solution," the teacher replied. "Keri would most enjoy being with the kindergarteners. The problem is, she wouldn't be able to keep up with them physically."

On the way home, Keri sadly stated she had no friends at day care. When I mentioned the names of some children she talked with, she said stiffly, "Those are not my friends. They are just other children who attend day care with me, not friends." Instead of going home, I took her to a playground, and we just swung and played for a while. She said she felt different—that she was not like the other children. Another day she came home, sat on the steps, and put her chin in her hands. Blond Shirley Temple curls surrounded her face and spilled over the tiny hands holding up her chin. The juxtaposition of cherubic innocence and grown-up angst was disconcerting as she flatly despaired, "I hate my life."

Something had to change, and it had to change fast.

Then the day care center came up with a solution. They put Keri with the kindergarteners for inside activities. She loved playing electronic word games and typing her name on the computers the older kids used. And during lunch she had a chance to chat away with the kindergarteners while cutting her food with a fork and a plastic knife. When it came time for playground and water activities, she went back with the two-year-olds.

Spring arrived, and her life was a lot more settled.

Keri put three caterpillars into a jar. She named them Bosco, Bosco, and Bosco. One caterpillar made a cocoon. "Now the caterpillar is a pupa," she told me. "A baby cricket is also a pupa." I asked her how she knew this, and she got out a story I'd read to her weeks earlier about ant life. She showed me a picture of the ants tending to the pupae, which were ant cocoons. Then she showed me the next page with a picture of adult ants hatching from the cocoons. She told me ants are insects, and so are butterflies and crickets. How did she remember these things, let alone make the connection?

We adopted two baby robins. Featherless, they were newly hatched and must have fallen from their nest during a storm. At first, I thought they were dead. We warmed them in our hands and took them to a veterinarian. The vet wanted us to raise them ourselves. He gave us special food to feed them every two hours during the day. Luckily, they slept all night.

Everyone helped with the birds, including Keri, who could be completely trusted to handle them with the utmost gentleness. I took them to work with me in a basket so I could feed them throughout the day. Twice a day, we took them outside for fresh air and to acclimate to the outdoors. We got books from the library on the care and development of baby birds.

Keri picked up worms from the yard, putting them in the birds' hungry, gaping mouths. She laughed as they made their fledgling flights. She happily said goodbye as they flew away from us. And just as the books said, they hung around nearby for the next year.

Raising these birds had an impact on Keri. It fulfilled a need in her to nurture. She fell in love with birds. Some day she would have a pet of her own, and she knew it would be a bird.

Table 4: Useful Lessons from the Toddler Years

- The best day care for some exceptionally bright, verbal, gentle, hyper-sensitive toddlers might be with another loving parent and just a few other children.
- Some of the best learning times often occur when doing simple things such as going on nature walks, gardening, snuggling, reading, and even enjoying the slow pace of bath and potty time!
- Just because professionals say a two- or three-year-old cannot comprehend time, eternity, and death does not mean this claim is true. Dealing with these concepts can be scary to a child.
- Each child's innate temperament needs to be accepted and compromises made.
- A simple solution to end arguments over radio selections, music, or noise in the car and at home is:
  - Anybody can veto the music selected. A veto supersedes anyone's desire to play the selection.
  - Anybody can request quiet. This supersedes anyone's desire for noise or music.

  For example: I choose something I like, but Keri cannot stand it so she says no. She finds some sleepy classical music, but Greg is driving and is afraid it will make him drowsy, so he says no. Some jazz is found, and nobody is tortured by it, so that is what stays on.
- Sometimes, the needs of the one really do outweigh the desires of the many.

Table 5: Characteristics: Age 2

- Developed frequent ear infections, accompanied by gunky eyes. Seasonal allergies. Occasional allergic hives. Frequent abdominal pain. Frequent low-grade fever. Low temperature, at times, when feeling sick.
- Stopped growing yet again, but just temporarily.
- Was intolerant of cold.
- Demonstrated below-average, but not abnormal, coordination and flexibility. (Placed in tots' gym classes to help physical development.)
- Had trouble sleeping at night and developed night terrors. Very disturbed sleep. Crying, moaning, and thrashing in sleep for about 3 hours per night.
- Exhibited sensory sensitivity (mostly to sound).
- Suffered from migraines with ataxia.
- Developed a gentle personality. Careful to never harm any living creature (plant or animal). Kind, sharing, chatty, creative. Rule-follower. Low tolerance for frustration. Low emotional flexibility. Biological, innate need for order and a gentle, highly verbal environment.
- Had near-daily screaming, raging tantrums or fits—unrelated to discipline or not having her own way—that seemed to come out of the blue. They occurred up to 4 times a day and lasted about 45 minutes, though many went on for several hours. During them, she would usually urinate on herself.
- Long-term, low-dose antibiotics, antihistamine, and decongestant reduced the intensity and frequency of fits.
- Began rudimentary reading and writing at age 2-1/2 after being placed at day care. Recognized all letters of the alphabet, read short-vowel words, and counted objects up to 40. Figured out it would be 4 more years before she would be 6. Knew her full address and phone number. Called friends and grandparents on the phone unaided, looking up their phone numbers in an address book.
- Alienated from children her age in childcare. Much happier with 5-year-olds, at least on a part-time basis.
- Close to age three, began taking 2-hour naps.

The Calm

Ages Three to Nine

A golden leaf falling
gently to the water,
tiny ripples spreading
into ever-growing
concentric rings
that eventually
hit the pond's edge,
reverberating back,
making a myriad
of ever-changing figures
on the water's surface.

— Jeanie

Chapter 4
Music and Montessori Mania

Keri was happier at the Montessori preschool, surrounded by other verbal children who could communicate with her. She made friends easily and they played at each other's homes. Keri was not quite three when school started, but although she was the smallest child, she was by no means the youngest. In fact, half of the children in her group would not be turning three until the middle of the school year. The older children at the school mentored the newcomers, teaching them to tie their shoelaces and showing them how to put on their coats more easily. Keri felt well taken care of by the big, curly-haired boy assigned as her mentor.

Greg and I enjoyed Keri's talkativeness, and at dinnertime we always got an earful about her day. She informed us the teachers were always saying "Shhhhhhh...." to her. She offered details about other children in the class: "Nora doesn't like cream cheese or apple butter but she does like apples; Jason cannot feed himself and needs help eating; Michael says I look like a baby. I told him, 'I'm not a baby!'"

Every day, Keri came home with interesting things she'd learned. "Adults should not drive cars when they are sick, because it could mess up their driving," she'd inform us. Or, "Vegetables lose vitamins A and C in water when they are cooked." She explained rules such as, "You must not talk when I am talking. You must wait your turn." She told us of her triumphs. "When I stood up for myself and told Ben 'NO,'" she boasted, "the teacher said, 'Good for you, Keri!'" She also learned new fun songs that made her smile and laugh. On car trips, she and Candace taught us amusing songs we could sing together.

I was quite impressed with the Montessori school.

I returned to work full time. Greg was no longer traveling much, so we arranged our schedules to maximize time with the children. I loved early morning hours, arriving at work around 6:00 a.m. Greg got the children up and off to school each morning before starting work, and I always called to say good morning and to give them my love. This routine allowed me to leave work earlier to be with the girls after school and Greg to arrive home later.

Listening to classical radio on the way home in the car, Keri fell in love with the sound of the flute. Of all the musical instruments she could distinguish in her beloved symphonic music, flute was her favorite. She begged me to allow her to learn to play it. Looking into it, I found it is not safe for the development of children's teeth for them to play flute before the age of 10. Keri was disappointed. She then asked if she could learn violin until she was old enough for flute. Investigating, I found there were violin classes for children her age and even a little younger.

Keri started Suzuki violin lessons. She thought it quite humorous that the parent was supposed to learn first while the child watched. I was awful, and even with practice, I got no better. Keri, on the other hand, took to the instrument with an odd mixture of seriousness and playful imagination. She assembled dolls and stuffed animals around her as an audience. She clipped a tiny stuffed animal onto her violin bow and pretended it was having a wild ride while she played. But when she was done, she always put on a serious face and bowed.

Now that Keri was in an environment she loved, did she cry less? Actually, the answer is no. She cried at school often, although not every day. But she almost always had a meltdown as soon as she left. She screamed so much in the car I used earplugs to protect my hearing. Often, the crying was not over by the time I pulled up in front of our house, so I either carried her inside, still screaming, or I left the car door open and sat outside, waiting until she calmed on her own. Sometimes, she fell asleep in her car seat, exhausted, the moment she stopped crying.

When she wasn't screaming and crying, she seemed to be very happy.

Keri explained she cried after leaving preschool because of all the things she didn't like during the day that she *hadn't* cried about. For example, she didn't like getting her hand stamped each morning with a letter of the alphabet, because she already knew all her letters, so she screamed about it on the way home. When I suggested she just not hold out her hand to be stamped, she got upset with me, saying, "The rule is . . ."

The teachers reported when they played music other than classical, Keri covered her ears with her hands and withdrew or cried. She refused to participate in some games that caused other children to laugh and have fun—those involving rough physical contact like rolling into each other.

Keri's frequent ear infections took a lot of fun from her life. Her eye allergies to random plants caused her conjunctiva—the thin, transparent layer covering the outer surface of the eye—to swell. The first time it happened, she was just two and a half and had been picking spring flowers. One eye swelled shut, with the clear conjunctiva so full of fluid it protruded between her shut eyelids. I rushed her to the emergency room.

These allergic reactions had to be treated with medicinal eyedrops, to which Keri protested vigorously. Luckily, by the time she was four, she not only allowed the drops to be administered without a fuss, she'd begun learning to put them in by herself.

The Montessori school had medicine on hand for Keri's eyes and for her migraines, to be given as needed. However, to do so they required a new permission note each day. I had a big stack copied and signed in advance. Every day we added the date to a note and sent it to school with Keri.

The scariest thing that happened the year Keri was three was the time she had a fever and was vomiting. Her pediatrician was out of town, so we saw her partner, who gave Keri a shot of Phenergan (promethazine) to calm the vomiting and make her sleepy.

After the shot, Keri became delirious, hallucinating even though her temperature was now down to 102.4°F (39.1°C). She was talking to Candace, who at the time wasn't there, and she was flailing and yelling not to give her water—but I wasn't offering any water. Every so often she would just whimper, "Help! Help! Help me, Mommy!"

Terrified, I phoned the pediatrician's office, reaching the doctor on call for after-hours emergencies. He first dismissed my concern with, "How can you tell a three-year-old is delirious?" Then he explained that hallucinations or psychosis were possible side effects of Phenergan. He advised me to stick her in a tub of room-temperature water to lower her temperature further, make her drink plenty of fluids, and wait it out.

I did as he advised, and after four hours of this terrifying ordeal, Keri finally went to sleep.

By the age of three and a half, Keri would start down paths of logic that had her sister alarmed and Greg and I stumped. One fairly innocuous line of thinking, about the differences between pretend and fantasy, possibilities and impossibilities, led her to announce there cannot be an Easter Bunny. The book about Peter Cottontail must be wrong. Candace got upset. Keri was too young. Candace tried to tell her that, of course, there was an Easter Bunny, but Keri concluded the Easter Bunny is pretend. She still hoped the pretend Easter Bunny came around, because it would still be fun.

One thought process of Keri's had my head spinning. We were out in our garden picking small rocks from the dirt. Even though she was only three, she remembered us doing the same thing the year before. She told me she read about farmers getting boulders out of their fields, and every year they had to get rocks out of their fields all over again. What we were doing was just like the farmers. She asked me where the rocks came from—why they were there again. I didn't know. She then told me that particles of the ground are solid but all together they act like a fluid, like water. The rocks from below must float slowly up to the surface, where we again have to remove them.

She continued with, "If you visualize really small, nothing is solid." I felt more confused as she talked. She described the rocks as being able to move through our planet the way our planet moves through the solar system and the solar system moves through the galaxy. Then on a small scale, molecules of water can go through particles of soil, and smaller things like atoms and electrons can move between the molecules, and we don't call a single atom a solid or a liquid. Then there are the grains of sand—each is solid, yet collectively they flow like a liquid. They move fluidly. Later, she showed me how Jell-O solidifies yet is still liquid, because after taking a spoonful out of a full bowl, the sides of the hole flow a bit back into the depression, as can be seen hours later. Where is the boundary between what we call solid and what we call liquid, or at least fluid?

Sometimes I felt God had given her to the wrong parents. I wondered if she would have been better off having been born to physicists, or at least, if she could have a smart mentor who could talk to her about the things she really wanted to discuss. Of course, these discussions came up at random times, like when she was sitting on the potty, out for a walk, or gardening.

I kept telling myself, *This child is only three years old. How will she be at six? At sixteen?* Every parent imagines what their child might be like in the future. I imagined Keri growing out of her allergies and fits. I saw her as an intelligent, beautiful young woman with curly hair surrounding a cherubic face. She would have nice friends. Maybe she would pursue her music; maybe she would study science. Whatever she chose, she would do it intensely, with passion, because this was her nature.

The one thing I knew for sure was Greg and I had our work cut out to provide balance in our daughter's life. We had to balance her intellectual drive with lighthearted, active play. We had to guide her to accept a wider world of people who might not want to talk about the things that fascinated her, while at the same time encouraging her to pursue whatever she desired. We had to teach her to understand diversity and to recognize the different gifts each person brings to the world. We needed to find ways for her to be socially happy while at the same time keeping alive her curiosity and enthusiasm for learning.

~~~~~~~~~~~

Going to the library was Keri's favorite outing. Of course, her reading and interest levels were far beyond books written for three-year-olds, and I found it difficult to find chapter books[7] suitable for such a young child. Between the ages of three and four, Keri wanted books about young sisters, dogs, family, and playing. She didn't want anyone in the book to get hurt or to do anything bad or mean. She loved the *All-of-a-Kind Family* books,[8] devoured the *Little House on the Prairie* series,[9] and then pounced on the *Anne of Green Gables* series.[10] All were aimed at 9-to-12-year-olds. Because she was so young, we stuck to hardcover books with their larger print.

One day when Keri was three and a half, I found my book, *The Works of Edgar Allan Poe*, opened to the poem "Annabel Lee."[11] *Odd*, I thought. *I don't remember getting out this book*, and I closed it and put it back on the shelf. The next time I saw the book, Keri was reading this poem out loud! She told me she loved the way the words of Poe's poetry "flowed, rhymed, and sang." I was a bit stunned she could repeatedly find this particular poem in a 750-page tome.

Could she really understand the poem? Keri explained it was a love poem from a man, about the woman he loved who had died. There were words in it I was sure she could not know the meaning of, such as *coveted* and *sepulchre*. But she did.

She especially enjoyed listening to me read another poem by Poe, "The Bells," because she could hear the sounds of the different bells in what she termed the poem's music. But because of the stories in the book I did not want Keri reading, I restricted her access to the book, limiting it to the poetry she so dearly loved. My father then sent her a book of poetry by Emily Dickinson. She loved Dickinson's poems for a

---

[7] Chapter books, which are split into chapters with few or no illustrations, are normally written for older children.
[8] Taylor, S., et al.
[9] Wilder, L. I.
[10] Montgomery, L. M.
[11] "Annabel Lee" was written by Edgar Allan Poe in 1849. It is believed that although artistic license was taken, it is most likely about the death of his beloved wife.

different reason—their depth of meaning and the morality behind the words.

Just as Keri turned four, we discovered she could speed-read, just as my father could when he was the same age. She read parts of Candace's seventh-grade textbooks, and one day she read Candace's old third-grade reader in two hours. *No way,* I thought, but when I asked her to tell me about stories in the book I chose at random, she could. She really *had* read it all!

At preschool, Keri was encouraged to bring books from home to read. She was also sent with the elementary students to check out books from the school library.

Keri's musical engagement with the violin came to an abrupt end when her physical inflexibility got in the way. The teacher tried to make her chin go farther toward her shoulder, and it hurt her. She didn't ever want to go back to him. "Okay," I said, while thinking how much I was going to miss her standing under the night sky, playing "Twinkle, Twinkle Little Star." Keri then wanted to know if she could learn piano instead, like her big sister—just until she was old enough for flute.

~~~~~~~~~~~

Keri was what might be termed emotionally inflexible, but we worked with her nature. An unexpected change in plans or routine, even if the change involved doing something enjoyable, could lead to a meltdown. Going to a dental appointment after being picked up from day care or school was peaceful, as long as Keri was told about it well in advance. A week ahead, we'd say, "Keri, next week on Tuesday, after being picked up from school, you'll go to the dentist before going home." Then we would tell her again the night before, the morning of, and remind her when she was picked up that afternoon. But if the change was due to something that came up that day, or if we forgot to properly warn her about what was happening, she sometimes just couldn't handle it.

As Keri got older, she learned to compensate for this part of her nature. It was still a part of her, but she became better able to cope by thinking through and preparing for possible outcomes. Because fewer events were then unexpected, she had more emotional reserve to handle the changes in plans and unforeseen occurrences that are a part of life. In other words, she matured, but this reserve took some years to develop.

Even at four, Keri had other peculiarities, some of which we brought to the attention of her pediatrician.

Her hands did something "funny," Keri said. She was constantly stretching them, and rotating her wrists and fingers. She explained her hands felt like they needed to move. Sometimes they also hurt. The doctor said perhaps Keri needed to exercise her hands and wrists to strengthen them.

I wanted Keri to get fresh air and exercise outside. I especially wanted her to play with her cousins in the snow and to come with me when I walked the dog and when I rode my bicycle. Keri loved tagging along when the weather was mild, but she balked in the winter months. Dressed in snowsuit, boots, gloves, and scarf, she had fun outside. But after just a short time, she always wanted to come in, fussing about her cold face, hands, and feet.

We discovered another curious trait we didn't think much about until years later. Despite a healthful diet loaded with fresh fruits and vegetables, sometimes Keri's bowel movement was such a huge, hard ball it was too big to flush. When I looked up this phenomenon on the Internet years later, I found a life-threatening condition called megacolon, which, thankfully, Keri did *not* have. That's when I began to say, jokingly, she must have a case of mini-megacolon. I had no idea her large stools might be a symptom of low thyroid or intestinal/immune system problems, or that they could indicate a problem with malfunctioning mitochondria (the principal energy source of cells). As it turned out, her mini-megacolon was no laughing matter.

Keri also had chronic and intermittently severe abdominal discomfort. The pediatrician said it was probably due to sinus drainage and to give her an antacid when she complained about abdominal pain. Later, some doctors postulated these abdominal complaints were due to migraines. Others suggested the pains were not real. Children with depression and other mental problems, we would be told, frequently complained of stomachaches.

Her perpetually bloated belly—even though her ribs were visible on her otherwise slim body—seemed to be just a part of her figure. One day after starting elementary school, Keri, tiny for her age, looked at her profile in the mirror, and asked, "Mommy, when will I lose my toddler figure and look like a child?" I reassured her that her figure was cute and reminded her she was still small. As she grew, she would naturally look less like a toddler. I also reminded her there is much natural variation in body shapes. Of course, all of my comments were true, but eventually we learned Keri's bloated tummy was also a piece of the puzzle.

Keri continued to have occasional, but notorious, fits. The teachers at her school felt these fits were the result of an immature nervous system that simply needed time to mature. Their conclusion sounded similar to the pediatrician's explanation of Keri's hiccups, which were still plaguing her. The term sensory processing disorder (SPD)—an explanation that might fit—had not even been coined, let alone a treatment developed to help rewire or train the brain to allow sensory input without overload.

We accepted Keri's fits as a part of her emotional makeup, stemming from her biology. We certainly did not consider them a behavior problem requiring discipline. Discipline for what? She obviously did not do it for attention. She didn't have a fit in response to not getting her way, or because she was being obstinate. And she was not destructive.

At the Montessori preschool, when a child displayed excessive crying, he/she was sent to the principal's office to calm down. This normally helped the child, plus it cut down on disruption to the class and reduced the distress of all involved. The principal was a kind, patient, older nun who had decades of experience with young children.

But Keri's crying, I was told, was different from that of other children. Although some sound and tactile issues could cause her to start crying, there usually was no observable trigger for her fits. And unlike other children who quickly stopped crying when removed from a situation, Keri continued to wail loudly for over an hour. The principal remained in the office with other crying children. When Keri was sent to her, the woman left the room. I understood why completely. Keri's loud wailing created a sense of distress in anyone hearing it. But she was not locked in. When she was done crying, she could go back to her class. I was grateful the school provided Keri with a place to cry in peace. This was all she wanted.

The teachers hoped I knew some magic to help Keri out of these fits, but other than leaving her alone until she was finished, I had no insights to offer.

As she got older, her fits abated, though crying at school stopped long before crying in the car and at home. When she was old enough to rationally discuss it, Keri provided her own perspective on how she could often seem fine away from home, yet have a meltdown as soon as she was with me. She often felt like crying away from home, she explained, but she felt vulnerable, so she tried hard not to. She felt overwhelmed by everything—sensations, sounds, frustration, tiredness, pain, and many other feelings. Once she could let down her guard, the anguish she'd held in all day exploded in a series of gut-wrenching sobs, screams, and loud wails.

Even at a young age, she understood the truth behind a saying she'd seen on a poster where I worked: "In order to survive a shark attack, *don't bleed*." Peers can be like the sharks. If you bleed—if you show vulnerability—you're likely to wind up as food in a feeding frenzy, a target for being picked on or worse.

When Keri was still just four years old, there were times we thought she might be hearing voices. Sometimes when she was alone, we could hear her talking and laughing. *With whom?* It sounded different than when she was playing pretend with her toys. Sometimes she would put her hands over her ears and say "Shut up!" when nobody was talking. Other times she'd agitatedly talk out loud to herself.

"*No, I don't!*" we heard from her room. "You were bad. You should be quiet when I practice." There was a pause, followed by the sound of Keri pacing about her room, saying, "I'm a *good* girl!" Then in a more plaintive voice, she pleaded, "Don't leave me. Please don't go. Don't hate me."

Greg and I froze, looking at each other in surprise tinged with fear. Since both of our mothers had schizophrenia, we were determined not to interpret Keri's behavior through biased eyes. We laughed at our paranoia and shrugged off our worries. After all, Keri was just a little girl.

In reality, our daughter *was* hearing voices. Years later, she told us she'd heard voices for as long as she could remember. She didn't know they were abnormal. They were a part of her, and most of the time they were as nice as she was, even helpful.

Sometimes her responses to the voices caused misunderstandings. One day Keri suddenly yelled "Shut up!" while her father was saying something to her. It seemed so out of character for such a polite child. But she had not yelled at Greg. She had yelled at *them*—the voices. *They* did not follow the rules of being polite and not talking when others were speaking.

Hearing Voices: Some creative, imaginative children hear voices. Many stop hearing them—with no interventions—within three years of when they start. Some do not. Some later manifest psychosis. Scientists and doctors do not yet know which of these children will need intervention, so getting the child's health tested is advisable (see Appendix B: Medical Tests).

If your child has any associated characteristics of autism, such as sensory overload, meltdowns, allergies, hand movements, etc., you may wish to consult with doctors and therapists versed in treating autism and sensory issues sooner rather than later.

If you suspect your child hears voices, try to keep his/her environment the way you would for any very sensitive child. Restrict television and video-game playing. Encourage active play and contact with nature. Provide good, wholesome nutrition, and throw out junk foods. Some foods/supplements, such as the long-chained omega-3 fatty acids found in cold water ocean fish and algae help protect the brain and may spur neurogenesis (growth of brain cells). Ensure excellent sleep hygiene and take care of allergies. Address sensory issues, both accommodating them and helping the child to overcome them (sometimes occupational therapy is useful). Watch for sources of psychological stress, such as teasing or bullying at school, excessive arguing at home, stress from a sibling, etc. Family therapy (also called family psychoeducation) to help express feelings in a constructive way may be helpful, and encouraging rules of respect for each other's needs is important.

For some, the voices are like helpful coaches. For others, they can become hurtful and negative. My daughter described them as feeling like she was sharing living quarters in her brain with roommates who were generally pleasant, sometimes not. At times they were overwhelmingly annoying, mostly due to the fact they got too noisy. Cognitive therapies are being developed to help deal with negative voices.

Chapter 5
Montessori Madness and Scalpel Success

When Keri turned five, she resented not being with her elementary school friends. But the way a Montessori program is set up, there is much to learn at any level. Also, as advanced as she was verbally, socially, and academically, she lagged behind her peers in written composition. Even using moveable letters and not having to write with a pencil, transposing thoughts into the written word was arduous for her. This seemed strange, since her verbal ability was such a strong point. She was getting increasingly frustrated, but, after all, she was only five! Keri's teachers assured me her writing ability would soon catch up with that of her peers. I had a nagging intuition it would not.

Other members of my family have writing disabilities, and I suspected Keri did, too. If this turned out to be the case, she might need formal instruction in writing, which the Montessori school did not provide. I wanted her to get help as early as possible, but I wasn't confident in my intuition, and I didn't want to be pushy or neurotic about it. Keri's Montessori educational professionals said to let it be, so I let it be.

Since my religious and ethnic background is Jewish, I now gave Keri the choice of staying in Sunday school at the UU church with her sister, or going to Sunday school at the synagogue. Keri fell in love with the rabbi's caring and compassionate wife, who would be teaching the kindergarten class at the synagogue. She was excited at the thought of having such a dynamic, jovial, and interesting person as a teacher, and she chose the synagogue. Keri connected with her new Sunday school teacher, relishing their time together while soaking up the world of Judaica through story, craft, and song. I split my time between the two religious worlds my daughters had chosen.

Midway through the year, I was asked to substitute teach a beginning Hebrew reading class. One afternoon a week, after her own school day was over, Keri had a one and a half-hour wait at the synagogue while I taught my class. Everyone got used to seeing this little girl sitting around, either on a bench in the front foyer or on the floor outside the classroom, reading big books. She plowed her way through *Little Women* by Louisa May Alcott. The book had many long, old-fashioned words, and Keri and I had some cozy nights curled up in bed with a heavy dictionary, looking them up.

At home, Candace and Keri still played with each other and were together a lot. Keri liked being with Candace while she did homework. One day I discovered that five-year-old Keri had been helping Candace with some of her eighth-grade homework assignments. With her ability to speed read, Keri could quickly find the answers in Candace's textbooks. But, Candace later informed me, Keri had actually begun occasionally helping her with homework back when she was in fifth grade, and Keri was two and a half.

In spite of ongoing problems with allergies, fits, migraines, and stomachaches, Keri was relatively content. Adding to her excitement about life in general was the opportunity presented to explore one of her passions—science.

Tom, the director of a children's summer program sponsored by a local university, was impressed with Keri and took a supportive interest in her. He talked to the out-of-state teacher who was coming to run a medical class for fourth- through sixth-graders. Based on Tom's recommendation, the teacher felt comfortable with a gifted five-year-old joining the class. She agreed to admit Keri for the three-week session.

But when the time came, the teacher took one look at Keri and changed her mind. "No way!" she said. Instead of the five-and-a-half-year-old she'd agreed to accommodate, what she saw in front of her was a child who looked like a toddler. The teacher marched us over to the director and told him the same thing—no way—but Tom talked her into giving Keri a try. If she still felt Keri should not be in the class by the end of the first day, Tom promised we would uncomplainingly not bring her back.

I was nervously awaiting their return when I saw the class walking toward me. As they approached, the teacher flashed a big grin and gave me a thumbs-up. Two older girls were holding Keri's hands. Apparently, they had adopted her. The teacher said Keri could handle a scalpel as well as the best of her classmates. She read and understood the exploratory and academic material and participated intelligently, thoughtfully, and maturely. In other words, she fit in just fine.

In the following weeks, the students saw a video of a live childbirth and toured a hospital and a medical helicopter. They dissected organs, including a cow's eye, which Keri brought home. They used microscopes and played science games. The teacher said the older kids treated Keri like any other student when it came to work and games, but they helped her with objects beyond her reach, and—because of her age and size—they held her hand when they went anywhere. This class was not just the highlight of Keri's summer; it was, perhaps, the highlight of her life until she was 11, when she was able to participate in a similar program.

Keri now said she wanted to be a pediatrician or a surgeon when she grew up, but she wanted to be a pilot and an astronaut, too. She asked if she could be both a doctor and an astronaut. I told her I thought this would be a great combination, but I had to reassure her she could be a mother as well.

~~~~~~~~~~~

The summer had been good for Keri's self-esteem, and she definitely had matured. Back at the Montessori school, she was assigned to the classroom for six- to eight-year-olds and she was self-assured and confident. But she was disgruntled, claiming the teachers were not following Montessori principles. She said they were separating the first-, second-, and third-year students,[12] and she felt like she

---

[12] Montessori classrooms group children in age ranges rather than by grade. Grade has the connotation of academic level. In a Montessori environment, children are supposed to learn

was in first grade. She had to sit in a group with kids learning to read. At least she was not crying about her problem. She was trying to solve it. She really *had* matured.

Keri wanted me to meet with the teachers, but I said no. If she wanted to be included with the second-year students so badly, I said, she would have to show her maturity by handling the matter herself.

She did.

She got on the computer and wrote the teachers a note requesting an after-school conference. They granted her request and, after the conference, agreed that she participate as a second-year student. The only areas in which she lagged behind were writing and spelling. Fortunately, students worked on these subjects individually, at their own pace. I was glad Keri had the opportunity to see she could initiate change and exercise control over her situation.

We found a joyful, playful violin teacher, Claire, whom Keri liked. So at six and a half, she started playing violin again. She had a lot of fun with her new teacher. Claire covered things she felt Keri needed to know, but they also had freestyle jam sessions, since Keri had a natural ability to play simple songs she had not been taught. (If she could hear the song in her head, she could play it.) I sat in on one of these sessions, and I could understand Keri's happiness as she and Claire jumped from one song to another, creating medleys.

Keri loved to play violin in the yard and along the creek that meandered behind our house. She played to the accompaniment of the ribbeting frogs, the gurgling water, and the chirping crickets. She played for me while I gardened, and she entertained neighborhood children and adults by having them call out the names of songs for her to play. She began to create original music, both on the piano and violin. Still, when referred to as a musician, she got huffy, saying stiffly she was *not* a musician because this was her hobby, not her

---

according to their individual achievement level. Thus, the children were referred to as being first-, second- or third-year students according to the number of years they had been in a group. At the beginning of the school year, the age range in Keri's class was from five and a half to eight. Traditional schools would have considered this first through third grades.

profession. After all, she was going to be a pilot/astronaut, pediatrician/surgeon, and a mother. She never wanted music to be her *job*. It was her *fun*.

Aside from Keri's ongoing health issues (mostly allergies), the meltdowns we accepted as being a part of her makeup, and her sleep disturbances (hours of moaning, yelling, and thrashing, along with nightmares and night terrors), life felt reasonably good.

While going for a walk with Greg and me, Keri met a girl riding a bicycle. The girl got off her bike to walk with us, and she and Keri started talking. Her name was Leslie. She was a year younger than Keri. She shared with Keri a passion for creative play, a love of nature, a kind disposition, and concern about the environment. She lived just a couple blocks from us. Leslie became Keri's best friend for years to come.

Table 6: Characteristics: Ages 3 to 6

- Displayed erratic growth pattern.
- Hallucinated when given a shot of Phenergan.
- Loved Montessori preschool, yet most days, she screamed and cried for a half-hour on the way home. (This behavior was less frequent after she reached the age of 6.)
- Compassionate; conscious of the needs of disabled children.
- Unable to cope with unexpected schedule changes. Meltdowns from sensory overload or frustration (*not* frustration from hearing "no" or not getting her own way, but rather from things such as her hands not doing what her mind wanted them to do).
- Complained of frequent stomachaches, headaches, back pain, ankle pain, and knee pain. Sometimes had trouble walking due to pain in her ankles and knees. X-ray of knees showed nothing wrong.
- Clumsy; fell frequently. Felt dizzy and fatigued. Frequently hurt from falling on stairs and bumping into things. Had numerous sprained ankles.
- Started having tics, though we did not recognize what they were at the time. Symptoms: She stretched out or splayed her fingers; lifted her eyebrows; tongued corners of her mouth; and made soft, hiccup-like sounds.
- Hypersensitive to cold temperatures, sounds, and touch (said people hurt her when she was just touched).
- Felt slowed and "spacey" on some days, staring into space. Felt as if her brain could not think.
- Hours-long fits of screaming/crying/wailing continued. Often, she would urinate during fits and sleep afterwards.
- Voracious reader—could speed-read third-grade books at age 4. Also learned to read Spanish while "playing."
- IQ tested at 175—99th percentile on Stanford-Binet IQ test.
- Played violin and piano. Excelled at playing music heard in her head. Composed simple melodies.
- Extreme difficulty writing. Reversed letters, transposed letters in words, omitted letters.
- Still had trouble sleeping at night. Night terrors continued.
- Sometimes talked to herself or heard "others" (hearing voices).
- Suffered from allergies, migraines, and frequent abdominal pain. Had intestinal problems.

Chapter 6
The Little Schoolhouse on the Prairie

When I fantasized about the perfect school for Keri, I imagined something like a home-school but taught by someone else. Tom, the director of the children's summer program who orchestrated getting Keri into the medical-oriented class the year before, made my dream a reality, at least for a year. Since he was between teaching jobs, he decided to create a school combining classes for full-time students with special classes for home-schooled kids. This tiny school would go through the sixth grade. Tom was a musician as well as a gifted educator, and he knew other children like Keri for whom this opportunity would be perfect. Keri was excited about attending. Going to this school promised to be as much fun for her as summer vacation.

During the summer, we visited my younger brother, John, and his family, who had moved to another city sometime before. Keri was happy to be with her cousin Roberta again. They played well together and shared similar interests. Roberta was turning into an excellent pianist, and each girl amazed the other. Roberta thought Keri had memorized the music she was playing on the piano, since Keri didn't use sheet music. Then Roberta found Keri was making up the music on the spot. Meanwhile, Keri marveled at the ease with which Roberta could read music and play it. Each learned from the other.

For the rest of that summer, and for many summers thereafter, Keri went to day camp at a nearby farm. Occasionally her friend Leslie accompanied her as a guest. At camp they rode horses, played in a stream, steered a tractor, and planted vegetables. They even got to plant pumpkins, which they harvested in time for Halloween.

Keri and Leslie both loved to pretend. They created fantasy worlds of fairies living outside under trees, in between rocks, and along the creek banks. Leslie enjoyed singing and dancing and was a willing audience for Keri's piano and violin playing. Each complemented the other. I was grateful Keri had found such a wonderful friend, especially now that Candace was almost 15 and no longer willing to play with her little sister. Leslie was tall, strong, active, athletic, and a bit impulsive. She was quick with a smile—full of laughter and exuberance. She engaged Keri in more physical activities, such as biking, skating, and catching fish and bugs in the creek. Keri, with her innate caution, kept them both out of trouble.

I was not surprised Leslie's mother turned out to be a down-to-earth, wonderful woman. We agreed to mother both girls as our own when they were in our care. As they grew older, they even attended religious functions together—Leslie going with Keri to our synagogue, and Keri going with Leslie to their church.

When autumn rolled around, Keri, turning seven, started at Tom's little school. Located in a rural area on the outskirts of town, it was just minutes from our house. The school used the lower level of a small stone church, set in a field surrounded by farmland. Since Keri had read and immensely enjoyed the *Little House on the Prairie* books, I referred to her school as "the little schoolhouse on the prairie."

The school was very close to the summer camp Keri had attended, and since Tom was a friend of the couple who ran it, the kids went on field trips to their farm, sometimes stopping to investigate roadkill along the way. At the farm, they rode and took care of the horses and had practical lessons in biology and mathematics. What a unique school day. Students and families went to the farm at night for bonfires and lessons on astronomy. Keri was allowed to play piano and violin at school. Along with the other students, she also was learning to play the recorder. In her midyear evaluation, Keri's teacher wrote the following about her progress in music class:

> *She has a good understanding of musical notation, and her work in aural theory is excellent (playing by ear*

> *and writing down melodies). Her musical facility has also been evident as she learns to play recorder.*

Officially, Keri was a third-grader, but she was given work tailored to her abilities. Her reading material for science, social studies, literature, etc., was between sixth- and twelfth-grade levels. For subjects other than math and writing, the teacher allowed Keri to answer questions orally. Mathematics was mostly at the third-grade level, but with a lot of fractions and percentages thrown in. We noticed something odd about Keri's math abilities: They fluctuated. Some days she flew through math calculations and did word problems with ease. Other days she could do only simple arithmetic and no word problems at all.

Although Keri was taking antihistamines and had a hypoallergenic bedroom setup at home, she started the school year with her usual fall allergies and screaming fits. I asked the teacher if he thought something was mentally wrong with Keri. He said no, so I dropped the subject. Both the allergies and fits eventually died down. By her February evaluation, the teacher wrote the following about Keri's work habits and social interactions:

> *Keri is an intelligent, thoughtful child who analyzes situations carefully. In the past month she has added to her intellectual ability a more serious attitude toward hard work.*
>
> *Keri is jovial and naturally kind. She is helpful at school.*

Keri was hopeful about getting into fourth grade at a public school magnet program for students gifted in the creative and performing arts.[13] Midway through the school year, she applied to be a violin major at this school, going through the auditions and testing that were part of the highly selective admissions process. She also had a private interview, the purpose of which was to ensure each applicant sincerely wanted to be in the program. Later I was told when Keri was

---

[13] Magnet programs or magnet schools promote greater diversity by drawing students from an entire county or other geographic area rather than solely from the district in which the school is located.

asked why she wanted to go to this school, she responded, "Because I want to be with children like me who love music."

She was thrilled when we got the letter accepting her for the coming school year. In the meantime, she was receiving formal typing lessons on the computer at her current school. Keri was frustrated trying to write by hand, and her teacher was having her practice handwriting both in school and at home. Writing caused her misery at school, but there were many other things about the place she dearly loved.

Unfortunately, along with Keri's springtime allergies came a recurrence of her meltdowns at school. Her frustration from trying to write, we felt, was a contributing factor. It seemed when she was feeling bad due to her allergies, she had no reserves for tolerating frustrations and annoyances she otherwise would have accepted without incident. I asked the teacher if he thought perhaps Keri should get special help for her writing, or maybe even psychological counseling. He did not think so.

Keri, always sensitive to sounds, became increasingly sensitive to the noise at school, which was causing her escalating distress. She also became less tolerant of the other children's boisterous antics, and a lot less forgiving of them.

While playing outside, a child the same size, but three years younger than Keri, picked up a broken tree limb and bonked her on the head. As with other little injuries Keri suffered, the tenderness at this spot on her head persisted. In the coming years, she felt extreme pain when other children playfully (because she was so tiny) bopped the top of her head with a book or binder while passing her in the hallway at school. A few hairs on the spot grew in white. These wouldn't be the only gray hairs she got before reaching adulthood.

One day Keri stunned her teacher by going berserk because a girl new to the school kept looking at her. There had been some verbal conflict between them earlier, and the girl was now glaring at her. Keri's distressed feelings quickly turned to anger and she started screaming, overwhelmed by emotion. Meaning to calm her, the teacher put his hand firmly on her shoulder. She responded by going wild. At home, Keri coped with out-of-control feelings by escaping to a quiet room—a safe place to calm down. We always left her alone during these times, respecting her need not to be touched.

At school, she had nowhere to escape. Like a cornered animal, she responded by becoming a tornado in the room. Tiny, well-behaved Keri threw chairs and even a heavy table, which the teacher was astonished she could lift, let alone throw. When he tried to physically restrain her, it caused her to rage against him. This little girl, who had never in her life shown physical aggression toward another living being, tried to fight him!

Keri's own emotional memory of this incident is one of total fury. Her rage was not directed at the teacher; she says it was focused on the girl who had purposely tried to provoke a reaction by irritating her. That the teacher was there and she fought against him did not even register. Keri is thankful this incident didn't happen at a public school today, where such behavior is criminalized. She might have been expelled from her school, labeled as a behavior problem, sent to an alternative setting, and treated accordingly.

Later, I was directed to a book, *The Explosive Child*,[14] which explains that some rage is common in frustration-intolerant, chronically inflexible children with sensory overload. The book did not reveal anything new to us or provide any new techniques to help Keri. At home we already allowed her what she needed—peace, quiet, and space to be alone and scream. In return, she was respectful, polite, and conscientious. It was at school she felt trapped.

For years I had been telling people about how bad these fits could get, with everyone (except my parents) telling me Keri was perfectly healthy and normal. Now the teacher suggested Keri get professional psychological help, commenting:

> As the year wore on, Keri seemed to wear out a bit. Some days she had a very low frustration level and could do little assigned work. Normally, she's a good worker.

---

[14] Greene, 2005.

And so it was that Keri began two types of therapy, one for her emotions—learning to understand and live with her own biology—and another for her writing.

For help with writing, we first took her to a large franchised tutoring program called Sylvan Learning, where she was given an extensive evaluation. To our surprise, we were told she had a real learning disability with writing and they could not help her. Keri already knew everything they could teach her, they said, but the knowledge in her brain wasn't being transmitted correctly, thus hampering her efforts to write. They suggested we take her to a tiny local tutoring facility.

This recommended facility, run by a former public school special education teacher, was the tutoring arm of a small, nonprofit, private school for bright children with special educational needs, such as kids with ADHD or learning differences. (I was glad to know that if Keri was ever in need of such a school, one at least existed.)

After being tested again, Keri was diagnosed as having a "specific language disability in written communication." The tutors patiently worked with her three times a week through the spring and summer months, ignoring the times she had meltdowns from frustration and sullenly hid under tables. By the time she started fourth grade, she had gone from struggling to write a single sentence to writing an entire page. It took her six hours to complete that page, but at least she could do so. To me, such progress was verging on miraculous.

For help with Keri's excessive crying and inability to express why she cried so much, we took her to a psychologist known for his work with highly gifted children. He had Keri (and the family) evaluated by a pediatric psychiatrist. The psychiatrist found nothing wrong, but his evaluation established Keri as his patient in the event we ever had a crisis and she needed a psychiatrist. Apparently, because of a dearth of child psychiatrists in our area, it could take a new patient an extended period of time just to get an appointment.

The psychologist found Keri to be delightful, well-adjusted, and without any obvious psychological problems. After a few sessions, he said that as much as he loved talking with her for his *own* pleasure, he felt she would benefit more from expressive arts therapy. He would act (for free) as a consultant with the expressive arts therapist. I felt good that together these three professionals—the expressive arts therapist, the psychologist, and the psychiatrist—would figure out how best to help my daughter. Acting as a team, they had a joint teleconference to formulate how to proceed. I was not charged for this additional conference; they did it because they felt it was the right thing to do. I felt truly blessed.

The goal of expressive arts therapy is to communicate and understand emotions through art as opposed to the spoken word. Instead of trying to gain Keri's trust solely by talking, the therapist started by creating a mask of my daughter's face. Keri had to trust the therapist as she applied plaster to her face. The following week, Keri painted and decorated the mask; the week after that she brought it home. For years afterward, she proudly displayed the mask on her bedroom wall. Other projects she worked on lasted for weeks, some even for months, which added to her eagerness to attend therapy sessions. Communication flowed more freely when Keri was simultaneously expressing herself with her hands. As time progressed, her projects became individualized, reflecting her personal interests, pain, joy, and suffering. It would take years for her to express verbally the complex feelings that erupted into some of her fits, but at least a foundation of trust and expression was being laid.

As for me, I felt I could not continue to meet Keri's needs while working full time. I requested a reduction in hours. If my manager refused, I was prepared to quit my job, even though this would mean losing the bulk of our collective income, a portion of which paid for Keri's therapies. My manager came up with an alternative. She suggested telecommuting, an idea ahead of its time. I was intrigued, but I didn't think I could put in the necessary hours for a full work-week even from home. She assured me the number of hours I put in wasn't an issue, as long as I completed my work. I agreed, and the company set up a home office for me, installing two more phone lines.

I was allowed to keep my office at work as well. This setup, which eventually became a permanent arrangement, proved invaluable.

As Keri headed off to fourth grade at the magnet school for the creative and performing arts, I felt I'd lined up as good a support system for her as I could.

Table 7: Additional Characteristics: Age 7

- Fluctuating attention, abilities, and spacing out.
- Very sensitive. Cried if given a stern or a "wrong" look. Extremely aware of other people's feelings, body language, and motives. Reacted to micro-expressions on people's faces.
- Had wailing fits that could last for hours. Seemed worse seasonally, perhaps due to seasonal allergies.
- At 7-1/2, started being tutored in writing. Was diagnosed with a written communications disorder.
- Went to a psychiatrist and a psychologist who recommended expressive arts therapy for her fits and hypersensitivity. No psychological or psychiatric problem was found; no diagnosis was given.

Chapter 7
Writing Woes and Dealing with Death

The creative and performing arts magnet school was very small—50 students each in grades four through eight. Keri liked her new teachers and her creative arts classes. She loved being a member of the orchestra, and she enjoyed the camaraderie of her fellow majors in string instruments. To our relief, she had no fits of wailing and agitation at school, though they did continue at home.

Teachers quickly made informal accommodations for her writing difficulties, accommodations that followed her through the sixth grade. She could answer essay questions on tests orally, and during fourth and fifth grades, I was allowed to partially type some assignments for her at home. Keri dictated stories and essays into a small handheld recorder while skating around the block. I had the arduous task of transcribing her dictation, which then allowed her to polish the paper to her liking without the monumentally stressful effort of typing it from scratch.

> Even a child not yet formally diagnosed with a learning disability (LD) may benefit from informal accommodations at school.
>
> Spending extra academic time to compensate for an LD, as well as time outside of school in therapies to overcome it, adds stress.
>
> Using accommodations to temporarily compensate for the LD gives the child a precious gift of *time* and lowers stress.
>
> Unfortunately, not all schools are flexible about these issues.

Never having learned to touch-type, I was slow at transcribing the dictation. Sometimes I wished Keri could just turn in the recording, but I had to admit this way was better. Once the story or essay was on paper, she could add to it, change it, and delete what she no longer wanted.

Slowly, Keri became more proficient at typing. By the sixth grade, she did all her own typing and was allowed a laptop at school, yet she still transposed some letters and omitted others entirely. Regardless of the method she used, the process of putting her thoughts into writing remained painfully slow.

Keri tried voice recognition software, then in the early days of development. It could not understand her little-girl voice and often misinterpreted her pauses and the slight extraneous sounds she made while thinking and talking.

> Using dictation software or allowing someone to type the initial paper may be helpful for some children. For others, dictating and being creative while being active is easier than sitting in front of a computer. Using a portable dictation device allows these kids to compose their thoughts while skating, running around, or jumping on a trampoline.

Keri's fifth-grade teacher proposed that Keri do her spelling homework on the computer. Unexpectedly, typing her spelling homework seemed to enhance her ability to hand-write the words correctly on weekly spelling tests.

All these accommodations were made without any formal testing, labeling, or written plans.

At the end of fifth grade, students received awards for being the best at various things. Expecting Keri to receive the award for "Best at Reading," I was surprised she got the one for "Best at English/Language Arts" instead. I asked her how she could get an award in English rather than reading. "Silly Mommy," she said. "You get tested in reading by having to *write*. You mostly get tested in English by having to *read*, and then you just answer some multiple-choice questions about what you've read."

Keri enjoyed her magnet school very much, but this period of her life was not without its tragedies. During her fourth-grade year, one of her teachers died. She also lost two of her grandparents: my mother and Greg's father, Larry. In addition, Napkin, the beloved family dog, died that autumn.

Larry, whom Keri had been close to since infancy, left behind a young 10-pound poodle named Mugsy. He had doted on the little dog, taking him on daily walks through the woods near his home in Michigan. In return, Mugsy had given Greg's father tremendous pleasure and exercise during the last year of his life. After the funeral, we had no choice but to bring the dog with us.

We were going to find him a good home.

It never happened.

Soon after we got back, Keri proudly walked down the sidewalk with Mugsy. Greg sat outside on the front stoop watching them. At a house down the block, where the gate had been accidentally left ajar, a big golden retriever ran out, grabbed Mugsy by the back, and shook him back and forth, inches from Keri's terrified face. Her screams brought the dog's owner, along with Greg and other neighbors who rushed to her assistance. Later, the retriever's owner said the dog killed muskrats from the creek in the same way she had tried to kill Mugsy, clamping her jaws around their backs and giving them a shake.

Mugsy was alive, but he had holes called sucking wounds around his back and abdomen, necessitating emergency veterinary care.

The outcome of this horror was twofold. First, Greg and I became friends with the family of the other dog, and Keri also made a new friend—the family's young daughter. Second, by the time Mugsy was healed from this ordeal, physically and emotionally, he had become part of the family.

Mugsy was extra precious to Keri. After all, he had been her beloved grandpa's dog. When he later started having seizures, the vet determined the dog had an inoperable liver shunt and didn't give him long to live. In the meantime, he had to eat a mostly vegetarian diet. Because of his continuing problems, Keri nicknamed him Boo-Boo.

I was concerned about Keri because of all these deaths in one year, but it turned out I needn't have worried. Like all of us, she grieved when faced with such losses, but she also displayed the natural resilience of youth and moved on with her life.

She continued to get support from her expressive arts therapy, and she received a great deal of love and support from family and friends. Keri and Candace had the best relationship I could imagine for sisters. At 16, Candace was no longer interested in spending much time playing with Keri, but they talked a lot about school, friends, family, poetry, books, art, and music. Keri still had the constant stressors of disturbed sleep and allergies, yet, other than the way she felt physically, she enjoyed her life the way it was, her music, her religious activities, and the curriculum and camaraderie at school.

One thing we could not explain was her declaration that on some days she felt as if her brain just couldn't function, a phenomenon we'd been noticing for a couple years. On these days of non-function, Keri couldn't concentrate or do even simple work. She felt spacey, she said, and often stared off into nothingness. If I'd been homeschooling her, these were the times I'd have let her do nothing.

The frequency of these episodes would increase in the coming years, but at the time, with nothing to the contrary forthcoming from the doctors, I thought this, too, was normal.

What I found alarmingly *abnormal* were the rare occasions when Keri did more than just space out. Like a soldier with a post-traumatic stress disorder (PTSD) flashback, she was suddenly fearful, as if responding to petrifying events only she could see. As she crouched, terrified, in a corner or under a table, I sometimes could use my body as a protective shield, lessening her distress. At other times, she was equally fearful of *me*. Coming out of the blue, Keri's brain seemed to suddenly interpret everything around her through a filter of terror. It reminded me of the time she became delirious from her reaction to Phenergan.

During these new fits, she urinated. After she was calm, I helped her clean up, acting nonchalant and comforting her in a quiet voice and low-key manner. Keri didn't remember her behavior during these episodes except at the tail end of them, when she felt confused and tired. We began to call these Keri's PTSD-like fits.

Keri had another type of fit—fortunately, also infrequently—that Greg and I termed "psychotic-like." One such episode occurred after she contracted a bad case of poison oak. Paranoid and scared, convinced of a conspiracy to do her harm, she refused to get out of the car at the doctor's office.

Her doctors did not seem concerned, for which Greg and I later blamed ourselves. Perhaps we hadn't stressed the severity of her fits, or perhaps we hadn't used the right terminology to describe them. If we had called them "occurrences of brief episodic psychosis" or "instances of delirium," would she have gotten better care, sooner?

Table 8: Characteristics: Age 8

- Continued expressive arts therapy.
- Continued tutoring for her writing.
- Continued to have migraines, tics, and allergies, as well as intolerance to cold.
- Had dry skin.
- Experienced fluctuating attention (spaciness), moods, fatigue, and dizziness.
- Had intermittent pain in joints and muscles and burning pain under her skin when excessively fatigued.
- *Loved* her new school (a public creative and performing arts magnet school).
- No longer had fits at school.
- Continued to have fits at home, sometimes urinating due to crying so hard. Had meltdowns when tired. Sometimes acted briefly psychotic. Did not remember rare PTSD-like episodes, which were sometimes accompanied by urination.
- Experienced disturbed sleep.
  - Trouble staying asleep.
  - Moaning for hours during the night.
  - Night terrors.
  - Bruxism (teeth-grinding).
- Dealt normally and maturely with four deaths in one year.

Before

Ages Nine to Ten and a Half

The feeling of being down,
Is a sun that gives no warmth,
And every leaf that rustles,
Vibrating in the cold brisk wind,
Adds to the sound of melancholy
Carried by the breeze.

Everyone looks the same,
and all seems very futile,
Everything not quite right,
Like a veil of distortion covering eyes,
And clouding minds.

— Jeanie

Chapter 8
School Scrutiny

As Keri was in the middle of growing up, better understanding herself, overcoming her writing problems, and becoming more emotionally mature, unexpected and misunderstood fatigue and depression would crash down upon her. Greg and I provided support through periods of success and blossoming independence, interspersed with bouts of bone-crushing exhaustion. The years between nine and a half and eleven and a half heralded a time of puzzling health woes, years when our daughter doggedly grabbed at life's pleasures in the slivers of time during which she felt well enough to pursue them.

The summer before sixth grade, Keri was increasingly exhausted and frequently ill. One day she pushed through her lethargy enough to start out for her best friend Leslie's house to play. She never got there. When Leslie's mom called to say Keri hadn't arrived, I felt a chill of panic. Leslie's mother began walking in my direction while I started toward her. I didn't have far to go.

Keri was in our driveway, crouched low to the ground next to the car, sobbing enough to break anyone's heart. She was sorry, she said. She just couldn't go to Leslie's to play. She knew her friend expected her, but she just couldn't.

Keri was in deep trouble. She obviously needed more help than her expressive arts therapy and a loving family could provide.

~~~~~~~~~~~

At nine years old, Keri had thrived in fifth grade. Her classroom teacher, who also led the speech and drama team, was a dynamic instructor. Keri looked forward to each of her creative arts classes.

And she especially enjoyed orchestra, which was not only her major but the source of her primary social circle at school.

In the main classroom, Keri felt frustrated socially, explaining she was sometimes excluded from group conversations. She also said the other children teased her at times, but she would not provide details.

The school's counselor was Keri's one-woman fan club. They were both tiny, and the counselor could relate to Keri on many levels, both academically and socially. To escape from the daily school bustle, she was allowed to take sanctuary in the quiet of the counselor's office whenever she needed. The office was also her refuge when she felt like exploding with frustration and anger at the other children, who were simply being children.

Academically, the material was easy for her, but completing her homework was proving to be a challenge. She often did the wrong assignments, and math took hours to finish. When Greg and I investigated, we discovered Keri's writing problems kept her from writing the directions fast enough when they were given verbally. And when the teacher wrote assignments on the board, Keri sometimes copied the page numbers incorrectly. Other students in the class had similar problems, so Keri joined a group of students in getting her assignment book verified. Sometimes mistakes still slipped through, but the teacher understood and was lenient.

At the beginning of fifth grade, Keri tested in the 97th percentile on a standardized math test. Much of her math homework was arithmetic involving large numbers, yet she knew some of the answers just by looking at the problem. Then she wrote down the answer, or part of it, in reverse order, transposing digits. Her problem was not in her ability to do the math; it was in the amount of time she needed to write down the numbers correctly.

The psychiatrist helped resolve Keri's math homework problem. He said she needed an accommodation that restricted the *quantity* of her math homework; instead, she should be graded on the *quality* of the homework completed. Since she didn't need all the repetition in the arithmetic being assigned, he suggested she be restricted to doing math homework for no more than an hour. Greg or I would then initial her paper, signifying she had worked for one hour, and the teacher would grade her on what was completed. Since Keri's tests in class showed she was doing fine in math, the teacher enthusiastically agreed.

> Limiting the amount of time a child spends on homework, especially when the child does not require the repetition, is reasonable. It cuts down on stress, which in turn cuts down on time lost due to meltdowns. Children may have more energy and think more clearly when they have less stress from homework and more time for active play.

Near the end of fifth grade, we requested that Keri be tested by the public school system for a learning disability in writing. Her problems would then be documented in school records, and the test results would formally establish the accommodations she required (and by law, would be entitled to). When a child is found to meet the federal or state requirements for special education and related services, an Individualized Education Plan (IEP) is developed to meet that child's educational requirements in the public school system. The IEP typically lists necessary accommodations, subject areas impacted by the student's disability, and special services that may be required.[15] Since her teachers were already making common-sense accommodations for her without the formalities, Keri had not yet needed a written IEP. Such documentation, however, could save her from future problems in other grades and other schools.

Testing wasn't done until sixth grade. By then, Keri was in the middle school wing of her performing arts magnet school, with many different teachers. Fortunately, these teachers were also accommodating her needs, even though she was having significant problems with her health and missing a great deal of school.

---

[15] Great ideas for accommodations and model IEPs can be found at Web sites such as "The Bipolar Child" (http://www.bipolarchild.com) and in books such as *Teaching the Tiger*, Dornbush and Pruitt, 1995.

Keri's tests results did not qualify her as having a learning disability (LD) in writing for the purpose of receiving academic assistance from the public school system. Her psychiatrist was outraged. By medical definition, Keri did have an LD, especially in the area of writing fluency. The testers noted it took Keri an inordinate amount of time— 1 hour and 20 minutes—to write a single paragraph of 12 sentences, but, they said, the *content* of her writing was at college level. The amount of time it took did not factor into the evaluation, only the quality of the final result.

Thus, Keri did not get an IEP. However, she was sufficiently covered under the school disability label OHI-Other Health Impairments, as well as a federal law providing educational support, Section 504 of the Rehabilitation Act of 1973. The 504 Plan is more general, having to do with civil rights and with the goal of removing barriers to the success of a student with disabilities.

The occupational therapist involved in the testing felt Keri *did* need occupational therapy, although given enough time, she compensated for deficits by completing tasks differently than the norm. Because some gifted-LD children are so good at problem-solving, it is common for them to develop strategies to cope with their areas of weakness, observed Linda Kreger Silverman of Denver's Gifted Development Center in her essay, "The Two-Edged Sword of Compensation: How the Gifted Cope with Learning Disabilities." In turn, such strategies can make learning disabilities in the gifted more difficult to recognize.[16] The occupational therapist gave us fun ideas for therapy to do at home, activities with which Keri happily complied.

As a result of the testing, meetings, and doctor's input, Keri received the following formal recommendations:

- *She should be graded on the quality, rather than the amount, of work completed. Keri and the teacher should determine in advance what is acceptable and establish a contract.*

---

[16] Silverman, 2000.

- *There should be a safe place in the school where she can go to recover her equilibrium when feeling overwhelmed.*
- *She should be allowed extra time to complete written assignments.*
- *In all classes, the teacher should provide Keri with a weekly syllabus with class assignments and expectations.*

At the time we requested testing, Greg and I were not aware such a request would put our daughter under a microscope psychologically. The first and only task accomplished before the end of the fifth-grade school year was that professionals in the field of psychology came to the school to observe Keri's social interactions with her classmates. The school counselor met with us to go over why the observation took place and to review the results. We were told the outside evaluators wanted to determine if Keri's grade placement was appropriate for her socially as well as academically. The school counselor laughed, saying she knew what they would find. She understood Keri's size created more obstacles for her than her age. She also voiced her opinion that Keri was sweet, kind, gentle, and honest, as well as quite mature and socially advanced for her age.

The outside observers reported Keri was actually *more* socially mature than her peers and displayed *more* socially appropriate behavior than some of the other fifth-graders. Her grade placement was completely appropriate. Keri did have some problems socially, but they were not due to behavior on her part. Just as the counselor had predicted, when the other children were standing in a group, talking, they had to look down to see Keri, who was only about three-quarters their height. It wasn't deliberate on their part, but because the other students weren't making eye contact with her, Keri was inadvertently excluded. Another problem was simply the immaturity of the other children. They sometimes teased Keri for things she could not help.

These "things," we soon found out, were motor and vocal tics mild enough for adults to ignore or misinterpret, but the other kids picked up on them. Keri had mild Tourette syndrome.

When Keri herself was asked about grade placement, she said, given the choice, she would be with children even *older*.

Chapter 9
Tic ... Tic ... Tic ...

On a visit to my brother's family, I laughed at John for not recognizing his daughter Roberta's facial movement for what it was—a tic—even though she did. Asked what she had just done, Roberta shrugged and said, "This? Oh, it's just a tic I have." I later had to apologize to John for laughing. Greg and I experienced parental blindness to the same issue in Keri when her therapist mentioned her tics. "Tics? What tics!?" I responded. We hadn't recognized Keri's movements as tics, either. Even Keri's pediatrician had misinterpreted them.

With a name for it, came confidence.

Keri felt relieved to have a word to attach to the things she did with her face, hands, fingers, and toes. She was especially glad to learn that a small, quiet, hiccup-like sound she made was actually a vocal tic. At school, some of the kids had mocked her when she made this sound. Now, having acquired a name for it, the next time a group of kids asked why she did that, she replied assertively, "It's a tic. I can't help it. It's like stuttering." To the credit of the other children, once Keri's actions were given a label and a simple explanation, the kids no longer felt a strong need to mock them.

After reading about Tourette syndrome[17] in a hefty but immensely readable book by David E. Comings, M.D., titled *Tourette Syndrome and Human Behavior*, I recognized Tourette genes coursing through the branches of my family tree. For years we thought Keri rotated her hands and splayed her fingers, sometimes in an undulating move-

---

[17] *The Diagnostic and Statistical Manual of Mental Disorders, 4th Edition, Text Revision (DSM-IV-TR)* contains the standard classification of mental disorders used by psychiatrists, psychologists, and other mental health and medical professionals in the United States. It describes Tourette syndrome (307.23 Tourette's Disorder) as starting prior to age 18 and consisting of both multiple motor tics and one or more vocal tics occurring many times a day (usually in bouts), nearly daily or intermittently, over more than one year.

ment, due to fatigue. Her hands *were* fatigued, but the fatigue was due to the tics; the tics weren't a result of the fatigue. Her toes did the same thing; they just weren't noticeable, hidden by shoes.

Another tic caused her to open her mouth wide and touch her tongue to each corner of her mouth. Looking over photographs, we found shots from age five that caught her in the middle of her mouth tic. I used to think her mouth tic was due to irritation when, actually, the irritation was caused by the tic. Not understanding the cause of her crimson, swollen lips, with chafing spreading out around them, I took Keri to a dentist and a dermatologist, and I layered on ointments. Making matters worse, the lip ointment I first chose contained propylene glycol, to which she was allergic.

This particular tic had caused Keri to lose a friend in fourth grade when it was misinterpreted. With determination, she modified it by substituting her fingers in place of her tongue. Later, after learning about cognitive behavioral therapy (CBT), a process that teaches a person to modify socially unacceptable or even harmful behaviors, including tics, I realized Keri was doing CBT *on her own*, to herself.[18]

> **Cognitive Behavioral Therapy (CBT)** diminishes undesirable behaviors while teaching alternate, more adaptive behaviors to replace them. Behaviors can be actions, thoughts, or emotional responses.

Later, when Keri acquired other motor and vocal tics, we recognized them for what they were. Understanding, for example, kept us from becoming annoyed when Keri suddenly released a screeching tic at the dinner table. In her own home, at least, she should be able to relax and not worry about expressing tics.

Determined to be socially acceptable, Keri hid the screeching tic at school. She said there were always times when groups of girls

---

[18] Cognitive behavioral therapy is usually done with a specially trained therapist and can be time consuming and costly.

screeched, so she held that tic in until other kids shrieked. Then she released it. Nobody at school even noticed.

I had to wonder about the energy Keri expended just controlling her tics.

An enlightening book for parents got me thinking about the way tics can be held in for a period of time, then released in a frenzy as if all the held-back tics were being unleashed at once[19] Could this description apply to pent-up emotions as well? The description of tic-release was very similar to Keri's description of her meltdowns after school. She often felt like crying at school, but since she'd seen other children belittled for crying, their weaknesses used against them, she heavily guarded her emotions. At home, where she felt comfortable and safe, she relaxed her guard, releasing the multitude of distressed feelings she'd held back all day.

Keri's ability to articulate all this was a major breakthrough. I thanked her expressive arts therapist for helping her develop this insight and find the words with which to express it.

Sometimes we get emotional support, insight, or just a different perspective from the most unlikely of sources, such as a random song, book, or poem. For me, I found it in a science fiction series by Nancy Kress collectively referred to as *The Beggars Trilogy* or *The Sleepless Trilogy*. Kress has deep insight into human society, which she projects into futuristic societies based on plausible science. In this particular series, genetically modified children are called the Sleepless—normal except that they need no sleep. Since they have more time to develop and learn, they grow into adults with superior intellect. The Sleepless then create a generation of children called the Super-Sleepless, whose intellectual abilities are greater still. Of course, rifts develop between the groups, but the gentle Super-Sleepless want to heal those rifts. The Super-Sleepless children were especially endearing to me because, like my little girl, they were smart and compassionate and had large heads and tics.

---

[19] Marsh, T. L., 2007.

In sixth grade, Keri's psychiatrist asked her if she would like not to tic. "Of course!" she exclaimed. What if he could give her a pill that might stop the tics or at least make them less noticeable to others? She liked that idea, but a suspicious look quickly came across her face. "What's the pill?" she asked.

"Risperdal," the doctor replied.

"Is it safe?" queried the always-cautious Keri.

"Relatively, yes," replied the doctor. "It's been used for Tourette syndrome for years, in children as well as in adults."

Keri asked to see the doctor's *PDR* (*Physician's Desk Reference*).

"That's a first for me," the doctor said, wryly, as he took his hefty *PDR* off the shelf and handed it to her. "I've never had a 10-year-old ask to look something up in the PDR before. In fact, I've never had a child of any age do so." Keri was not satisfied with the information about Risperdal (generic name, risperidone) in the *PDR*. She asked the doctor if he minded if she told him her answer at the next appointment, because she wanted to find more information about the drug on the Internet.

When she next met with the psychiatrist, her answer was "No." Yes, she badly wanted not to tic, but she felt the potential side effects of Risperdal (a long list, including death) outweighed the possible benefits of alleviating her tics. She'd rather live with the tics.

> Triggers for tics and obsessive-compulsive behaviors may be stressors, which may include illness or psychological stress. Also being researched is the possibility of our own immune system attacking the brain (referred to as an auto-immune reaction) in response to some infectious agents such as Group A beta-hemolytic streptococci, the bacteria that can cause "strep throat." Thus, some cases are currently being treated with medical interventions such as antibiotics.

Chapter 10
Depression

At the end of the fifth grade, Keri was nine and a half and excited about the long summer vacation. She could go out to the farm camp when she wanted, stay home when she wanted, read, create art, immerse herself in her music, and play with neighborhood friends. Mostly, she wanted to play at camp—ride horses and lie around on an inner tube in the creek.

But each time she went to the farm she got sick from allergies, making her unable to return or even to play with her friends at home for two or three days. She was already getting allergy shots and taking prescription pharmaceutical antihistamines. The allergist had nothing more to offer and, at the time, we knew nothing about alternative and complementary treatments for allergies such as dietary changes, probiotics,[20] or nutritional supplements.

> **Pharmaceuticals,** patented medications sold by pharmaceutical companies, are government-approved to treat diagnosed conditions. They are also referred to as *traditional medicines*. Some nutritional supplements are also pharmaceuticals.
>
> Nutritional supplements, vitamins, minerals, roots, and herbs, are considered foods when used to enhance health or to combat a disease process in the body. They are euphemistically referred to as **nutraceuticals**.
>
> When a nutraceutical is used in lieu of one or more pharmaceuticals, it is termed an *alternative treatment*. When used in addition to pharmaceuticals, it is referred to as a *complementary treatment*.

At first, Keri was dejected about the allergies, but decided one day of fun at camp wasn't worth several days of feeling awful. She had plenty to do at home and around the neighborhood to keep her hap-

---

[20] Vliagoftis, H., et al., 2008.

py, including some wonderful books she'd set aside for the summer. However, when trying to read the small print in the thick paperback novels, she was soon complaining of blurred vision. When neither the optometrist nor the ophthalmologist could find anything wrong with her eyes, she ultimately abandoned her summer reading in disgust.

She still had plenty of other options, but much of the time she felt too tired to do anything. Playing at a friend's house left her feeling exhausted, and she said her head hurt. Sometimes she'd agree to play with friends and then later call to cancel.

Keri started following me around the house, sitting near me lethargically while I worked. Her friends urged her to rollerblade or bike with them, to explore along the creek, to play in the backyard playhouse. She stayed indoors instead. When friends showed up at the door, she sent them away.

Her actions were not due to a lack of desire, Keri explained. She *wanted* to be with her friends, but didn't have it in her to follow through and actually play. Her fatigue soon segued into depression. She cried but didn't know why. She labeled her feeling as "despair" but said there was nothing she despaired *about*. She couldn't understand such feelings without thoughts to be feeling sad about. Neither could Greg nor I.

A visit to the pediatrician revealed nothing. After a cursory exam, she said that other than Keri's allergies, she was physically fine. She had no explanation for the tiredness and lethargy. Perhaps she was just feeling depressed, the pediatrician postulated, and remarked it was a good thing Keri was already in therapy. The therapist, on the other hand, said there was nothing actually bothering her, nor were there any depressing factors in her life.

I scheduled an appointment with the psychiatrist. He could see her in a few weeks. (Had Keri not already been established as a patient at age seven, the wait could have been several *months*.)

While we waited, summer was waning. Keri started crying so hard she wet her clothing. Her sleep, which had never been good, got even worse. She started slapping herself across the face while screaming. I tried to be comforting, but she seemed to be unaware of my presence. As if she were in a world of her own, she robotically hit herself until I intervened by restraining her. This caused her to scream harder, but at least it got her to stop slapping herself. When I let her go, she ran to her room and screamed until she fell into an exhausted, fitful sleep.

Keri had plunged into deep, incapacitating depression.

Neither Greg nor I knew what to make of this new turn of events. Greg missed doing things with Keri on weekends, and he felt distressed that his little girl was crying so much. All we could do was offer comfort. I understood feeling depressed about situations, and I knew some children were sensitive and prone to depression. We made up reasons why Keri might be depressed.

Greg and I both went with Keri to her appointments with the psychiatrist. My husband's supervisor was not very understanding about him taking time off from work, but family had always come first. Greg wanted to be sure Keri had support from both her parents and that he had the knowledge he needed to be the best possible father for his daughter.

The doctor said Keri did not have a situational depression, defined as a reaction to a situation or event. Her depression was not psychological; *psychologically*, she was a normal, healthy child. Rather, he explained, she had an intrinsic or biological depression, also referred to as clinical depression. There was something chemically wrong inside her brain, but a medical test had not yet been developed to determine the underlying cause. I know now there is a long list of known, testable, and diagnosable medical problems that can cause depresssion, but tests for these problems, even though such tests *do* exist, are usually not prescribed, just as they were not prescribed for my daughter. (For more information about specific tests, see Appendix B: Medical Tests.)

That summer, Keri had no medical tests at all, but she did receive a psychiatric diagnosis of major depressive disorder (MDD), which is considered a severe mental illness. I didn't know it at the time, but this diagnosis would have a significantly adverse effect on her future medical care.

To treat her symptoms of depression, the psychiatrist prescribed a low dose of Zoloft (sertraline), a type of antidepressant called a SSRI (see box). She began taking it just in time to start middle school.

> An **SSRI**—selective serotonin re-uptake inhibitor—increases the brain's neurohormone serotonin (5HT) level by slowing down its removal rate. Other neurotransmitters in the brain, such as norepinephrine, dopamine, acetylcholine (ACh), glutamate, and gamma-aminobutyric acid (GABA), may be involved to different degrees in different individuals' depressive illnesses.
>
> Pharmaceutical medications affecting brain chemicals are collectively referred to as **psychotropic medications**.
>
> Some nutritional supplements also are used to protect brain neurons, help boost brain chemicals the body can synthesize, and/or boost neurogenesis. These include tryptophan, folate, B_{12}, omega-3 fatty acids, melatonin, trimethylglycine (TMG), and SAM-e.

Table 9: Characteristics: Age 9

- Migraines, allergies, and sensitivity to cold, touch, sounds, and odors continued.
- Complained about her knees, ankles, back, and neck hurting.
- Stomachaches, headaches, migraines, dizziness, and intestinal problems continued.
- Having her involuntary physical movements labeled tics helped confidence and self-esteem.
- Learning disability (LD).
- Dry skin much worse.
- Exhibited attention problems/spacing out.
- Had blurred vision when trying to read small print in books.
- Suffered from frequent fatigue.
- Diagnosed with major depressive disorder. Prescribed Zoloft, an SSRI antidepressant.

Chapter 11
Getting On the Roller Coaster

I was amazed at the immediate impact of even a small amount of Zoloft (half of the lowest-dose pill), but Keri's astonishment exceeded mine. Although she continued waking up during the night, for the first time in her life she quit screaming, moaning, thrashing, and crying for hours in her sleep. Greg and I could finally get a refreshing night's rest. It was as if a switch had been flipped in her brain. Suddenly she could tolerate popular music without the sensory overload that in the past caused meltdowns. She began to listen to the same music as her peers. Talking to friends and classmates about bands and lyrics provided a greater social connection with them.

Most stunning to Keri was her happiness. When a local news station approached her psychiatrist about children using antidepressants, Keri readily agreed to be interviewed. At the time, children using antidepressants was a fairly new concept. Understanding the controversy and misconceptions about "drugging" kids with antidepressants, she eloquently stated during the television interview that her antidepressant was not a happy pill. Zoloft did not *make* her happy, she explained. Rather, it *enabled* her to feel happiness, if that was the emotion to be felt in a given situation. She movingly went on to say she felt the antidepressant saved her life.

Some people were shocked by Keri's revelations. These people find it hard to believe a child can have serious depression that is not emotionally based and, as such, cannot be resolved solely with psychotherapy or family counseling.

Coming out about her depression on TV, and talking openly about it afterward at school, started discussions in Keri's classes about other students' problems and the medications they were taking.

Yet, as her physical condition continued to deteriorate, there seemed to be a huge disconnect between Keri's happy school and social life and her general health.

Keri still complained of blurred vision when reading. Then one day, she said colors looked different. She kept closing one eye and then the other, marveling that colors appeared different depending on which eye she used. Testing at the ophthalmologist's revealed she had lost some color vision in her left eye, a condition called acquired unilateral dyschromatopsia. Losing partial color vision was so bizarre the doctor assumed it must be a side effect of the Zoloft. He reported it to Pfizer, the drug manufacturer. Pfizer said this side effect had never been reported before.[21]

As time passed, it became apparent that Keri's minor color vision loss was permanent. She took the loss well, even making light of it. The world looked more interesting, she said, when she could slightly change its colors by closing an eye.

For years Keri had had problems with sprained ankles and with her knees going out. This year, in sixth grade, she broke her right arm when serving in volleyball at school, even though the ball was one designed specifically for children and she was using the proper form. It's a good thing she had her laptop; while she healed, she couldn't write for two and a half months.

Another of Keri's persistent problems was insomnia. Although she felt extremely tired during the day and fell asleep quickly after going to bed, she woke during the night, unable to resume sleep for an hour or more. If she woke towards morning, by the time she got back to sleep it was time to get up for school. She was no longer depressed, but she often lacked the energy to do things she wanted.

Keri, now age 10, seemed to be getting even less tolerant of weather extremes—especially cold. Her tics became more numerous. She had frequent viral infections—colds as well as sinus and ear infections. Even her migraines became more numerous and more intense.

---

[21] Impaired color vision has since been added to the list of possible side effects.

Peering out from sixth-grade photos is the pallid, pinched face of a little girl with dark circles under her eyes and her arm in a cast. Her doctors referred to the dark circles, common in children with allergies, as allergic shiners. Her skin was dry and cracked. Her hair was more dry and brittle than ever. She often felt cold and fatigued. She bruised easily, and she developed red pinpricks of broken blood vessels called petechiae from minor pressure against her skin.

To me, the most surprising illness Keri developed that year was pleurisy (pleuritis), a painful inflammation of the pleural membrane, which lines the rib cage and allows the lungs to freely expand and deflate. When this membrane is inflamed, every breath hurts. Keri's case, we were told, was the result of a mildly contagious virus. I'd thought only elderly people got pleurisy.

I was called to the school frequently because of Keri's migraines. Luckily my workplace was a five-minute drive away, so I could get there quickly to administer ibuprofen with a small amount of caffeine, as directed by her doctor. If it was early enough in the day, she had time to recover and remain at school.

Several teachers complained Keri was spacing out. She was well-behaved and she was not fiddling around, they said, yet two teachers described her as "staring, doing nothing for moments." One teacher suggested Keri either had ADD (attention deficit disorder, the inattentive type of ADHD without the hyperactivity) or she was having absence seizures. When I saw the same thing at home and in the car, I called her name. She didn't even blink.

Thinking Keri was again becoming depressed, the psychiatrist increased her antidepressant dosage. This made her more animated, but it also made her very anxious. She began to have anxiety attacks with hyperventilation. Her brain seemed so exquisitely sensitive to stress that little, everyday things became catalysts for future post-traumatic symptoms. Keri developed phobias. She became afraid of certain bugs, including spiders. It didn't help that she got some minor spider bites at home and that at school a teacher was bitten by a highly poisonous brown recluse spider.

> During an **absence seizure** (formerly known as a petit mal seizure), a person may appear to be blankly staring into space while devoid of facial expression. He/she may exhibit eye blinking or purposeless mouth or arm movements, or may even take aimless steps while appearing out of it. Seizures of this type, which can last from seconds to a minute or so, are more common in children; many youngsters grow out of them during adolescence. Absence seizures are usually treated with antiseizure medications.

In addition to her other physical problems, Keri experienced an episode of something even more bizarre—a prolonged, severe bout of hypersomnia. Essentially, she slept for three straight weeks. After several days of this behavior, I hauled her to the pediatrician, who sent her for a mononucleosis (mono) test. She was not the least bit anxious about the blood draw, but during it she passed out. This vasovagal response (becoming light-headed) or syncope (fainting) had never happened to her before. We searched for a psychological reason—a trigger—to explain it and decided it was because a previous phlebotomist had had trouble drawing Keri's blood, making several attempts before she had success.

As time went on, many other phlebotomists continued to have difficulty inserting needles into Keri's veins, and she developed a phobia of blood draws that lasted for the next four years. Finally, when she was in her mid-teens, we learned how to ease the process. Because she was so cold and had low blood pressure, not only did she need to drink a lot of water before blood draws, she also needed to bundle up. To prepare her veins, she wore a jacket and gloves indoors until it was time for blood to be drawn.

When her blood test for mono came back negative, the pediatrician concluded Keri must be sleeping due to her MDD (major depressive disorder). Yet she didn't *seem* depressed. The only time she cried was when I tried to get her out of bed. When she got up to eat or use the bathroom, she stumbled around in a daze, bumping into things and falling down, hurting herself. Nevertheless, we were told her problems were mental, and the psychiatrist again increased her Zoloft dosage.

By the end of sixth grade, Keri had missed 40 days (two full months) of school. Some ill students receive homebound instruction through the public school district from a teacher who comes a few times per week to the student's home. Keri's absences, however, except for her three-week-long sleep episode, were sporadic. During her few extended absences, homebound instruction would have been futile, since both her brain and her body were incapacitated. I was grateful for the understanding of several of Keri's teachers and for the fact the school counselor intervened, as needed. Although Keri already knew much of the material being taught, she had multiple makeup assignments to do on top of her new work. Rather than feeling overwhelmingly stressed, however, she took the situation in stride. When I asked about homeschooling her, she wasn't interested. She loved being at school, she said, and besides, she didn't want to be taught by me; she needed me to be just her mommy.

The use of nutritional supplements was still in its infancy, but in desperation I began a very cautious and hesitant experiment with their use. I heard of an antioxidant called Pycnogenol. Although it had anti-inflammatory and anti-allergic properties, I was primarily interested in the fact that it might help treat rough, dry, cracking skin. Keri tried it and loved it. She alternated taking Pycnogenol with grape seed extract (resveratrol), another super-antioxidant. No miraculous results, but at least her skin became smoother and softer.

Then I heard about the use of fish oil for attentional problems and started her on a low dose of this supplement, as well. Then I learned it, too, has anti-inflammatory properties. Later, research on this substance generated an explosion of information about its efficacy in helping problems from autism to asthma and from ADHD to schizophrenia.

Keri's Views on Stress

As an older adolescent, Keri reflected on the reaction of her biological sensitivity (or wiring) to various external and internal input (stressors).

External stressors—from school, home, and the world at large—helped her become a mature, independent adult with a strong sense of self-esteem and self-confidence. These were her *good stressors*. Her body itself, she felt, was her *bad stressor*.

Sensory stressors such as migraines, allergies, Tourette's, body aches, sleep problems, and those horrific, ongoing nightmares were damaging for Keri. Her own unique biology—nature, immune system, neurology, metabolism, chemistry—was her most significant underlying stressor.

Her fits and psychotic-like episodes were also huge negative stressors. She felt as if her brain circuits were neurologically or chemically shorting out. The missing piece—the silent stressor—was whatever was affecting her biology to make her brain short out.

Chapter 12
Socially Secure and Spreading Her Wings

At 10, Keri's doctors interpreted her deteriorating health, more frequent migraines, sleep episodes, and the newly added phobias and episodes of anxiety, as a progression of her mental illness. Yet despite feeling physically awful, she was optimistic, excited about life, and, when feeling well enough, full of creativity.

This was the year she got the pet she'd wanted since she was two years old—a bird. Keri researched and made her choice carefully. She named the baby, a Goffin's cockatoo, Chieena and visited him weekly until he was old enough to be brought home. She kept a baby book journaling his development. Chieena soon learned to say his name, sat with Keri as she played the violin, and bobbed his head when she played piano. He even laughed when she laughed.

At school, she was full of confidence. In spite of her deteriorating physical state and frequent absences, her sixth-grade school year was wonderful in many ways. She loved her middle school classes, and she was both socially and emotionally happier than she'd been the year before. She remained a violin major; for her minor she chose drama, where she learned practical skills she put to immediate use. What she learned about drawing stage perspectives, she used to design a playground for her bird. With her father's help, she turned this idea into reality by building the playground from sketches she'd drawn to scale. She also learned costume design, including fabric selection. Often she enjoyed these tasks more than acting.

She especially loved being on the school's speech and drama team, which competed with other schools around the state. For her part on the team she considered poetry reading, excited about the possibility of reciting "The Bells" by Edgar Allan Poe. She read the poem out loud several times, while plunking on the piano as I worked in the kitchen.

Suddenly I realized she was *playing* the poem! I could actually hear it in the music. Surprised, I ran into the living room. "What were you playing?" I asked.

Keri laughed. She had always heard music in Poe's poetry. It was part of the allure his poetry had held for her since she'd discovered it at the age of three. Now she had put one of his poems to real music.[22] I laughed as well.

Ultimately, Keri chose not to compete in the poetry-reading category. Instead, she and a classmate partnered in duo-acting. They had a blast; they also qualified for the state finals.

Keri became more creative in writing, crafting a captivating tale of historical fiction involving time travel for her creative writing class. And for the first time, she wrote lyrics for one of the melodies she'd composed at the piano.

Seemingly out of character, Keri wanted the experience of entering a Miss Preteen pageant. I grew up as a tomboy. I don't wear makeup. I only dress up under duress, and when I *must* dress nicely, other people pick out clothes for me. With a mother like this, Keri was definitely on her own; preparing for a pageant was totally out of my range of experience. For the dressy portion of the event, she wore a long cream-and-lace dress handed down from an aunt and inexpensive gold-colored shoes. Being at the creative and performing arts school had already taught her about makeup—especially stage makeup—so she was able to put more of her school-taught skills to use.

Keri entered the talent show as the only contestant with music and lyrics she'd written herself.[23] Hers was not at all like the popular pieces that year—those from *The Little Mermaid* and *Pocahontas* movies—but in my biased mother's mind, her simple tune was beautiful, a haunting melody that stayed with me, running through the corridors of my mind. She didn't win, but that wasn't the point. What she wanted was the *experience* of participating in a pageant, and that she got.

---

[22] "The Bells," composed by Keri Cross, Sept. 1, 1997.
[23] "Running Through Time," lyrics and music by Keri Cross, 1998.

Unfortunately, about a month before the end of the school year, a group of students started teasing Keri about her tics again. The school counselor intervened and had a talk with the popular boy who had instigated it. It turned out he actually liked Keri and had meant the teasing to be a sign of friendliness. When other students followed his lead and took up the teasing, he'd been horrified. He apologized to Keri and did his best to get the other kids to stop.

By then, Keri was planning to leave the performing arts magnet school. She loved music, enjoyed playing the violin, and was continuing with piano. She'd also added flute to her life, fulfilling a desire she'd had since the age of two. But she wanted to do all of this outside of school. She was looking forward to returning to her Montessori roots by attending a small Montessori middle school for seventh- and eighth-graders.

Chapter 13
A New Psychiatrist, a Fresh Look

Midway through sixth grade, Keri's pediatric psychiatrist moved away. The school counselor recommended another she knew to be a strong advocate for his patients. I can't say my daughter warmed up to him right away. Greg and I didn't, either. This psychiatrist was the man who would be diagnosing, treating, and helping Keri for a decade to come. But first, we had to get to know each other and build a partnership based on mutual trust and respect.

We exchanged reading material. Since at the time, everyone involved believed Keri's physical symptoms to be an extension of her psychiatric issues, we addressed only the problems considered mental. I was of the opinion that these problems were the result of her high IQ and sensitive nature, aggravated perhaps by her Tourette's. Being overly sensitive to stimuli is a frequent trait of highly gifted individuals. So is appearing OCD-ish, inflexible, and intolerant of others who are bad, unfair, unjust, and unconcerned about issues important to the child. Early reading and problems with writing are also common in highly gifted children. I wanted this psychiatrist to see my daughter as a whole person, not just a bundle of symptoms.

I was willing to learn and be guided by this new doctor, but only after I was assured he understood the world of highly gifted, sensitive children. Fortunately, we were willing to learn from each other.

The new psychiatrist started out assuming that if Keri had mental problems, they were due to Greg and me not knowing how to parent. He had us read a book on old-fashioned, common-sense parenting and typical childhood milestones. In turn, Greg and I had him read a book on parenting gifted children, including gifted children with learning disabilities. I gave him articles describing the fact that many children who are both gifted and learning-disabled can suffer from a mix of symptoms, such as sensitivity to touch and sound, and how such children can be easily overwhelmed by emotions.

As he got to know us and Keri better, he ruled out parenting issues but wanted us to read articles about autistic spectrum disorders (ASDs). Something about Keri's behavior—a few characteristics—niggled at the doctor, reminding him of autism or an autistic spectrum disorder such as Asperger's.[24] Is this what he thought Keri had?

"No," he said. Keri had none of the diagnostic symptoms of ASDs, such as impaired ability to communicate, use social cues, understand facial expressions and body language, or use imaginative play. Nor did she have a limited range of interests. In contrast, her level of social awareness was very high. She was expressive, highly adept at reading faces, body language, and social cues and was considered much more socially mature than other children her age. Her range of interests was broad, including astronomy, aerospace, biology, medicine, science fiction and fantasy, art, music, drama, poetry, history, birds, and, of course, playing with friends.

Yet the authors discussed other symptoms that were eerily familiar—rages, meltdowns, and tantrums—as well as the potential contribution of bowel or intestinal problems to psychiatric conditions. The articles also examined the potential role of vaccinations, including the possibility of individual hyper-autoimmune reactions to the vaccines. None included a list of physical symptoms that might have caused me to investigate further, but even if they had, there was little information available.

The psychiatrist then brought up hyperlexia, a condition in which a child has incredible rote reading skills at a very young age. But rote reading is defined as reading without comprehension. This description did not fit Keri.

---

[24] Discussions are now underway on revisions to the *The Diagnostic and Statistical Manual of Mental Disorders (DSM)*, the 5th Edition of which is anticipated to be released in 2013. One such proposal would eliminate a specific diagnosis of Asperger's in favor of the broader austism spectrum disorder.

Other symptoms within the realm of autistic spectrum disorder did fit, such as Keri's need for routine and predictability and her oversensitivity or abnormal responses to sensory stimuli. The difficulty she had in describing the feelings behind her meltdowns and fits was another match.

> Filtering out noises and other irrelevant stimuli is a largely automatic process known as **sensory gating**. A deficit in it is considered a **neurobiological marker** and is indicative of a genetic underpinning associated with bipolar disorder and schizophrenia spectrum disorders.

There was no information about mitochondrial dysfunctions and autism in the material the psychiatrist provided. If there had been, the similarity in physical symptoms—symptoms I later discovered ranged from fatigue and migraines to changes in brain function and even vision problems—might have made me gasp.

The Limbic System

Our next area of investigation was into sensory integration disorder (SID), also referred to as sensory integration dysfunction or sensory processing disorder (SPD). I learned Keri's limbic system might be hypersensitive. The limbic system is a label for the complex interaction of those parts of the brain involved in perception, emotion, and reaction to stimuli. SID/SPD could explain Keri's sensory overload, including her inability to tolerate hard touches and certain sounds, as well as some of her fits.

One reason we suspected the involvement of the limbic system was that some of Keri's oversensitivity to stimuli seemed to stem from an inability to filter out sensory input others disregarded. She could not ignore sounds, other conversations, or people glancing at her, or even the fleeting facial expressions most of us unconsciously dismiss as having no relevance. I had been fascinated by the immediate, profound effect the SSRI antidepressant (Zoloft) had on Keri's ability to tolerate sound stimuli she previously had been unable to bear. This made more sense after I read that SSRIs affect the limbic system.

The parts of the limbic system of particular interest to me were the amygdala and the hypothalamus. The amygdala, sometimes referred to as the primitive brain, regulates our automatic fear responses. Reacting immediately to certain stimuli by bypassing the analytical, thinking part of the brain, it is responsible for our fight-or-flight reactions and is also the source of phobias.

The hypothalamus is responsible for the production and release of hormones affecting various bodily processes, including blood pressure, heart rate, the sleep/wake cycle (circadian rhythm), metabolism, emotions, growth, body-temperature regulation, sexual development, and hormonal cycles.

The hypothalamus sends signals produced by its neurons to a part of the pituitary gland called the anterior pituitary. These signals act to physically stimulate or inhibit the pituitary's production of hormones such as adrenocorticotropic hormone (ACTH), thyroid-stimulating hormone (TSH), growth hormone (GH), prolactin (PRL), follicle-stimulating hormone (FSH), and luteinizing hormone (LH).[25] As shown in figure 1 and table 10, these hormones affect the activity of glands and systems throughout the body, including the brain.

All this superficial learning was well and good, but I still had nothing to run with—nothing I could actually use to help my daughter. If I had probed a little deeper, I might have understood that glitches in the hypothalamus can cause a cascade of problems throughout the endocrine system and that nutrition also influences the brain and glands, supplying building blocks for the conversion of hormone precursors into chemical forms the body can use. I would have understood sooner that problems in the endocrine system can

---

[25] Some of these substances, such as FSH, PRL, and LH, are often thought of as female hormones. They are important in males as well, although some of them work on different glands in each sex. Testosterone, commonly known as a male hormone, is also important in females.

result in a host of symptoms which can mimic or exacerbate mental, psychological, or psychiatric disorders. And I would have discovered endocrine malfunction can cause a host of bewildering physical maladies, many of which Keri was experiencing.

Figure 1: Pituitary—The Master Gland

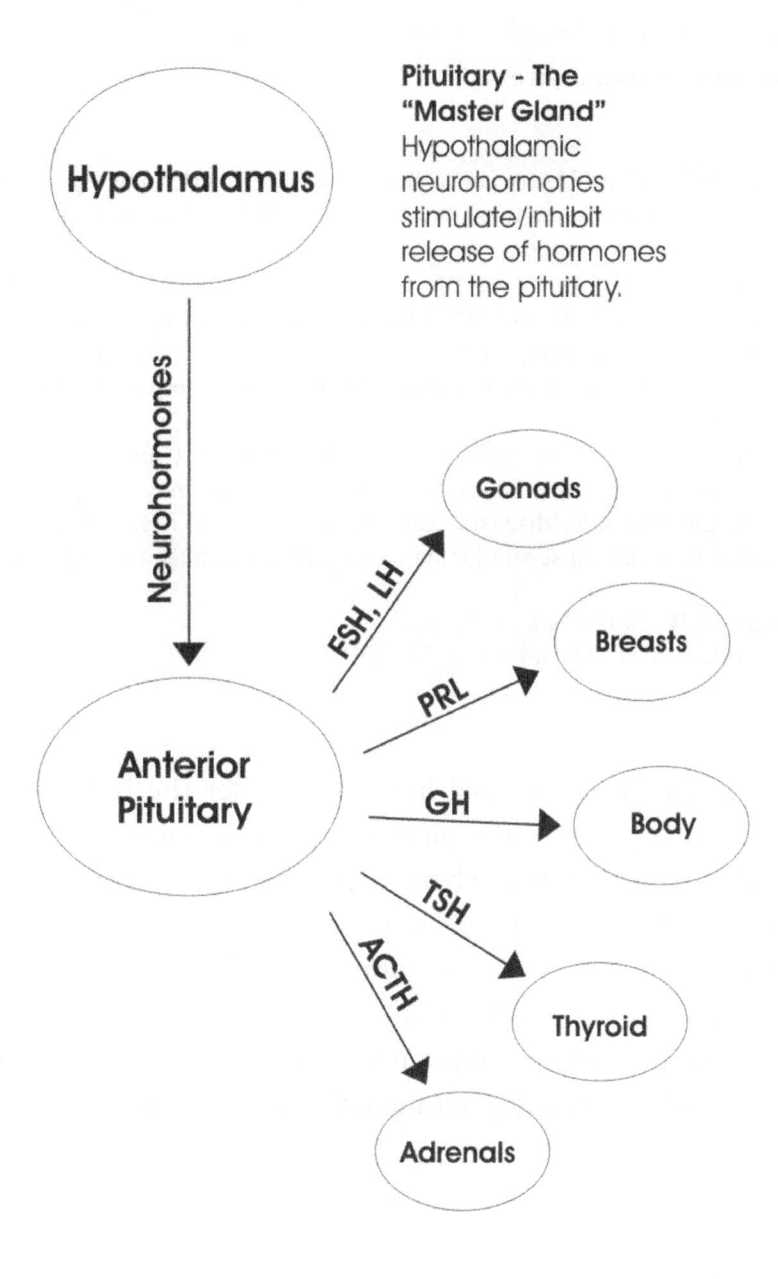

Pituitary - The "Master Gland"
Hypothalamic neurohormones stimulate/inhibit release of hormones from the pituitary.

126   It's Not *Mental*

In fact, her list of symptoms grew with each passing year: depression; low energy and fatigue; joint and muscle pain; erratic growth; dry, cracked skin; thin, dry, brittle hair and nails; low blood pressure; low immunity; trouble sleeping; horrific nightmares that sometimes continued after she woke, causing terror and confusion; intermittent ataxia and falling down; migraines; staring spells; feeling cold; easily broken blood vessels; vulnerability to stress and PTSD; and gastrointestinal distress.

> Many different problems can cause similar or overlapping symptoms. A person can have more than one problem. And one disease process can cause or exacerbate others.
>
> Iron deficiency anemia (low iron level) can cause fatigability (easily physically exhausted), impaired thermoregulation, impaired cognition, immune dysfunction, GI disturbances, attention problems and frustration intolerance ("poor effort intolerance"), impaired growth, and delayed puberty.[a]
>
> Disorders involving inflamed bowels (such as Crohn's disease and celiac) can increase the risk of developing iron deficiency anemia.[b]
>
> On the flip side, diseases causing an excess of iron (such as hemochromatosis) can cause similar symptoms due to damage to the pituitary.
>
> [a] Agarwal, R., 2007; Clark, S. F., 2008.
> [b] Conklin, L. S. and Oliva-Hemker, M., 2010.

Table 10 lists a few crucial hormones under the influence of the hypothalamus by way of the pituitary gland, along with some of the things that can happen when these hormones are affected by dysfunction in the hypothalamic-pituitary-adrenal axis. In this incredibly complex world of hormones, where the level of one hormone (or nutrient) affects the levels or functioning of others, everything is intertwined, and one malfunction can produce a host of symptoms that are *anything but* mental or psychological in origin.

Table 10: Glitches in the Hypothalamic-Pituitary-Adrenal Axis

Hormone Affected by a Glitch	Some Symptoms of a Glitch
Cortisol (produced by the adrenal glands)	<ul><li>Irritability, anxiety, depression, psychosis</li><li>Fatigue</li><li>Low/high blood pressure</li><li>Hypoglycemia, hyperglycemia</li><li>Muscle and joint pain</li><li>Intolerance to stress, vulnerability to PTSD</li><li>Compromised healing and immunity</li><li>Amenorrhea (not menstruating)</li><li>Nausea</li><li>Weight gain, weight loss</li><li>Slowed growth rate (in children)</li></ul>
Thyroid Hormones (T3—triiodothyroxine and T4—thyroxine)	<ul><li>Irritability, anxiety, depression, psychosis</li><li>Fatigue/weakness</li><li>Weight gain, weight loss</li><li>Constipation</li><li>Thin, dry, brittle hair</li><li>Intolerance to cold</li><li>Muscle pain and headaches</li><li>Dysmenorrhea and amenorrhea (menstrual problems)</li><li>Impaired cognition</li><li>Learning problems, lowering of IQ, short stature (in children)</li><li>High cholesterol and triglyceride levels</li></ul>
Reproductive Hormones (sex hormones)	<ul><li>Fatigue</li><li>Mood swings, depression, anxiety, and irritability</li><li>Change in bone density</li><li>Delayed or premature puberty</li><li>Lack of breast growth and lactation, or unusual breast growth or lactation (even in males)</li><li>Amenorrhea and dysmenorrhea</li><li>Weight gain or weight loss</li></ul>

Hormone Affected by a Glitch	Some Symptoms of a Glitch
Growth Hormone	- Depression and anxiety - Fatigue and weakness - Sleep problems - Decreased growth (in children) - Insulin insensitivity and impaired glucose tolerance - Bone loss - Impaired cognition, decreased concentration - Increased sensitivity to heat or cold

Chapter 14
Rituals and Routines

Someday, Keri imagined, she would be a physician, a pilot, possibly an astronaut, and a mother. She loved medical science, planes, and astronomy. She also loved babies—human, animal, and even dolls. Gentle, compassionate, and empathetic, at the Montessori preschool she used to lag behind when the other children ran outside to play. She didn't want the one special-needs child to walk out to the playground alone. Now that she was 10, she loved interacting and working with some of the severely mentally and physically disabled children who were integrated into her regular sixth-grade classroom. She had the patience to listen while they haltingly talked, as well as the kindness to wipe off drool. Since she often displayed little tolerance of her able-bodied, able-minded peers when they impulsively did or said things she considered stupid, this patience puzzled me. I questioned her about this discrepancy. "*They* have no excuse," she said of her able-bodied peers.

In the cozy expressive arts therapy office, stuffed with flourishing plants and filled with crafts, sandboxes, and an assortment of small plastic people, animals, houses, and trees, Keri created her own miniature worlds. She crafted Native American villages, woodland houses, and fairy kingdoms. In each fantasy world she included disabled children, along with accessibility for wheelchairs. She developed lifts for the children to go up into the trees. She even attached chariots to insects so disabled fairies could fly along with their families and friends. In Keri's worlds, people with disabilities were helped—never excluded. No one ridiculed, hurt, or was mean to others. No one purposely broke things, hit, stole, lied, cheated, or littered. No one intentionally harmed the environment. These were things Keri did not do, and she had a hard time coping with the fact that others did. It was one reason she was so particular in choosing her friends and why those friends were so very special to her.

For example, lying did not fit Keri's view of a right and orderly world. She recognized the chaos and randomness of the world at large and alleviated her discomfort with it by controlling and ordering what she could in her own life.

> Therapy helped Keri to find adaptive ways to self-soothe—adapting to an innate biology that caused her to feel a greater degree of distress at the inequities of life.
>
> Some people have a genetic variation that reduces the level of a neurochemical called Neuropeptide Y (NPY). Low levels of NPY cause a stronger and more emotional reaction to even minor stressors, such as viewing an image of a threatening facial expression.
>
> NPY-level variability can help to explain differences in children's resilience in stressful situations.
>
> A low level of NPY also can decrease an individual's ability to tolerate muscular pain.
>
> "Scientists Find Genetic Factor in Stress Response Variability," NARSAD, 2008.

According to the books I read on child development, the fact that Keri did not lie was considered abnormal. In fact, lying in order to hide instances of misbehavior from those who were unlikely to know about them was considered a sign of intelligence. I sometimes lied in my youth, but when I became a parent, I promised myself that, come what may, I would *never* lie to my children or in front of them. I might withhold information, but I would never lie. As hard as this was, I kept my promise. Over time it became a learned skill to answer questions I did not want to answer without actually providing false information. Is this why Keri didn't lie? Or was her behavior yet another symptom, since the books said *all* normal children lie?

When asked something she did not wish to answer, Keri might cry, but she wouldn't lie. It wasn't that she did not understand the concept of lying. She said that some kids at school lied so much it became a habit. They lied even when there was no reason to do so.

Keri understood lying as one of the survival mechanisms in middle school, so she became adept at answering evasively in order to not hurt feelings or create controversy. Her psychiatrist assured me that contrary to what I had read (and saw on an educational TV program about child development), *not* all normal children lie.

Keri had expectations for people according to their roles, and she felt distressed when they did not live up to those expectations. Greg, who was the steady rock of the family—quiet, serious, and reserved—did not wander as far from her expectations as I. I was more exuberant, more passionate about everything, qualities that conflicted with Keri's view of the way a mother should act. "There's a double rainbow outside," I'd exclaim loudly as I ran through the house, urging everyone outside to see. In the privacy of our home, this was okay. Outside, my laughter and exuberance were met by the disapproval of Keri's crinkled brow.

Over time, Keri did lighten up. One day she commented that as she grew older she felt like she had grown younger.

As a toddler, Keri had a strong need for order and routine, and over the years, she created bedtime and morning practices that relieved stress and chaos. Her rituals incorporated caring for the dog, herself, her dolls, and her belongings. She kept her room neat and organized, with clothes she laid out the night before according to the weather forecast. She cleaned her toys and put them in order. At first, these activities were merely an extension of her nurturing pretend-play and did not concern us. However, after she started on the antidepressant, the need grew exponentially—perhaps obsessively—with increasingly elaborate routines consuming hours of her day. Each night and each morning, she *had to* tend to things. Sometimes she became so tired she could hardly function. If we suggested she skip her rituals in favor of going to sleep, she would cry for hours, making her lose even more precious time.

Keri's new psychiatrist insisted she was displaying symptoms of obsessive-compulsive disorder (OCD). I did not perceive Keri's rituals, routines, and caring pretend-play to be OCD, at least not the OCD I'd seen portrayed in movies, books, or on television. There was no repetitive hand washing and no repetitive checking. In fact, I saw no repetition at all, except for the repetition of performing the ritual of cleaning and caring each day. In my eyes, using the term OCD to describe routines performed every day would be tantamount to diagnosing *everyone* with OCD. Don't we all have a daily morning ritual of washing our face, brushing our teeth, showering, eating breakfast, kissing a loved one good-bye, and then doing it again the following day?

Mitzi Waltz's book on OCD in children and adolescents had not yet been published.[26] If it had, I may have felt differently. I would have seen that OCD, like depression, does not always look the same in children as it does in adults. I would have recognized my daughter in the opening pages under "What OCD looks like," where Waltz describes a little girl obsessed with Furbies, fuzzy talking electronic toys. This was normal child behavior, but taken to an extreme.

Some obsessions are normal—we call them hobbies. Our passions add spice to our lives. Sometimes the abnormal is only normal taken to an extreme. In Keri's case, one extreme was the degree of frustration she experienced if prevented from satisfying what she perceived as her needs. She absolutely could not cope with any attempt to intervene. She *had to* do what she felt she had to do. At the time, I may not have recognized this as OCD, but at least I knew her resistance was *not* what today might be called oppositional defiance.

Keri frowned in anger at the psychiatrist when he suggested her routines were obsessive-compulsive. "This is my *therapy*. It makes me feel better," she declared angrily, crossing her arms in front of her. "It's *not* a disorder!"

I sympathized with Keri's point of view. For her, it *was* therapy. And if Keri was right, then the doctor must be wrong. I realized her actions weren't quite normal, but I had no label for what they might be.

---

[26] Waltz, Mitzi. *Obsessive-Compulsive Disorder: Help for Children and Adolescents*. Ed., Linda Lamb. Sebastopol, CA: O'Reilly Media, 2000.

When the doctor saw Keri working on her homework, he tried to prove his point to me another way. "Imagine you've made a big smudge on the paper," he said. "What would you do?"

"I would carefully erase it," Keri replied.

"What if the smudge got worse, and when you tried to erase more, the paper got a small hole in it. What would you do then?"

"I would start again with a clean sheet."

The psychiatrist persisted. "What if you didn't have time to do it over?"

"I wouldn't turn it in," Keri said. When the doctor reminded her she would get a zero if she didn't turn it in, she said she'd rather get a failing grade.

"But what if you *had* to turn it in just as it was, with a smudge and the hole in it?" he asked.

Unable to cope with such a scenario, Keri began to cry. The doctor apologized, explaining that he had to ask these questions so her mother could see something.

I grudgingly acknowledged the psychiatrist's point, but was not convinced Keri's actions were undeniable proof of a brain disorder. The doctor had shown Keri had trouble coping with the stress she felt from even *thinking about* the presented scenario. I agreed to accept that, *maybe*, Keri had OCD, that her behavior wasn't just, as I called it, OCD-ish. The treatment for OCD, he said, was an SSRI antidepressant, which Keri was already taking. We dismissed the fact that the OCD had only become a disruptive issue in Keri's life *after* starting on the antidepressant, since we interpreted this new problem as an *escalation* of her mental illness in spite of appropriate medication.

To this day, Keri disagrees with the diagnosis of OCD (the symptoms of which later dissipated). She says her methods of play were neither obsessions nor compulsions. Rather, they were the coping mechanisms she used to deal with the nature she was born with, exacerbated by what she was feeling at the time (possibly due to a side effect of the medication). I was left wondering, "What is mild OCD, anyway?" In Keri's case, it seemed both she *and* the psychiatrist were right.

Table 11: Diagnoses: Age 10

Actual Diagnoses:
- Highly gifted-learning disabled (LD).
- Allergies.
- Migraines.
- Tourette syndrome.
- Obsessive-compulsive disorder (OCD).
- Major depressive disorder—not otherwise specified (MDD-NOS).

Suspected Issues:
- Attention deficit disorder (ADD) – inattentive type of attention deficit hyperactivity disorder (ADHD).
- Absence seizures.

Significant Medical Issues:
- Pleurisy.
- Migraines of increasing severity.
- Broken arm without significant cause.
- Sudden partial loss of color vision in one eye.

Significant Medical Issues—Not Diagnosed or Assumed to be Mental:
- Pallor and weight loss.
- Three-week sleep episode.
- Severe intermittent dizziness.
- Intermittent ataxia (suddenly falling down).
- Muscle and joint pain; abdominal pain.
- Severe, intermittent feelings of fatigue; increasing lethargy.
- Insomnia (waking too early, difficulty staying asleep).
- Problem focusing on small print.

Table 12: Characteristics: Age 10

- Antidepressant (Zoloft) made her more functional. No longer cried in her sleep throughout the night. Tolerated noise better. Tolerated popular radio music for the first time.
- Social & confident. Excited about life. Good self-esteem; happy between bouts of depression.
- Continued with expressive arts therapy and became more able to talk about complex feelings and issues.
- Ongoing insomnia—waking up at night and waking too early.
- Possible absence seizures—spaced out. Afterwards, startled if someone was in the middle of trying to get her attention. Teachers complained she either had ADD or was having seizures.
- Increasing tics interfered with typing, and hands fatigued quickly when writing.
- Broke arm simply from hitting a ball.
- Body pains:
  - Back and neck—chronic muscle spasm in one part of her back.
  - Joint and soft tissue pain in knees and ankles.
  - Very sensitive to pain and injury.
- Recurring depression, meltdowns, and psychotic-like episodes, especially during the evenings and when not feeling well.
- Episode of hypersomnia that lasted several weeks.
- Missed about 40 school days due to doctors' appointments and various illnesses, including pleurisy, depression, migraines, fatigue from insomnia, and hypersomnia.
- Became pallid, thinner, and looked sickly. Often dizzy. Frequently fell down stairs. Dry, cracked skin continued.
- Developed phobias and began to have anxiety attacks.
- Lost some visual acuity and some color vision in her left eye.
- Overly sensitive to heat, cold, sounds, smells, and touch.
- Was diagnosed with mild obsessive-compulsive disorder (OCD).
- Was given the label other health impairment (OHI).

The Brewing Storm

Ages Ten and a Half to Twelve

Come the wind, come the rain
the fury will not abate
until the dark destructive clouds
exhaust themselves and dissipate.

Scattered above our world

Stillness revealed in a clear bright night,
a landscape devoid of form
a morass of violent destruction
and descending upon us—another storm.

Changing—all remains the same.

— *Jeanie*

Chapter 15
All Seems Well . . .

Animated with sheer joy, Keri, who in the fall of eighth grade was not quite 12, skipped and twirled across an almost-empty parking lot. She stretched her arms upward, as if to embrace the huge blood-red harvest moon hanging low and full in the darkening autumn sky. All the way home, she chatted happily. Then she lit candles on our front stoop and settled in among the flickering flames. She sat in rapture, watching the stars in their infinitesimally slow progression across the night sky.

The scene of Keri twirling beneath that crimson-colored moon marked the beginning of one of the most wonderful months of her young life. Yet one day I would shudder at the memory of that moon, looking back on it as the beginning of the end, like an omen from a Stephen King novel.

~~~~~~~~~~~

We'd known Keri was going to love seventh grade at the Montessori middle school. Over a year earlier, when I first visited the school, a student had met me at the door and shook my hand. With an ease belying his young age, he'd politely informed me the teachers were busy, but he'd be happy to show me around. He was not unique. Almost all the students acted in much the same way, their maturity exhibiting less of a separation between the children and adults.

The school, made up of fewer than 30 seventh- and eighth-graders, was nestled in an old church in a busy area of downtown. Students could walk to the city's main public library, parks, the courthouse, and other places of enrichment. Physical education class consisted of fun activities such as going to parks, rollerblading, swimming, and visiting the YMCA.

Students cooperated on community projects and took extended field trips, which helped to build friendships and enhance self-esteem. They saw alligators in swamps, rafted on the Colorado River, camped in a desert, gardened, and fixed up old cemeteries. When one of the students had a party, all were invited.

Keri made friends at this school. Here nobody teased her about her tics or anything else, except for friendly joshing about her small stature and the fact she did not maintain normal body temperature. They dubbed her "the reptile" because, like a cold-blooded animal, she was prone to both hypothermia and hyperthermia. Keri didn't mind a bit. One day I commented to a teacher how strange it was that at Keri's last school she was teased about her tics, yet here the students never even noticed them. The teacher looked at me with surprise. "*Of course*, the kids notice them," she said, "but it would be rude to comment about them."

Early in seventh grade, Keri took the SATs, the national college entrance exams, which had been scheduled by her previous school as part of Duke University's Talent Identification Program (TIP). With an average score for a student entering college, Keri qualified for Duke University's summer program for high-scoring seventh- and eighth-graders. She excitedly chose Ocean Camp in California as her three-week educational excursion.

No longer involved in organized in-school music classes and orchestra practice, Keri had more free time, which she used with increased creativity. She played piano, violin, and flute with joyful abandon, some days playing whatever was in her head for hours, just for fun. Claire, one of her violin teachers and a long-time friend of mine, mentored her. With Claire, Keri could learn more of what she wanted—less traditional fare such as fiddle music, or any beautiful or fun song that struck her fancy.

Keri also loved fashion and costume design, staying in theaters after movies to watch the credits and see who designed the costumes.

She designed and created a unique black and gold dress that she wore to a piano recital, a school party, and her grandma Sylvia's birthday party. She also combined her passion for fashion with photography, dressing dolls in costumes of her creation and then posing them in various settings to photograph. She began drawing and experimenting with media such as charcoal, pencil, pastels, watercolor, and oils. Although not a natural artist, she was determined to learn and was strongly motivated to practice.

She also did something remarkable about her poor penmanship. She began to write nicely, albeit with painstaking slowness. She said she could feel herself put her brain into art mode, which allowed her to *draw* the letters and words. Not only was her penmanship better, but the words were more likely to be spelled correctly and less likely to have dropped or transposed letters. When she had to write quickly or take notes, her penmanship reverted to what I called chicken scratchings. One thing art mode did *not* cure was her tendency to reverse letters. In fact, I've fondly kept some doodle artwork she did for me using my name. The first letter is backward, yet it looks so artistically "right." The backward letter made me love the piece all the more. It was *so* Keri.

~~~~~~~~~~~~

Keri started seventh grade with her usual fall allergies, but I never expected the school to call saying she was coughing up blood in what turned out to be her first bout of pneumonia. Coming on the heels of pleurisy the spring before, her illness was again puzzling, but she recovered uneventfully.

Although doing well academically, Keri was having problems with organization. She had to redo lost work. She lacked focus and had problems staying on task. How she felt, emotionally and physically, fluctuated from one day to the next. Correspondingly, so did her ability to complete assignments. She also continued to complain about her eyesight. When she played the violin, she had trouble seeing the music. Even Claire commented that Keri wasn't focusing—not playing the notes on the page.

I was getting tired of the word *focus*. At the synagogue, Keri's teacher poked at the page with his finger, telling her sternly to *look* at it and *focus*. "She just won't look at the page and focus on what she's supposed to read," he complained to me. As he emphasized the words *look* and *focus*, he jabbed his index finger into the palm of his other hand.

Keri was still on a low dose of fish oil, which was advertised as being helpful for focus, but it didn't seem to be helping her. When I mentioned her teachers were frustrated with her, Keri reiterated that she couldn't *see* well. I took her to the eye clinic again. And again we were told, other than the partial loss of color vision in one eye, her vision was fine.

Keri's tics, both vocal and motor, were increasing, but she was determined to hide them from her schoolmates as much as possible. She also tried to disguise the fact that her energy was limited. When she was overheated, her body ached and she felt a fiery burning on the surface of her muscles, just under the skin of her legs and sometimes her arms. The pain continued until she had time to rest and cool off.

She still had occasional spacing-out episodes, during which she stopped all activity, stared, and was unresponsive. Afterward, she didn't remember them.

Her sleep-related problems continued. She fell asleep quickly but woke in the wee hours of the morning. Unable to go back to sleep, Keri sometimes started her day at 2:00 a.m. Oddly, these were often good days, times when she cleaned, did homework, and played with friends.

On bad days, she felt cold and tired, crying easily. Her head hurt. She was extra-sensitive to sounds and touch. Her body was in pain, and a touch felt like a blow. Once in a while, she thought someone had suddenly hit her or she smelled odors or heard sounds no one else did. At times a feeling of paranoia or fear came over her. She just wanted to sleep.

Even more disturbing, on two occasions Keri slapped herself while screaming. Slapping episodes fall under the umbrella of self-harming behaviors and normally occur when a child feels extreme stress. But it *wasn't* stress that was making her feel the way she did, Keri insisted. Rather, *the way she felt* made her stressed. Just before each of these slapping episodes, she had a vague, uncomfortable feeling of not feeling right inside her body and mind. Her feelings then exploded, as if her brain had short-circuited.

The psychiatrist again increased her antidepressant. She was now taking close to the maximum-allowed adult dosage.

One of Keri's teachers had an odd observation about her attention-related problems:

> *Keri does not really have a problem with attention span, but she is highly distractible. We have noticed that Keri has acute hearing and notices what everyone is saying in all the conversations around her. Keri has difficulty doing work at a table with others and will sometimes go into a hallway to concentrate. Even when she is across the hall with other students, Keri hears what we teachers are quietly discussing amongst ourselves.*
>
> *I suggest that Keri be tested for ADD. I am open to trying ideas. Perhaps headphones might help her to block out extraneous input.*

Keri was unable to ignore all the things she shouldn't be hearing or noticing. The instances of extraneous input most people wouldn't have noticed, even if they'd wanted to, were stimuli she just couldn't filter out.

I came across the book *Teaching the Tiger: A Handbook for Individuals Involved in the Education of Students with Attention Deficit Disorders, Tourette Syndrome or Obsessive-Compulsive Disorder* by Marilyn Dornbush and Sheryl Pruitt. Here were ideas for helping children with fluctuating abilities, attention, and energy levels at school. I gave Keri's teachers copies of the sections that applied to her, with specific items highlighted. Although the teachers already were doing what the authors recommended, they said the information helped them to understand Keri even better. Based on my family's experiences, I found the book applicable to children with symptoms of depression, bipolar disorder, and schizoaffective disorder.

Toward the end of seventh grade, Keri began to contradict us, make belittling snide remarks, and neglect her chores. When I asked her gently to do something, which was all that had ever been needed in the past, she wouldn't do it. I tried using a stern tone of voice. This she interpreted as me yelling at her, which caused her to fall apart, crying for hours. Other parents said such behavior was normal for her age; that we just needed to lay down the law. Greg and I discussed the issue at length and decided in favor of patience, even at the risk of having a spoiled brat. Because her behavior was so out-of-character, we chose not to react to it as willful or defiant. Instead, we assumed the cause was biological; something was wrong physically—possibly a side effect of her medication.

Keri's psychiatrist referred to her brief, intermittent psychotic symptoms—paranoid delusions of conspiracies to kill her and hallucinations of smell and taste—as her temper spells. Since they were followed by hours of sleeping, they could indicate a type of epilepsy with complex partial seizures in a location of the brain called the temporal lobe. He explained such seizures are often associated with hallucinations of smell, sight, taste, and touch and can produce episodes of fear like those Keri experienced. Seizures in this part of the brain can be very difficult to diagnose. Epilepsy also has a high correlation with migraines, so Keri's severe and frequent migraines could be part of the picture. Before the psychiatrist labeled Keri with another psychiatric diagnosis, he wanted her to have a thorough neurological evaluation, including an electroencephalogram (EEG) with nasopharyngeal electrodes[27] to check for temporal lobe seizures,

---

[27] The article "Nasopharyngeal EEG recording in psychiatric patients," by B. K. Gupta, B. Yerevanian, and M. Charlton in the *Journal of Clinical Psychiatry* (July 1989, 50(7): 262–4), explains that an EEG recorded with nasopharyngeal electrodes can reveal temporal lobe activity that a regular EEG may not be able to detect. The authors conducted a study showing EEGs with nasopharyngeal leads are more effective than scalp EEGs in detecting epileptiform

and a magnetic resonance imaging (MRI) scan of her brain. He referred her to a pediatric neurologist at a hospital medical center.

The neurologist had Keri walk, stand on one leg, and touch her nose. She angrily contradicted everything I told him about hallucinations and delusions. This doctor quickly decided her problems were not neurological. He dismissed her as just having "some psychiatric issues" and declined to run the tests requested by the psychiatrist.

Lacking medical evidence to the contrary, the psychiatrist determined Keri met the criteria for ADHD—Inattentive Type, which is attention deficit without impulsivity or hyperactivity. Keri laughed as she told the psychiatrist her ADHD should be called attention *surplus* disorder rather than attention *deficit* disorder.

We agonized over whether Keri should try a small amount of the stimulant Adderall. Rumors were just emerging that stimulants prescribed for ADHD might exacerbate or even precipitate bipolar mood cycling and psychotic illnesses in some children. The psychiatrist had heard such rumors, but he felt confident Keri did not have a psychotic disorder.[28]

Evidence was also accumulating that administering stimulants and antidepressants without a mood stabilizer such as lithium, an atypical neuroleptic, or some antiseizure medications could cause greater mood instability in children and aggravate bipolar illness, thus increasing mood cycling.[29] (In fact, some scientists believe mood cycling *itself* can induce *more* mood cycling, a theory known as "kindling.") Keri was taking an antidepressant without a mood stabilizer. But she had never been diagnosed with bipolar disorder, only with depression and now with ADHD, so treatment with both the stimulant Adderall and the antidepressant Zoloft seemed completely appropriate for her.

Keri weighed in on the decision. Even though the medication could increase her tics, if it could possibly fix her brain, she was willing to

---

abnormalities. However, this method is currently out of favor in deference to less invasive techniques.

[28] Many years later, the FDA issued warnings suggesting stimulants might be best avoided by individuals with a family history of psychotic disorders.

[29] Goldberg and Ernst, 2002; Papolos, D., and Papolos, J., 1999. *The Bipolar Child* (p. 53).

take it. It was agreed she would start on Adderall before starting eighth grade in the fall.

Things were looking up.

Ocean Camp

That summer, Keri nervously but happily made the cross-country trip to California by herself in order to go to Ocean Camp under Duke University's program for gifted youth. Prior to the start of camp, she spent a week with my brother Sam and her cousins. She also stayed with my cousin Dan, who delivered her safely to the camp. I was a bit worried about her depression and other problems, but my family was great with her, and the people running the camp assured me that issues such as depression, Tourette syndrome, ADHD, etc., were amazingly common among the high-IQ kids for whom the camps were designed.

The psychiatrist once opined Keri lacked emotional resilience but proffered no advice on increasing her resiliency. Seeking guidance, I read a book by Robert Brooks and Sam Goldstein titled *Raising Resilient Children,* but it did not address children like Keri. Nothing in it related to how Greg and I parented or to Keri's problems with lack of resilience. Years later, I read a description of stress cascade in the literature on schizophrenia,[30] which resembled Keri's apparent "lack of emotional resiliency." The author discussed how seemingly mild stressors can have a profound effect on people with this disorder and that their heightened susceptibility to stress could be caused by difficulty in filtering out external stimuli.

Actually, Keri *did* have resilience, which she showed by using her maturity and foresight to adapt to her nature. By now, she had come up with ways to compensate for her need for consistency, for being unable to cope well with the unexpected, and for needing to know

---

[30] Corcoran and Malaspina, 2001.

schedules in advance. Keri's preparations for her trip to California reflected how much she had grown in independence and confidence.

In the weeks before leaving, she made numerous phone calls to her uncle Sam, gathering information about everything she would be doing with his family. She wrote down the activities he'd planned for each morning, afternoon, and evening and recorded the type of clothing she would need for each.

Choosing her words carefully to explain her need to know as much as she could in advance, Keri said, "Life is so full of the unexpected that I try to plan as much as possible for what *can* be planned for. This reduces stress for me. I feel like I have a limited amount of energy to cope with the unexpected. So I'm trying to reduce the amount that's unexpected and increase the expected. This makes me more likely to have the emotional reserves to cope with the unexpected parts."

I felt such insight was quite thoughtful for an 11-year-old, especially one who was trying to deal with a God-given temperament that was naturally inflexible and who, since birth, had been unable to cope well with the unexpected minor stresses of a normal day.

I was proud of my daughter for preparing for this trip by herself and for dealing with her needs more independently and assertively. She was exhibiting the internal strength and responsible attitude that would help her attain her goals as an adult. Whatever her teen years might hold, whatever trials were ahead as she went through the normal stages of separating from parents and struggling to find her place in the world, her trip to California proved she would be okay. In fact, I could already see in her the self-assured, competent adult she had the potential to become.

The time Keri spent at Ocean Camp was one of the highlights of her childhood. She had the exhilarating experience of swimming in the ocean with a great white shark (she was in a cage). She studied marine life, learned to snorkel, and had one minor mishap—bonking her head on some rocks. She experienced real dangers, achieved real successes, and returned home glowing with confidence.

Your Eyes are in Your Head

After returning from Ocean Camp, Keri's vision complaints escalated. This time at the eye clinic I was told the problem was in her *head*, not in her eyes, and that she should have psychological testing.

The psychiatrist sent Keri for psychological testing. "Have you gotten her *vision* tested?" asked the psychologist after the testing. I felt like exploding with exasperation. The psychologist suspected Keri truly couldn't see well. She gently explained, "Most doctors and optometrists only check children for nearsightedness. I suspect Keri may be farsighted, which means she might not see small print well. It's also possible her eyes aren't focusing together. Unless a parent *specifically requests* a child's binocular vision (the way the eyes see together) be tested, eye doctors usually don't check."

In disbelief, we returned to the eye clinic with the recommendation they check Keri's vision more thoroughly. Keri was not only farsighted, but when she tried to focus up close she had a convergence insufficiency. Her left eye—the same eye in which she'd lost some color vision—drifted outward, resulting in further blurring of small print. Not only did she need reading glasses to correct her farsightedness, they had to have prismatic lenses to help her eyes properly converge. She'd been right all along. She really *couldn't* focus!

Why hadn't she been checked for this sooner? The clinic said they don't expect children to be farsighted, and they only check binocular vision if they suspect a problem. *Given her vision complaints, why had they not suspected a problem?* I was steaming! Later, when the ophthalmologist running the eye clinic asked for permission to use Keri's case as a teaching tool in order to avoid such mistakes in the future, we were happy to say yes.

With her new glasses, Keri took up reading long novels for the remainder of the summer. When school started in the fall, she was looking forward to being able to see and to being on medication for her ADHD. Hopefully, she would be able to block out distractions and not lose her homework. No more lack of focus. No more spacing out.

Chapter 16
Maybe Not So Well

One day Keri solemnly told me she could not imagine life without her music. She and her music were one. Even if we had been poor, she would have found a way to have her instruments and to play. I was delighted so many things brought her joy. She had her art, her music, her school, her grandfather's dog, her bird, her family, and her friends. After years of struggling with depression, tics, sensory sensitivities, fatigue, illnesses, and migraines, life was *good*. Really, really, *good!*

Too good, maybe?

Less than a month into eighth grade, shortly before turning 12, Keri was content, twirling under the full autumn moon and playing her violin under the twinkling stars. She was on a high dose of Zoloft, the SSRI antidepressant and had started on Adderall, the ADHD stimulant medication. She was energized. In the evenings, she zipped through her homework and still had the energy to clean her room and the rest of the house as well! She worked on the side taking care of people's pets. She took on extra household chores, organizing the kitchen, bathing our pets, and working in the yard. Keri declared we needed to have family meetings and family game nights. And because she organized them, we did.

The term hypomania, defined as an energized state a step below mania during which people seem to be at their most energetic and creative, never entered our minds. Keri just seemed more herself than ever; we felt we were getting a glimpse of her without the fatigue, pain, depression, mood fluctuations, and sensory sensitivities of the past.

This was the last full year of school before her bat mitzvah at age 13. Keri eagerly joined the b'nai mitzvah class to prepare for this life passage. The classes were filled with study, laughter, camaraderie and the philosophical discussions she relished. She liked her classmates, got along well with her teachers, and was looking forward to being able to lead prayer, read Torah, chant haftarah, and generally take her place as an adult in the Jewish religious community. Since she now had prescription prismatic reading glasses, she could see the small Hebrew text and was enthusiastically learning what she had missed the year before. She often sang prayers in the car on the way home from class. At home, she played the religious tunes on her violin.

Keri was in a creative frenzy. One day she sat in my office and crafted a family—mother, father, children, dog, and cat—out of ordinary office supplies. She created awesome 3-D miniature junk collages in different color schemes using items from around my office. Her music took off. She played violin in the sunshine along the creek behind our house, harmonizing with the babbling brook. She played flute outside in the moonlight. She played for hours—haunting melodies of her own creation, never to be played the same twice. She wanted to learn to play the harmonica, and she did. She started to learn guitar.

Keri and her Goffin's cockatoo, Chieena, had bonded as friends. While Keri played violin and flute, Chieena cheerfully accompanied her. When she sang to him, he sang along with a soft crooning sound. While she played the piano, Chieena was an enthusiastic audience, sitting nearby, swaying and bobbing to the melody.

When Keri brought home two old paperbacks she'd found on a bookshelf at school, it seemed only slightly odd that she urged me to read them but wouldn't say why. Since Keri had, in the past, given me books to read that struck her fancy, I thought little about it. One of the books was *I Never Promised You a Rose Garden*, by Joanne Greenberg. The story is told through the eyes of a Jewish teenage girl who has severe, chronic delusions and hallucinations. The other was *Lisa, Bright and Dark*, by John Neufeld. Lisa was a smart 16-year-old who seemed successful and normal but was actually becoming increasingly psychotic until eventually the psychosis became severely disabling and obvious to everyone.

Almost as if she didn't want anyone else to see them, Keri refused to return the books to school. That was peculiar. Was my 11-year-old trying to tell me something, or was my child merely being a child? At the time I didn't sit around analyzing her motives.

Keri was sleeping less and less. The week before she turned 12, she hardly slept at all. The night before her birthday, she slept an hour and a half. The following night she dozed for no more than 30 minutes. By the next day . . .

Screaming!!!

Keri was screaming for the voices in her head to shut up and leave her alone.

The doctor had given us a benzodiazepine medication,[31] Ativan (generic name lorazepam), to give Keri in case of emergency. In the past, an emergency was when she had nightmares that wouldn't stop even after she woke up, or when she became briefly psychotic or delusional, as she had the time she had poison oak. The last time I'd given her one of these pills, many months ago, she had fought it, thinking it was poison. Surely the liquid I was offering was not water, but a toxin. I was trying to kill her. Surely the doctor had prescribed the pill only to ensure her death.

Today she took the pill without a fight.

When Keri calmed down, I gave her something to eat. Once she was tranquil, calm and secure, we talked about the voices. Keri explained she hadn't known *they* were what the psychiatrist was talking about when, some months earlier, he'd asked if she heard voices. She thought he meant voices from across the room, not voices in her head.

"The voices," she said, "sometimes say I'm bad and I should give up. But sometimes they calm me or make me laugh. Sometimes they warn me of danger and help me. Other times they are mean, and sometimes they're just too noisy." To her, the voices—*they*—weren't something

---

[31] Benzodiazepines are anxiolytics, commonly used for short-term relief of severe, disabling anxiety. Some well-known benzodiazepines are Ativan (lorazepam), Valium (diazepam), and Xanax (alprazolam). In addition to being used as an anxiolytic, lorazepam is sometimes used as an emergency medication to stop severe seizure episodes or to stop the severe agitation associated with acute psychotic episodes.

abnormal, because, as far back as she could remember, they had always been there. Only occasionally were they bothersome.

She then slept for 16 hours.

Screaming. More screaming. Loudly sobbing. Calling out for Mommy. Keri was hysterical, lying on her bedroom floor, thrashing and screaming as if in agony. It took two hours before either Greg or I could understand her words. She was yelling for *them* to stop hitting her. She pleaded for her mommy and daddy to "Make them stop!"

They were bashing in her skull and trying to rip off her limbs—and they were succeeding. They were dismembering her. They were no longer just voices inside her brain.

Greg was ashen, shaking as he told me this was the exact hallucination his mother used to have. He wanted to howl "Noooo! Not my child!" Instead, he tried to remain calm, attempting to explain to Keri that no one was there. *They* did not exist. No one was hitting her. There were no voices. Keri became more frantic and hysterical.

My thoughts flashed to my mother's deep frustration with our stupidity at not believing her and for dismissing what her senses told her to be true. Taking a different tack, I insinuated myself into Keri's hallucination, attempting to protect her from within the hallucination itself.

In my sternest, most authoritarian voice, I loudly demanded *they* quit hurting my child. "GO AWAY!" I commanded, as I pushed and pummeled at the beings surrounding her—beings invisible to me but so very real to my daughter. Announcing firmly that Keri was "my baby," I stated emphatically that I would not allow anyone to hurt her. Gathering her into my arms, I used my own body as a protective bubble against them. It worked! Keri slowly began to calm down, at which point she promptly fell into a deep sleep.

Greg and I felt as if we'd been hit over the head with the proverbial two-by-four. Could our younger daughter have a mental illness? Like *my* mother? Like *his* mother? I clung to the hope that these latest episodes were brought on by nothing more than her accumulated lack of sleep. I was confused. How could a kid act psychotic for a few hours and then be fine? Did she need a sleeping pill, an antipsychotic medication, or a therapist? I could think of no other choices. The idea that her symptoms might be caused by improper medications, fluctuating hormonal imbalances, or nutritional problems, did not occur to me. And although I did consider she might need a sleeping pill, I had no idea to what extent her sleep problems could be contributing to psychiatric symptoms. At the time, the whole situation just seemed crazy.

Keri's psychiatrist once told us something he'd learned in medical school, "When you hear hoofbeats, think horses, not zebras." In other words, when trying to come up with an explanation for symptoms, think first of the most likely one (the horse), rather than a more uncommon one (the zebra). I completely understood and agreed with this analogy.

Over the years I had read the opinions of many experts, from T. Berry Brazelton to Richard Ferber to John Rosemond. I often wondered what common-sense advice Rosemond would give. He seemed to be a proponent of the think-horses motto. Think behavior. Think discipline. But I couldn't see how to apply discipline to help a child who usually was self-disciplined—obedient, caring, kind, cautious, and self-motivated—but who had these "episodes." I did not believe Keri's actions were manifestations of a behavior problem or that they required disciplinary measures. After all, before Keri was even three, she knew to go to another room when she felt the need to scream and cry. She hadn't screamed and cried for attention, or because she wasn't getting what she wanted, or out of vindictiveness. She *wanted* to be left alone, to sob until, as she later explained, she was "done."

Two different psychiatrists had ruled out anything wrong in the parenting department and had said Keri's problems were not behavioral. Testing had shown her problems weren't psychological, either. Instead, she appeared to have a biologically based psychotic disorder. In other words, the hoofbeats must be those of a zebra.

Stopping Keri's episodes of frank psychosis—hearing voices, feeling pain, experiencing olfactory and tactile hallucinations—was essential, the doctor said. Additionally, doing so should put an end to what we'd been calling her psychotic- and PTSD-like fits, episodes of sudden screaming with extreme sensory hypersensitivity accompanied by unprovoked feelings of terror. Also, she should get relief from what looked like nightmares that continued even while awake, once the psychotic episodes were stopped.

The next logical step, he continued, was to treat Keri pharmaceutically. Greg and I agreed. Without any medical diagnoses to treat, the drugs of choice were psychopharmaceuticals, also referred to as psychotropic medications—substances that directly affect brain chemistry. Greg and I passively accepted that a mental diagnosis was just like a medical one (not true) and that its biological cause cannot be determined (only sometimes true). In our stunning naïveté, we looked forward to Keri taking the little pill that would make her all better.

Chapter 17
What the . . . ???

Keri didn't want to take medication to get rid of the voices. To her, that meant they would still be there, but she would not be able to hear what they were saying. Losing her ability to hear the voices would make them angry and frustrated. As strange as this reasoning seemed to me, from Keri's perspective it made perfect sense. Having grown up with them, the voices were *real* to her. They were powerful entities—not a symptom, like a rash, that would disappear with treatment. I tried to explain they really *were* a symptom and to trust what I was saying. Keri took the pills.

The medication prescribed by the psychiatrist to make the voices go away was called Risperdal (risperidone), one of a category of drugs collectively referred to as second-generation or atypical antipsychotics or neuroleptics. Ironically, this drug was the same medicine offered to Keri two years earlier to help stop her tics. At the time, she'd declined the offer because of the drug's potentially serious side effects. She'd read that the older neuroleptics (referred to as first-generation, or typical antipsychotics), including Haldol (haloperidol) and Thorazine (chlorpromazine), were notorious for causing terrible side effects, including severe movement disorders characterized by extrapyramidal symptoms (EPS) such as tardive dyskinesia (TD).[32] Another major side effect of this category of drugs was the potential for elevated prolactin levels, which could cause lactation (milk production), breast growth (even in males), and osteoporosis (thinning of the bones). Still other possible side effects included drooling, feeling like a zombie, weight gain, sedation, and even premature death.

---

[32] Other extrapyramidal symptoms include Parkinsonian movements, akathisia, and dystonia.

Since the newer neuroleptics affected more specific brain receptors than the older ones, they were considered safer, especially for pediatric use, although they were more likely to cause weight gain. Risperdal, considered fast-acting, was the most *similar* to those of the first generation, but it was also the most extensively researched for children, since it was being used to treat children with Tourette syndrome.

This drug, like any other medication, works differently on different individuals. In making treatment decisions one must constantly weigh risk versus benefit. However, without more information about risks and benefits for a specific individual, rather than for a statistical collection of individuals, we are still evaluating and predicting without all the data needed.

We had to rely on the psychiatrist's wisdom. Much less data existed about the use of neuroleptics for pediatric patients than for adults, and most of the pediatric data available was from open-label or chart-review studies, which are not placebo-controlled clinical trials. Children may be more sensitive to dosage levels than adults, may need to start at a lower dosage, and may need to have the dosage increased (titrated) at a slower rate. They may also be more apt to suffer from movement side effects, weight gain, insulin resistance, and other identified issues than adults; yet, as we learned later, they may be less at risk for developing chronic tardive dyskinesia.[33]

Keri took the pills, but she did not get better.

> Whether one type of neuroleptic is actually safer or even more effective than another is open to debate, not well-researched in children, and may vary by individual.
>
> **Psych Nurse** told of a patient doing well for decades on Haldol without side effects, having a good life and holding a job. When a new doctor switched the patient's medication to a newer, theoretically "safer" atypical neuroleptic, the patient destabilized and lost his job.

---

[33] Correl, 2006.

Some days she was clingy and anxious. She bawled and hung on to me like a toddler. Intermittently her muscles and joints hurt unbearably. With pain, her distress and inability to cope were amplified. Some days she acted like a person with PTSD, reliving events such as nightmares, pain, or unpleasant interactions with other people. She pleaded with me to help her "stay in the present." On these days, even if it was warm and sunny, Keri felt very cold, wearing her heaviest winter coat and gloves on her frigid hands, in a desperate attempt to feel warm. We called these her bad days.

I could tell it was a bad day as soon as I heard her voice. On mornings when Keri awoke "off," even if not yet delusional, paranoid, and psychotic, her voice sounded very different, with a higher pitch—more childlike. She sounded scared and whiny, and she lisped. The words most mothers love to hear, the softly whispered, "I love you, Mommy . . . soooo much!" were shortly followed by Keri completely falling apart. Each time I saw this scene begin to unfold, I knew what was about to happen but had no way to stop it.

One day she woke from a nap slapping at the maggots she felt crawling on her body.

Because of her poor sleep and general feelings of agitation, the doctor had recently raised her dosage of Zoloft again. Keri wanted it lowered. She couldn't give a logical reason, but she just felt the dosage was too high, that the antidepressant was making her worse. Over the next couple months we slowly reduced the Zoloft while trying to raise the Risperdal in minute increments. The tiniest dose of Risperdal made Keri's body ache horribly and caused her to sleep the days away. It also increased her appetite, causing her to gain weight.

At the Montessori school where she had previously felt so at home, she now felt alienated. Her language arts teacher complained about her lack of participation in class during discussions about the book *Catcher in the Rye*.[34] The school advisor suggested I discuss the situation with Keri at home.

---

[34] Salinger, 1951.

The book focuses on a character named Holden Caulfield, Keri explained, a boy who is obviously suffering from untreated depression and getting no support. When she offered this description in school, the other students did not understand the difference between feeling depressed and suffering from depression. One boy even argued there was no such thing as "depression," that a person can only "be depressed." When Keri tried to explain depression is an actual illness (after all, that's what she'd been diagnosed with), the teacher did not back her up.

Keri went on to say that Holden is upset by people he perceives as being phonies. Keri could relate to this perception. "Many of my classmates are like the phonies in the book. But the ones most like those phonies are the ones who defend the phonies in the book as being the good guys. I can't say what I *really* think or I'd be kicked out of school!"

"The students say they don't like the book. They don't like Holden, the main character, either; they call him nuts. At least I *understand* him. My classmates do not, and cannot, understand his suffering and depression. However, since I have to get along with my classmates yet satisfy the teacher's mandate that I contribute more to class discussion, I will try to contribute superficial, inoffensive comments that won't leave me open to ridicule."

Keri felt distressed and even physically ill in that class. The students repeatedly called Holden Caulfield nuts. Being "nuts" was very, very scary for her. I wanted the language arts teacher to understand why my daughter was not participating. I wanted him to allow her to tell him once about the whole book and then leave her alone. But only one teacher she dearly loved, and who doubled as the school counselor, knew what was going on in Keri's life. We'd been advised not to tell her other teachers.

I began keeping detailed notes about how Keri was doing because I was so puzzled by the rapid changes in her. When I later read about these frequent and rapid mood changes, called ultradian cycling, on discussion boards at the Child and Adolescent Bipolar Foundation

(CABF) Web site (http://www.bpkids.org), they were often described by other parents as a bumpy roller coaster ride, but without any of the fun. The description was apt.

In the span of a single day, Keri could go from happy and singing when she first awoke to depressed, anxious, and hyper; to screaming and crying; to calm and contented; to a state of sensory overload; to scared and panicky, ending her day so distressed she needed to sleep in our bedroom. Here is an example of changes over the course of a typical Saturday.

- *Saturday morning: Goes to volunteer work at vet clinic (as part of school project).*
- *1:00 p.m.: Walks back happily from vet clinic with me.*
- *1:30 p.m.: Whiny. Congested while frustratedly trying to express her screeching tic. Acts like a two-year-old in need of a nap.*
- *2:30 p.m.: Crying inconsolably but does not know why.*
- *3:15 p.m.: Vomits.*
- *3:30 p.m.: Totally calm. Says she peed in her clothes and wants a hug; asks father to please bring her a change of clothes. Showers.*
- *5:00 p.m.: Works on a project for Sunday school. Cheerful. Eats. Plays piano.*

Keri had times—we called them her "sleep days"—when she felt bad and slept for one or two days. She didn't have a fever, but her body ached. She felt dizzy and stumbled trying to walk. Oddly enough, on the day following these sleep days, she felt fine. So much was going on I made a habit of putting all symptoms in writing for the psychiatrist. I wrote the following when Keri was taking 0.75 mg of Risperdal *b.i.d.*,[35] telling him of her severe stomachaches and excessive sleeping, as well as her having been in tremendous physical pain the night before from tight, aching muscles and joints.

> *Can Risperdal cause the symptoms she has been having? The fact that these symptoms are not every day, yet she takes the Risperdal every day, makes me think it*

---
[35] *B.i.d.* is Latin for *bis in die*. It refers to administering a dose twice a day.

> is not the Risperdal. But if it is not the Risperdal, I still don't have a clue as to what is going on with her. This is reminiscent of her hypersomnia of two years ago, except that lasted for three weeks, rather than a day or two at a time, and was supposedly due to depression.

The Risperdal made Keri feel better mentally and emotionally, but her body could not tolerate even the low dosage she was on. In addition to hurting all over and stumbling intermittently while walking, she was nauseous. Her spells of dizziness became more frequent. Even when she wasn't dizzy, she suffered another side effect from Risperdal, a frequent and dangerous lack of coordination—the doctor called ataxia—which caused her to fall at random when standing or walking. She'd occasionally suffered from ataxia in the past, but usually in association with migraines or a sleep episode.

At the sound of an ominously loud thud, Greg and I bolted up the stairs. Keri was lying face up, unconscious, on the cold tile of the bathroom floor. A moment later, she opened her eyes in confusion, wondering what had happened to her. Except for a small lump on the back of her head, she appeared to be uninjured. While we put ice on the lump, she pondered what had taken place. Was her fall the result of ataxia? Did she pass out from hitting her head when she fell? Or did she fall and hit her head because she passed out? She had no idea.

On another occasion, she fell down a small flight of concrete stairs, head first. She'd just been standing on the landing, talking to a friend.

Then came one night when she was in agony, every muscle in her body tense and in pain. This was another EPS side effect of the Risperdal called acute dystonia or a dystonic reaction. As directed, we gave her the antihistamine Benadryl (diphenhydramine HCl), but it did not ease her pain.

When the psychiatrist lowered Keri's Risperdal dosage to 0.50 mg, she felt better physically, but the voices came back with a vengeance. This time the voices were mean and disturbed her at school, so the doctor decided to switch her from Risperdal to another atypical neuroleptic, Zyprexa (olanzapine). Using a method called cross titration, we would lower the dosage of Risperdal while increasing the dosage of Zyprexa. Everyone hoped Zyprexa would be a better choice, but I was concerned about one of its possible side effects—amblyopia, commonly known as lazy eye. After all, Keri already had eye problems.

~~~~~~~~~~

Autumn turned to winter.

Finally, Keri had an MRI (without contrast) and a brief EEG. Neither revealed any problems. The negative EEG, we were told, did not rule out seizures.

Next the pediatrician sent Keri to a pediatric endocrinologist who focused exclusively on her short stature rather than her combination of symptoms. He had Keri's DNA tested for Turner syndrome or Turner mosaic, and he checked the functioning of her thyroid gland. The DNA test was negative for Turner, and her thyroid seemed to be functioning normally. And that was the end of that.

> Testing thyroid function often consists of measuring the thyroid-stimulating hormone (TSH), produced by the pituitary gland, as opposed to measuring actual hormones produced by the thyroid and available for use. Designed to detect primary hypothyroidism, such testing can miss cases of hypothyroidism due to causes other than a malfunctioning thyroid gland.

The endocrinologist's hard-copy report of the visit addressed Keri's short stature only. At 12 years, 3 months, she fell below the 5th percentile in height for her age. Her bone age was a year behind her chronological age,[36] due, according to the report, to "some constitutional delay." If Keri's growth fell further behind, the endocrinologist said, he could reevaluate her.

We were told to expect her adult height to be 4 feet, 10 inches (1.47 meters), which was significantly shorter than her relatives.

---

[36] The bone age of a child refers to the stage of bone maturation (i.e., calcification of the growing ends of the bones), as seen on an x-ray. Prediction of adult height is often made by using a child's bone age in conjunction with his or her current height.

> **Growth-hormone** (also referred to as somatotropin) deficiency can be a bit complicated to diagnose and may require several different tests.
>
> One test, requiring repeated blood draws, involves checking how the pituitary responds to growth-hormone-producing stimuli.
>
> The process of growth-hormone production, which mostly occurs at night during deep sleep, may be altered in children who have grossly disturbed or fragmented sleep. In this case, a better indicator may be obtained by measuring growth hormone present in blood samples obtained overnight. This requires overnight hospitalization.
>
> Hospitals or clinics with neuroendocrine units are better prepared to conduct the testing required.

Changing Meds, Evolving Diagnoses, and Insights

As Keri completed the switch from Risperdal to Zyprexa, the psychiatrist gave us forms on which to list her medications and dosages and to chart her sleep. We were to note total hours of sleep, awakenings, night terrors, and sleepwalking (although Keri did not sleepwalk). We were also to track her fluctuating anger, energy levels, and mood. I added short notes to explain her anger episodes, such as when she was upset about going to the doctor and getting blood tests. I also recorded times when she was simultaneously depressed, anxious, and exceedingly hyper, a combination the doctor referred to as a "mixed state." Her daily sleep now ranged from 7.5 to 18 hours.

A few months earlier, both the psychiatrist and I read the recently published book, *The Bipolar Child*.[37] I was amazed at how often the authors portrayed experiences that matched my daughter's. Not sleeping as an infant, temperature dysregulation, night terrors, irritability, and sensory sensitivity, all problems Keri had faced, were noted as issues connected to the hypothalamus and the limbic system, parts of

---

[37] Papolos and Papolos.

the brain the psychiatrist had already discussed with us when Keri was in the sixth grade.

The authors went on to describe even more of Keri's symptoms: depression, sleep problems, nightmares that didn't end when a normal person's would, moodiness, psychosis, even characteristics akin to ADHD. Could Keri have bipolar disorder? Would all the pieces of this puzzle finally come together?

There were, of course, other symptoms that did not fit. Keri's fits or rages were never caused by the word "no," as described in the book and by many parents of children with pediatric bipolar disorder; rather, they seemed to come out of the blue. In fact, in sharp contrast to most children with this condition, she handled "no" quite well. And her rages, instead of involving aggression or violence against others, were more like meltdowns.

Keri's doctor did not change her diagnosis to bipolar disorder just because he read *The Bipolar Child*, but it did give us greater insight into Keri's problems, along with ideas on how to treat her. It also set me off in a positive direction to learn more about my daughter's brain, how to help her deal with her problems, and how we might use nutritional supplements to potentially augment the effectiveness of her medications.

As part of my investigation, I studied the use of essential fatty acids (EFAs) from cold-water fish (fish oil) for mood regulation and treatment of depression or dysthymia (a milder form of depression). One non-prescription EFA supplement, OmegaBrite, had been proven in a double-blind, placebo-controlled clinical study to be helpful in the treatment of mood disorder, especially when used in conjunction with lithium. This type of study, which paralleled the rigorous standards used by pharmaceutical companies in order to obtain FDA approval for new medications, was the only type my daughter's psychiatrist would accept as proof that a supplement might be beneficial.

> Some medical insurance will pay for prescription nutritional supplements even when intended for off-label use, such as when fish oil is used for mood disorders.

Moreover, Keri displayed some of the physical symptoms of EFA deficiency: dry skin and dry, thin hair, a learning disability, vision problems, mental deterioration, immune-system dysfunction/susceptibility to infection, slowed growth, and behavioral changes. And so, armed with a "prescription" from her psychiatrist, Keri started to take OmegaBrite, highly concentrated and purified fish oil, as a medication. Since the fish oil was to be used with antioxidants, she also was put on vitamins E and C.[38]

> Submitting a prescription order or letter from a physician denoting the need for a supplement, along with a sales receipt, may allow the supplement to be paid for with pre-tax medical spending accounts.

Since Keri's symptoms seemed similar to those of my biological mother (as well as to those of Keri's paternal grandmother), the psychiatrist had an idea. At his suggestion, I asked my brother Mark, who had managed our mother's medical care, to obtain her medical records, and I talked to my mother's siblings and other relatives about her symptoms. Perhaps insight into my mother's illness and medication history might help Keri.

After great difficulty, Mark was able to acquire the sketchy records. We learned my mother had once been on lithium, a mood stabilizer, which apparently helped but also caused life-threatening side effects. Most of her life she was not on medications yet was able to live alone and rarely required hospitalization. She died from cardiomyopathy and we'd been told her children were at greater risk of this disorder as well. Having just the positive symptoms of hallucinations and paranoia without negative symptoms—lack of affect or motivation, her last psychiatric diagnosis was paranoid psychotic disorder. Before her death, during a time I remember her as being calm and without paranoia, she'd been on Haldol, one of the older neuroleptics.

---

[38] Antioxidants help lower lipid (fish oil) peroxidation rates.

What was she like as a child? Everyone said she was beautiful, "a wonderful child" and "so smart!" Some remembered her occasionally acting like a "spoiled brat"—whiny, childish, and throwing tantrums—although she was extremely sweet, gentle, loving, and affectionate. She also had migraines. She was labeled at various times as suffering from major depression, schizophrenia, and "some kind of personality disorder."

I admired the way my older brother, Sam, was raising his own special needs child, with unflagging devotion and understanding, coupled with the determination to get his son appropriate help. Above all, I admired his patience! So, feeling sandwiched between two generations of this illness, I reached out to my brothers with my thoughts:

> *I have been getting to see our mother reincarnated in the form of my daughter.*
>
> *I am understanding our mother's behavior, her curses, etc., because I am getting glimpses of it in Keri.*
>
> *I see more and more of our mother's illness in Keri, and I know without a shadow of a doubt that Keri has the same illness, whatever it is, that our mother had. I accept that. But I do not accept the outcome. I am trying to get Keri all the help I can to achieve a different outcome.*
>
> *I feel angry at the medical community. I'm not angry at her psychiatrist, but I do feel frustrated and angry at the general level of knowledge after all these years.*
>
> *If you want to understand both our mother and your niece better, read* The Bipolar Child *by Papolos and Papolos. Even if what they have is **not** childhood-onset bipolar disorder, so much in that book describes Keri. The book is absolutely fascinating. It goes into the chemical make-up. One physical finding is so weird because some of us share it—low body temperature, and also fluctuating body temperature.*
>
> *I've read genetic illnesses sometime skip a generation. What usually happens with children like Keri is that they get a double dose of genes that contribute to bi-*

polar disorder or to the psychotic disorder.[39] *Of course, Greg's mom has symptoms nearly identical to our mother. Disturbingly, she, too, had a poor outcome from ECT, as far as being left with hallucinatory problems.*

The book The Bipolar Child *addresses early symptoms that Keri had, such as sleeping little and only in small chunks of time, as well as crying inconsolably when away from me (Sophie would remember that well!). It addresses the raging fits and why Keri even cried so much in her sleep when she did sleep. The book explains why such a child may act bossy and oppositional—because they are inflexible. The book describes why, biochemically, these kids are the way they are and how it can impact their normal childhood development and their developing personalities.*

The book says the disturbed sleep, crying, and thrashing most of every night is because of a problem with dreaming. You and I can wake up when the dream gets too bad, but these kids don't! Can you imagine? These ongoing terrors affect the kids too, and sometimes you won't know it until years later, I guess like PTSD, which is often exactly how Keri acts—like she has PTSD.

Given the internal environment these kids have to grow up with, I am amazed they are as sane as they are!

I think a lot about money and my kids' futures. Even with good insurance, we spend thousands of dollars a year out of pocket on mental health and medications.

I love you guys very much. If you want to read The Bipolar Child, *I will be happy to send you a copy.*

I'll let you know if and when Keri gets a solid diagnosis.

The last line of this letter haunts me to this day. I had no idea how elusive a solid diagnosis could be. Like blind men trying to describe an elephant by the part they were touching—trunk, ears, legs, or tail—

---

[39] Evidence has emerged that some individuals with bipolar disorder and schizophrenia share some of the same genes ("Evidence of genetic overlap of schizophrenia and bipolar disorder," 2005).

each doctor attempted to diagnose Keri based on the constraints of, and observed symptoms relating to, his or her own specialty.

~~~~~~~~~~

Keri's psychiatrist made a valiant attempt to explain the differences between bipolar disorder with psychosis (a mood disorder accompanied by psychosis), schizoaffective disorder (psychosis accompanied by a mood disorder), and schizophrenia (a psychotic disorder that can include symptoms of mania and/or depression). Nevertheless, I really had a hard time with the explanation and wondered how doctors could ever decide on the final diagnosis. I still felt confused after reading the DSM-IV descriptions, but finally I got it sorted out (see table 13).

Table 13: A Non-Medical Explanation of the Differences between Bipolar Disorder with Psychotic Features, Schizophrenia, and Schizoaffective Disorder

Disorder	Explanation
Bipolar disorder with psychotic features	If you stop the *mood symptoms*, you'll stop the psychosis. Psychosis only appears as *part* of the mood disorder. This does not mean, however, that antipsychotic drugs are never used.
Schizophrenia	If you stop the *psychosis*, you'll stop the mood symptoms. The mood symptoms only appear as *part* of the psychosis. This does not mean, however, that antidepressant drugs are never used.
Schizoaffective disorder	If you stop the *mood symptoms*, you'll *still* have the psychosis. If you stop the *psychosis*, you'll *still* have the mood symptoms. The mood symptoms and the psychosis must be treated as if they were two separate illnesses.

All three conditions are possibly on the same spectrum, potentially sharing overlapping genes and/or underlying physiology. They also may be affected by some of the same environmental influences.

Unwilling to assign any of these diagnoses to Keri, the psychiatrist instead diagnosed her as having "mood disorder—not otherwise specified (NOS)." He prescribed lithium as a mood stabilizer, saying that five days after starting this drug, Keri would need a blood level. Since she had developed a severe fear (phobia) of blood draws, we planned for her to take lorazepam to calm down enough for the blood draw. The doctor hoped the lithium would reduce her phobia and anxiety to the point she would no longer require lorazepam for future blood draws.

Armed with a prescription for lithium and a lengthy informational printout, I left the psychiatrist's office feeling relieved. *Keri will be okay once she's on a mood stabilizer*, I thought. *Lithium will be the magic bullet.* I delayed the start of the lithium by a few days to ensure I could get Keri to the blood draw precisely five days after starting on the new drug. I don't think avoiding this delay would have changed what happened next.

Table 14: Characteristics: Age 11

- Learning disability and vision problems:
  - Had trouble with computations.
  - Developed a technique to better enable her to overcome her writing disability by putting her brain into "art mode."
  - Still complained about vision problems. Music teachers questioned whether she could see well.
  - Music teachers also wondered whether she might have dyslexia because of mixing up hand direction and fingering when playing written music.
- Vision problem verified:
  - Underwent psychological testing that ruled out a psychological basis for her vision problem.
  - Eye testing indicated she needed reading glasses with prismatic lenses and correction for farsightedness.
- Contracted viral pneumonia.
- Played flute, piano, and violin. Composed music.
- Became more interested in visual arts—photography and drawing.
- Liked her new school (a Montessori middle school for seventh- and eighth-graders).
- Episodically acted psychotic—as if she had PTSD. Was afraid; thought people were bad and scary.
- Had episodes of lack of concentration/spacing out. Put on the stimulant Adderall for ADHD-Inattentive Type.
- Happy, happy, happy for a month; started sleeping less and less, then not at all. Became acutely psychotic the day after turning 12.

Hell

Age Twelve

Liquid Red

Standing alone,
 arms outstretched
Colors around me
 blur to red
Liquid
Only for a moment
Before
 this beautiful world,
 this empty red void
 forms around me
And I stand
 in the middle
So small
As each scream
I make
 echoes all around
In this red,
 translucent,
 glassware world

– Keri

Chapter 18
Blindsided

The week after her psychiatric visit, Keri was in a terrific mood, with an upbeat attitude toward life in general. Each day I picked up a happy, talkative child from school, her big green eyes sparkling. At home she socialized with friends, did homework, listened to music, and played with the pets—all normal activities for a 12-year-old.

On Thursday, she got into the front passenger seat, fastened her seat belt, and brushed away a few curly auburn hairs that had escaped from her ponytail and were tickling her thick dark lashes. She began chatting happily about her day, but as I drove through town, her speech became increasingly agitated and disjointed. My brain swirled with escalating alarm and confusion.

Suddenly, Keri unlatched the car door and tried to jump out! Thank heavens she was still wearing her seat belt. Keeping one eye on the road, I reached across her and yanked the door closed. Then I grasped the seat belt clasp firmly, to keep her from releasing it, and eased the car to the side of the road. I felt torn between wanting to calm her and wanting to scream at her. I carefully kept my voice calm, with just a note of concern and surprise. "What are you *doing*?"

Her reply was near panic. "I need to get out of the car—*now*!"

"NO!" I replied sternly, hoping she would respond to my tone of authority.

We were only about a mile's drive from home, and most of that was through a park. I grabbed her right arm, trapping her left arm beneath it, and proceeded to drive ever-so-slowly toward home. My heart was pounding. *I just need to get her home*, I thought; *I just need to get home*.

Once inside the house, Keri remained extremely agitated. She yelled at Chieena and shook his birdcage, screaming he was evil and she didn't like the way he was glaring at her. She screamed at Mugsy, her precious Boo-Boo, because he was staring at her malevolently. In fact, she thought we were all evil, conspiring in a plot against her. When the little dog looked up at her with puzzled eyes, she lunged forward, shoving him away with her leg and screaming at him to *stop looking at her!*

An all-out kick could have killed the nine and a half-pound (4.31 kg) poodle. Yet even in her psychotic state, my daughter's innate gentleness was still there. She didn't have it in her to actually injure the dog, although she was truly terrified, believing he was out to do her harm. Mugsy, who had scurried back, startled, was confused and scared. So was I. So was Keri.

Next, she ran to the kitchen, yanked out the tableware drawer, and overturned it, scattering the contents across our kitchen table. I watched in a state of mounting fear as she grabbed a steak knife, not knowing whether she intended it as a defensive or an offensive weapon. I was wrong on both counts. "I need it!" she yelled, frantically.

"To use against us." It was more of a statement than a question.

"*No*," was her surprising response. "*Against ME!*"

Keri was so out of control, so agitated, that I easily plucked the knife from her grasp. Of course, once I did, she tried to grab another.

While this bizarre scenario was unfolding in the kitchen, I could hear my friend Claire in our finished basement, a space she used once a week to give violin lessons, playing a happy duet with her student. The whole scene felt surreal.

I pinioned Keri's arms to keep her away from the knives, pulling her into the living room while talking to her softly. She became furious when I restrained her, but I explained, calmly but firmly, that I could not let her harm herself or the pets. "I'm going to let you go," I kept repeating, "but you need to stay in the living room." I assured her I loved her; I just needed her to stay where she was safe.

Finally Keri stopped struggling. I released her and backed away, but when I looked in her eyes, what I saw there was unrecognizable—

maybe a hard glare of fury, hatred, or something else. She leaped at me, grabbing me around the throat as if to choke me. I was shocked, but even in the moment I realized that just as her attack on the dog was restrained, so was her attack on me. Like a cornered animal, she needed to strike out in self-preservation, yet her still-gentle nature didn't want to inflict harm.

But if Keri was attacking out of self-preservation, why was she so determined to get to the knives and kill herself? Possibly, in her mind, escape by death was better than facing whatever evil she felt around her.

For someone so small, at that moment she was surprisingly strong. (It's a good thing she was doing only a halfhearted job of trying to choke me.) I needed to protect myself, but at the same time I was determined not to hurt a single square centimeter of my daughter's body—no violence. Keri felt trapped; she just wanted to get away. I pulled her hands away from me as I stepped aside as if to let her pass; then I slipped behind her, grabbing her arms into an X shape across her body. I pulled her to the floor and wrapped my legs around her. She was now immobilized, but so was I. With my body wrapped around hers, I couldn't reach the phone to call for help. I could only wait, either for Greg to come home or for Claire to come upstairs. Time passed with agonizing slowness.

Forty-five excruciatingly long minutes later, Keri was no calmer. My strained muscles quivered with fatigue, but in the minutes I'd been acting like a human strait-jacket I'd had plenty of time to think things through. Finally Claire said goodbye to her last student and came upstairs. "Call the hospital," I gasped out softly, so as not to further agitate Keri, "and let them know we need to bring in a psychotic child."

After calling the hospital, then calling Greg so he could meet us there, Claire got Keri a change of clothes, pajamas, toothbrush, toothpaste, and hairbrush from her bedroom, all of which she put into a bag along with Keri's medications.

Since my car was equipped with child safety locks to prevent the back doors from being opened from the inside, Claire and I hustled

Keri into the backseat. Claire drove while I sat with Keri, my arms still wrapped around her, keeping her safe.

Chapter 19
At the Hospital

At the hospital, Keri was no longer violent and aggressive, but she was still agitated and episodically tried to run, or rather, escape. At least she was no longer attacking! While the hospital verified her stay would be covered by our insurance, they allowed us to be locked up with her on the *inside*, rather than having us remain with her in the waiting room while trying to control her. Claire comforted Keri while I filled out numerous forms with insurance, medical, and personal information. The entire process was gruesome, but without Claire's assistance it would have been far more difficult.

This particular facility was a behavioral hospital. There, when a presumed psychological illness occurred in a child, the mental health workers assumed either the parents and/or some psychological trauma were to blame. Parenal-caused behavioral problems would be due either to lax or inappropriate discipline or to emotional or physical abuse. Since the behavioral hospital's approach presumed family was the cause of the child's behavior problems—his or her mental illness—visitation and communication were curtailed. Real hospitals do not have this restriction on visitation and phone calls.

> **Psych Nurse** observes that there are multiple valid reasons for separating relatives from their agitated family member. In some cases, emotionally laden, intensely personal family interactions can further agitate a child who is already in an emotionally volatile state.
>
> Horrified reactions from family members also can exacerbate situations.
>
> Even parents trying to clarify events in front of their child, contradicting the child's paranoid or deluded perceptions, can serve to further frustrate their son or daughter.

Sometimes, if the child is furious at a parent for bringing him/her to the hospital, it *is* best for the parent to leave. But Keri was no longer angry. She completely understood why she was there and was frightened by what was happening to her brain. She wanted to be fixed. She was horrified by the feelings that ebbed and flowed unbidden and seemingly not at her command.

Looking back, I shake my head at the insanity of taking a child whose brain is so obviously affected by *something* anywhere other than a *real* hospital. If something is so wrong that a child's brain is malfunctioning, the cause should be investigated. Of course, a medical hospital would have just sent us on our way to a psychiatric hospital, and the only psychiatric hospital our insurance would pay for was this behavioral facility. But there was nothing behavioral about what was happening to my daughter. Whatever the cause of the malfunction in her brain, it was not something that could be fixed by psychological or behavioral methods.

At the time, however, I was simply grateful for our generous insurance policy. I didn't yet recognize the absurdity of separating the brain from the rest of the body.

Finally it was time for an interview with the nurse-administrator, who wanted to hear what had happened in Keri's words as well as in mine. Seeing Keri's medicines she said, "Your daughter is too young to be on so many medications." I wondered at what age it became appropriate for a sick child to take medicine. It is hard enough to get most children with any condition, from diabetes to cancer to bipolar disorder, to be compliant with treatment without a nurse coming along and making such an asinine statement. Yet what provided me with amusement for years to come was Keri's reaction to this remark. I didn't have to say anything. Keri suddenly became focused on the nurse-administrator and sternly expressed her own analytical outrage and anger. I was amazed at the manner in which she was switching between clarity and delusion.

The nurse-administrator then asked what had brought us to the hospital. I related how Keri had acted aggressively toward the pets, tried to jump out of a car, and had attacked me, albeit halfheartedly. I explained Keri had acted in delusional self-preservation and desperation, lashing out in fear and paranoia, thinking we (pets included) had all turned evil. This, along with Keri's desire to harm *herself*, was why I'd brought her to the hospital. The nurse-administrator must not have been listening, since her next remark was that our home situation must be awful for Keri to harbor such extreme anger toward me. I was dumbfounded. Our home life was good! Keri was *usually* a loving individual. This was psychotic. This was delusional.

By this time, Greg had joined us. The nurse-administrator now had all four of us (Keri, Claire, Greg, and I) trying to make her *listen* to what we were saying without twisting it through the interpretive filter of her own prejudices.

The hospital staff notified Keri's psychiatrist, and after a strip search and removal of her shoelaces, Keri was admitted. Twelve years old, tiny and prepubescent, she was placed with children younger than she.

It would be weeks, we were told, before Keri would be able to come home. In the meantime, according to hospital rules, visitation was restricted to one brief period each weekday and twice each day on weekends. We were instructed to withdraw Keri from her current school, as she would go to school at the hospital. Again, I found this confusing. If she was well enough to go to school, why would she need to be in a hospital?

What we did not yet realize was this mental-health hospital—the only one authorized by our insurance company—was not meant for children with *real* psychiatric disorders at all. It was meant for children with *behavioral* or *emotional* problems, not for those with problems affecting a body organ—the brain—and certainly not for children with a psychotic disorder. The teenagers in residence were there mainly because of drug abuse, running away from home, and delinquency. Thank heavens Keri was being housed with the younger kids!

It seemed so wrong that although our daughter was sick and scared, we were not permitted to stay with her. Keri wanted her mommy; she wanted support from those who loved her. Yet instead of flowers, gifts, cards, and visitors, she was to get isolation and group therapy to work out her supposedly behavioral problems.

Keri's psychiatrist was wonderful. Each day he came to spend time with Keri and with us. He explained that there was no hospital within a hundred-mile radius of our city that was appropriate for a child with psychosis. Moreover, he worried that keeping Keri in a hospital for behavioral problems might actually make her illness worse. He wanted her discharged as soon as possible, which would be at the start of the following work week.

That Friday, Keri went to the hospital school. Later, she told us the schooling was a good idea. In her current state, in stark contrast to just days earlier when she had been operating at a college level, she was having difficulty grasping even basic third grade material, but at least the staff was *trying* to make her think. The teacher gave her a simple math sheet as homework, but she was not allowed a pencil to take with her. On Saturday, Keri asked for a pencil at the nurse's station to do the math sheet. The nurses looked at each other, wondering what to do. The children were not allowed pencils; they could be used as a weapon or self-destructive device. However, since Keri seemed so mature and at least externally calm, they gave her one to take to her room.

The heavy window curtains in Keri's room completely blocked the sunlight, making the room dark and depressing. Keri thought this was wrong. If children weren't depressed when they entered the hospital, they soon would be if kept in dark rooms where heavy curtains blocked the sunlight.

Standing between the curtains and the window, Keri could see it was bright and cheery outside, the sunbeams reflecting off the crystalline surface of the snow like millions of tiny prisms. But there were no ropes or cords to tie back or open the curtains, since such things could be dangerous.

Keri thought of a way to bring the sunlight inside. Using strips from the scratch paper left over after doing her math homework, she tied back the curtains. "Not allowed . . ." sputtered one nurse after another, until each realized the curtains were held back with nothing more than scrap paper.

Mostly, though, Keri was quiet and withdrawn. The nurses labeled this behavior "being good." In reality, Keri was usually quiet and withdrawn when she was scared; when the auditory hallucinations were bad; when she was holding in her fear and other emotions, just trying to survive.

Several nurses commented on our daughter's maturity and intelligence. We were told that in group session, when each child was asked to tell why he or she was there—what he or she had "done" to be admitted to this hospital—Keri said she was there because an illness was causing a chemical problem in her brain that resulted in delusions and hallucinations. One nurse remarked our daughter knew more about mental illness than most of the nurses on staff.

Keri was discharged on Monday, but during the time she was a patient, her blood was drawn to test her lithium level. To avoid the protests of a phobic child, the blood draw took place at four in the morning, while she was still half-asleep.

Keri left the hospital with a diagnosis of bipolar disorder. Later, because psychosis was Keri's most salient symptom regardless of mood, her psychiatrist changed this diagnosis to psychotic disorder–NOS (not otherwise specified), an action that did not please Keri. "Psychosis-NOS," she said, "only describes a symptom, not the medical condition causing it." In her opinion, it wasn't a *real* diagnosis. At first I didn't understand what she meant. "It's like going to the doctor with a headache," she explained, "and the doctor diagnosing you with 'head pain–not otherwise specified.' This diagnosis says nothing about *why* you have a headache." In the same way, Keri's diagnosis labeled her symptoms (hallucinations), without specifying a reason for them. What could I say except "good point"?

Chapter 20
At Home

Now that Keri had a diagnosis of bipolar disorder, we thought the puzzle was complete. We knew there were pieces left over, but we decided they were superfluous, or perhaps part of a separate puzzle altogether. We soon discovered how wrong we were; there was a lot more to learn.

Keri's migraines increased, only now they were preceded by bizarre prodromes or auras[40] including, at different times, visual and perceptual changes, depressive symptoms, paranoia, confusion, aphasia (being unable to speak), and ataxia. She displayed ongoing psychotic symptoms, even when her mood was normal. She woke more frequently during the night and often needed to sleep during the day.

Keri continued to take Zyprexa, but she had side effects from even a tiny amount of it. She slept 12 to 16 hours a day, yet she was still tired and lethargic. She was itchy, constantly hungry, and suffered from stomachaches. She felt agitated and anxious, for which she used lorazepam *p.r.n.*[41] And she had depression and agitated sleep that now lasted through the night. Her night-time, terror-like screaming was back, starting about three hours after falling asleep and continuing for about three hours more. The word *nightmare* doesn't really describe the dreams Keri was experiencing. She'd had nightmares when she was younger, ones that didn't stop when they should have, but these episodes were far worse. She was living through traumatic horrors in

---

[40] The prodrome stage of a migraine is characterized by a preliminary set of symptoms preceding the actual headache. A migraine aura is sometimes considered to be separate from the prodrome stage. Not all migraines have prodromes or auras, and one or both of these symptoms can occur without progressing to an actual headache. Migranes with auras are called classic migraines. Ataxia, aphasia, severe depression, and paranoia are considered less-common features of migraines.

[41] *P.r.n.* is Latin for *pro re nata* and refers to administering doses as needed.

her sleep as if they were real; it felt, she said, as if her brain was hallucinating the nightmares. When she awoke screaming, wide-eyed and terrified, the horrors paused. She ran around her room frantically, trying to keep them at bay, but each time she stopped, her eyes closed and they returned. We called these episodes Keri's "dreams while awake," and the only thing that seemed to banish them was lorazepam. The drug didn't stop the trauma she felt or her desire to keep screaming in horror. What it did do was act like a chemical straitjacket to prevent her from acting on her residual anxiety and agitation.

Lorazepam, we found, could also stop Keri's fits, but each time she used the drug, her body was left feeling as if she'd been hit by a truck. She hated how lorazepam made her feel physically, but she said the trade-off was worth it.

One night she awoke hallucinating she was being whipped. Over and over, the heavy leather lash came down on her back, arms, and legs, ripping open her skin as she screamed in agony. To Keri, it didn't matter that there was no lash, no sadistic flayer, no blood; *she felt every bit of the pain.* The only difference between her hallucination and reality was the absence of physical scars. Mentally and emotionally, the experience left her traumatized. Is it any wonder she later went through the house gathering every belt, leather strap, and dangly toy—anything reminiscent of a lash—and threw them into the yard?

Keri was experiencing post-traumatic stress disorder (PTSD), just as if she really had been whipped. How "sane" would I be if I'd been through this experience? I waited until she was not around to retrieve the discarded items from the yard, but I kept them out of sight for months.

Keri's psychiatrist was silent about these episodes. I knew bipolar children often had vivid, horrific nightmares that didn't stop when a normal nightmare would, but I never read about terrifying dreams that continued even after the child awoke, or about children who used frantic motion to hold their nightmares at bay. I once again searched the Internet for information, hoping to discover at least a term for Keri's behavior. The closest things I found were descriptions of dreamlike, hallucinatory experiences one has while falling asleep and waking up called, respectively, hypnagogic and hypnopompic states. These vivid, brief experiences, which Keri did (and still does) have occasionally, are more common in people with the neurological sleep disorder called narcolepsy. But they did not describe her waking nightmares. The first thing I found that seemed close to what we were observing was *REM while awake*.[42] Later, I read about a similar phenomenon occurring in patients with Guillain–Barré syndrome (GBS), a viral infection that can cause mental status changes, including psychosis. The GBS sites termed these *wakeful dreams* and said they were caused by temporary, narcoleptic-like changes.[43]

Needless to say, Keri was anxious and extremely emotionally needy. Many days she clung to me all day. Or, if she wasn't actually touching me, she at least needed to be in the same room. I called these her Velcro days—the days she was afraid to be alone, even to go to the bathroom. She wanted someone with her at all times, except when she would suddenly become afraid of us, screaming in paranoia and fury for us to get away.

The voices she heard were no longer limited to the distinct few she'd always had in her head. Now other voices joined in, sometimes with a soft mumbling, other times with a jumbled, deafening roar. She heard people behind closed doors. She heard voices behind her when she was alone in a room. She heard and saw other things that weren't actually there, though at the time she didn't recognize these auditory and visual phenomena as hallucinations. To Keri, they were as real as anything else perceived by her senses. They confused her. They frightened her. She was uncertain whom she could trust. She wanted out of the nightmare her world had become.

The walls in Keri's room were adorned with posters and cheerful Winnie-the-Pooh decorations, but during her rages she ripped them down, one by one, until all that was left were holes, gouged plaster, and scuffed and chipped paint. Clothes, books, and debris began to

---

[42] REM stands for rapid eye movement and corresponds with the period (supposedly of sleep) when the brain is dreaming.
[43] Cochen, V., et al., 2005.

pile up on the floor, yet she couldn't tolerate the thought of anyone touching her stuff. This was okay with me; cleaning her room was certainly not on my list of priorities!

As the winter dragged on, Keri's mood kept changing. We got her a light box to use when she woke up in the morning to help alleviate depression. It didn't make her feel less depressed, she said, but she did feel more awake. One sunny day, when it was slightly warmer, we took her out to a farm for a few hours with the horses. She was still anxious and clingy, but she smiled. She even *laughed*! Back at home, she was scared again, needing me to stay with her while she showered.

We took her to school as much as we could, but often she was there for just a few hours before the anxiety or the voices would become too overwhelming and we had to pick her up. We continued to be grateful she was not enrolled in public school, with its rules about mandatory days of attendance, excused absences, and makeup work.

In addition to her anxiety and nightmares, Keri was always hungry, another side effect of Zyprexa. But this was different from normal hunger. She acted like she was suffering from hypoglycemia (low blood sugar). Whining like a toddler in need of food, she would turn pale and slump to the floor. Neither the doctor nor the pharmacy offered any solutions. Instead, I found tips on the Internet from other parents who'd dealt with the same issue. They suggested I put her on the same type of diet I would if she had diabetes—no refined sugars and few refined carbohydrates. Increasing Keri's activity level and choosing foods with a low glycemic index might reduce her glucose-insulin fluctuations.

In an effort to stave off Keri's intense hunger, I learned to boost her protein intake in the morning. I cooked breakfast meats, and since she loved pancakes and French toast, I added protein powder to whole-wheat pancakes made with milk and eggs and soaked whole-grain breads in the egg mixture for French toast. I stored extras in the fridge so Keri could eat immediately if I didn't have breakfast already cooked when she woke up.

In spite of my efforts, she became slightly overweight, though not obese. In her current emotionally fragile state, even this modest weight gain contributed to more distress, frustration, and instability. Her clothes no longer fit, but she couldn't tolerate the crowds, noise, or stress of shopping. My solution was to buy overalls, which luckily were popular at the time. They were comfortable and cute, she looked good in them, and they hid her figure.

The one side effect of Zyprexa that became insurmountable was itchiness. Despite the fact Keri was taking the anti-allergy drug Benadryl (diphenhydramine HCL), the itchiness grew worse and ultimately led to anxiety attacks in and of itself. The Zyprexa had to be abruptly discontinued.

Keri had had severe adverse reactions to small doses of two different atypical neuroleptics: Risperdal and Zyprexa. When taking Zyprexa, her anxiety and agitation had escalated to the point she was taking lorazepam at least once and sometime multiple times each day. Since lorazepam worked so well for her, the psychiatrist decided to put her on a daily dose of Klonopin (clonazepam) instead of another neuroleptic. Clonazepam, like lorazepam, is a benzodiazepine, but it is longer acting. We could still give her extra doses of lorazepam as needed.

Keri required constant vigilance, and both Greg and I were exhausted. I was able to do some work from home, but often only late at night and very early in the mornings. I was feeling the strain. My husband was feeling the strain. Our marriage was feeling the strain.

We hoped the doctor was right about the change in medications. But with Keri *off* the Zyprexa and *on* the clonazepam, Hell got even worse.

Chapter 21
Monsters

Keri's body temperature plummeted. She shivered too much to sleep. When covered with an electric blanket, her temperature rose too much. She was awake all night, as were we, trying to make her comfortable. Toward morning, after we gave her a small amount of lorazepam, she finally slept. When she awoke that afternoon, she was happy and hyper and I took her to school.

The next morning, Keri was still energized. It had been months since she'd been this giddy and animated; she'd even been scolded at school for talking too much. But at six-thirty that evening, as if someone had flipped a switch in her brain, she became intensely angry. These feelings scared her; she couldn't think of anything she felt angry *about*. Before long, this combination of anger and fear escalated into a state of severe anxiety and then to psychosis.

Monsters were outside the house. Keri could see them through the window, huge beasts clambering about in the cold darkness, looking for a way in. She could hear their long claws scraping across the windows and siding, seeking any small opening they could widen to accommodate their massive bulk. Once inside, they would kill her because she was a bad person—a person filled with anxiety and fear. She knew she would soon die.

It was useless to tell her the monsters weren't there. When people are in the midst of a psychotic episode, their hallucinations are as real to them as anything you and I can see, hear, taste, smell, or touch. If you tell them you can't see or hear the things they do, to them this means *you* are deficient—something is awry with *your* senses—or, as in Keri's case, that the monsters were there for her and not for me.

I can only imagine what my daughter must have felt, but I could see the terror wrenching her face and smell the acrid stench of it. In the past, she had depended on me to protect her. This time, she knew the evil was out to destroy her specifically, and she had no expectation that *anyone* could protect her, even her mother.

I gave her a dose of clonazepam, along with some lorazepam, hoping one or both would work soon. In the meantime, I needed to help her deal with the monsters.

Years before, her grandmother Sylvia, an artistic jeweler, had given Keri a very special gift, an intricate shield of David[44] she'd designed and crafted from gold. When the piece was finished, Sylvia had broken the mold so Keri would have a one-of-a-kind creation. Keri wore her beloved necklace day and night.

I had never lied to either of my children, and I did not feel it was a lie now to tell Keri the monsters could not succeed. I said her shield of David, given to her with so much love, would protect her, that while she wore it, the monsters could not harm her. I also told her she could say the *Shema*, a special Jewish prayer. Even without the necklace, I explained, the monsters could not harm her while she repeated this prayer. I held her protectively in my arms while she said the words over and over until she felt less afraid and the lorazepam had had time to take effect. After a while, she even started to feel defiant toward the monsters.

Later that night, while occasionally yelling at the monsters, Keri made a bed in the bathroom between our bedroom and hers. She brought in all her dolls and lined them up against the wall near her head. She also brought in her CD player. Finally, with classical music blaring from the player and clutching the necklace in her hand, she fell asleep.

The next morning, Keri insisted she had not been psychotic. The monsters had been real; she was just glad they'd given up and left. She felt exhausted and cold, and her voice was high-pitched and whiny. Emotionally, she seemed like a four-year-old. By noon, she was cold,

---

[44] A shield of David is also referred to as a star of David, a Jewish star, or Solomon's seal (after the biblical King Solomon).

but she'd begun to act normally and her voice had returned to a normal pitch.

I dropped her at school in the afternoon and drove to work. Once at the office, I closed the door and cried. I was at an emotional breaking point. Perhaps it wasn't enough that Keri had therapy once a week to help her cope with her illness. Maybe I needed therapy as well. I picked up the phone and made an appointment for *me*.

Keri's moods continued to change frequently throughout each day. Each evening she felt happy. Sometimes she was so happy it was scary. Then, as if someone had flipped a switch, she'd go from ecstatic to angry, despairing, or even psychotic and delusional. Greg was avoiding out-of-town business trips so he could be home each night. It was a good thing, because I felt exhausted and frayed.

To cope with her increasing symptoms, the psychiatrist cautiously prescribed another atypical neuroleptic, Seroquel (quetiapine). Seroquel was new and the last of the three atypical neuroleptics available at the time. (Clozapine, a fourth atypical neuroleptic, was considered quite dangerous and a medication of last resort.) If the Seroquel didn't work, we were told that one of the older, typical neuroleptics, such as Haldol, would be tried. But Risperdal, the atypical neuroleptic most like Haldol, had earlier caused Keri intolerable side effects at even tiny dosages. Furthermore, Haldol was notorious for causing severe and lasting side effects such as tardive dyskinesia, which really frightened us. We wanted desperately for the Seroquel to work, and we carefully followed the cautionary adage: *Start low; go slow.*

Seroquel was reputed to be weaker and slower-acting than Risperdal or Zyprexa, but it also was supposed to be more benign (safer). The average dosage at the time was 300 mg; Keri started on 12.5 mg. The plan was to dose her twice a day, increasing the dosage by 12.5 mg every two days until we reached a dose that was effective. Because one of the main objectives was to avoid side effects that could cause this medication to fail, it could take months before we reached a dosage that actually worked. When looking at a lifetime, however, the effort seemed more than worth it.

In addition to Seroquel *b.i.d.* to control hallucinations and psychotic episodes, Keri was now on the following medications: lithium for bipolar disorder, clonazepam for anxiety, lorazepam for when the clonazepam wasn't enough, and fish oil/antioxidants to help protect her brain cells, ease depression, and improve the effects of the lithium. The Zoloft and Adderall had long since been discontinued.

Hell continued unabated.

Some days Keri couldn't get out of bed, and her head hurt. Some days she could manage a couple of math problems; other days she couldn't remember how to do simple arithmetic. Her mood changed from pleasant to angry to psychotic over the course of a day. Sometimes she was quite pleasant. Other times she was whiny and complaining, like a young child in need of a nap. Often, she got so angry at the bird for making noise that she screamed and attacked his cage.

One evening, Keri was hyper happy at seven forty-five. At eight thirty she was insane. The switch had flipped again. Our child, who normally abhorred vile language, was holed up in her room spewing vile hatred toward us, screaming we were assholes and cussing up a storm. Simultaneously, she begged us not to leave. Greg and I stayed calm, ignored the cussing, and remained close at hand outside her bedroom door. The screaming went on for two hours, during which time Keri urinated on herself, the bed, and the floor. Finally calmer, she allowed me into her room, accepting assistance in cleaning up her bed and the floor. In the meantime, she'd taken off her soiled clothes but wouldn't clean herself; instead she followed me around naked. Suddenly she accused me of making fun of her. When we offered her medicine, she became agitated again, claiming the medicine was poison and we were trying to kill her. Still, she was so terrified she didn't want me to leave her side. Having someone around she hated, she said, was better than being alone. A half hour later, she was curled up on the floor asleep.

At 5:30 the following morning, Keri woke up vomiting. She wanted me to stay with her as she drifted back to sleep. When she woke again a few hours later, I helped her into the shower. She felt dizzy and showered sitting down, afraid of falling. Afterward, she needed help getting up and dressing.

By afternoon, she was feeling fine. She went to her therapist and later took a walk with Greg and Mugsy. But by evening, she was extremely dizzy and feeling angry again. She had wanted chicken for dinner but now could eat nothing. "Just make it better," she begged me repeatedly. When I asked what she wanted me to do to "make it better," her answer was simple: "Kill me."

In addition to Keri's dizziness, cognitive impairment (not being able to think well enough to do her schoolwork), and abrupt mood swings, and her paranoid delusions that we wanted to kill her, she was becoming increasingly agoraphobic. Despite taking the clonazepam, which was supposed to ease her anxiety, she now had a fear of leaving the house. Even when I managed to get her into the car, she was afraid to get out of it.

The psychiatrist increased the dosage. Her anxiety escalated. Soon she was afraid to leave the house at all. Then she became afraid to leave the upstairs. Finally, she wouldn't venture beyond the confines of her bedroom. I had read that a person suffering from agoraphobia has a zone within which he or she feels safe, and as the condition progresses, that zone shrinks. Keri's zone was shrinking rapidly. Within days, not only was she afraid to leave her bedroom, she wouldn't get out of bed!

This was the point at which she said, thoughtfully, "Mommy, I think it's the Klonopin that's causing me to feel so afraid." Clearly, the drug wasn't helping, but could it be possible that clonazepam was *causing* some of her problems. I contacted Keri's psychiatrist to let him know she was discontinuing the drug. Within three days, the agoraphobia had disappeared completely, and she was left with the same level of anxiety she'd had before starting to take this drug.

In discussing these results with the psychiatrist, we learned a new phrase. Keri had had a *paradoxical reaction*, which is what happens when a medication designed to alleviate a symptom actually exacerbates the symptom it is supposed to help.

One morning, Keri was cussing, scared of us, and screaming for us to leave her alone even though she was upstairs and we were downstairs. She then came downstairs yelling about how we couldn't be trusted, saying over and over, "Leave me *alone!*"

I'd had enough of this silliness. It was one thing to be upstairs yelling away, but coming downstairs and following us around while yelling at us to leave her alone was ridiculous. "Go back upstairs," I told her, "and leave *us* alone."

Her reaction was baffling. "Don't hurt me! Don't hurt me!" she screamed while running up the stairs. I didn't understand what had happened. We could hear her upstairs, wailing like an infant, when she suddenly started yelling, "Help!" Both Greg and I ran to her, alarmed. But my approach was met with complete hysteria. Keri told her father I had *hit* her! Apparently, when I told her to go upstairs and leave us alone, she felt or saw me strike her.

This was a good day for Greg to stay with her.

Until this incident, I'd never even considered sending Keri away to a residential treatment center (RTC). I knew that a hospital or other facility could not care for her better, keep her safer, or help her any more than we could. I agreed with her psychiatrist that she was better off at home. But when she hallucinated I hit her, I was distraught. Mommy had always been her source of comfort. A mommy was supposed to protect, not inflict pain. I'd rather send her away and have her hallucinate strangers hitting her, rather than the mother she desperately needed as her source of unconditional love, nurture, and comfort. Later I sobbed in Greg's arms, telling him I was ready to give up.

On days Keri didn't wake up whining, paranoid, or psychotic, her moods usually followed a specific pattern. She was pleasant in the morning, whiny in the afternoon, and by dinnertime (around 6:00 p.m.), either happy and laughing or psychotic. If she was incredibly happy around sundown, we knew to brace for the worst. The switch in her brain would flip—sometimes in the middle of a sentence—and she would feel intense anger, agitation, hate, and paranoia. Greg and I shook our heads over the irony of bracing for the worst each time Keri seemed happiest.

One night after the usual switch to agitation and paranoia, Keri was in her room screaming and cussing at us while we listened to her trashing what little had not been already destroyed. Suddenly, it was deathly quiet. When we opened the door to make certain she was all right, we found her dangling out the window, a two-story drop to the concrete driveway below. We grabbed her just in time. Was she thinking of suicide? Actually, she wasn't thinking clearly about anything. She had just wanted to jump. "To your death?" we asked. That was okay by her. Mostly, she was thinking, "*Stop* what's happening to me; *end it* and *escape*." Escape from her nightmares. Escape from everyone, including herself.

After this incident, Greg and I nailed the windows in Keri's bedroom so they could be opened only a few inches. Realizing that windows nailed closed could be dangerous in case of fire, we carefully weighed the risks against the benefits. The windows, newly installed the year before, could still be opened easily by pulling inward on the tops of them, but Keri didn't know this. We decided the risks were worth it.

Another night, neither Greg nor I could calm our daughter. Certain we wanted her dead and therefore were trying to poison her, she refused to take the lorazepam. Finally, terrified and agitated, she ran into the night.

I ran after her, frantic at the sight of my little girl sprinting toward the large park and nearby train tracks, but I soon lost sight of her. She could hide anywhere, behind a garbage can or parked car or in a shadow. I called to her, trying to be reassuring, begging her to come back, but there was no answer. I returned home in fear and failure.

My hands shook as I made my first 9-1-1 call. Thinking of my little girl's scared, twisted face as she dashed away from us, I tried to explain calmly to the 9-1-1 operator that my 12-year-old daughter had run away, toward the park, and that I was very scared for her because she was psychotic and delusional. I heard the sudden tension in the operator's voice. "Does your daughter have a weapon?" she asked.

What did she mean? "Of course not," I replied in confusion.

I tried again to explain that Keri was terrified. *She* was the one in danger. She would hide from the police because she was paranoid. She would never hurt anyone. I was calling because I was afraid *she'd* be hurt. I answered the operator's question about the clothes Keri was wearing: overalls because she'd gotten pudgy, a red short-sleeved shirt with matching red socks, white sneakers. When I answered the question about her height and weight (about 4 feet, 5 inches [135 cm] tall and 85 pounds [39 kg]), I could hear a change in the operator's voice. "Oh," she exclaimed, "a *little* girl."

It was then, with abject horror, I realized the police would consider *Keri* a monster—a threat and a possible danger to others just because she was psychotic. My fear mounting, I became a bit hysterical. Keri was terrified of evil—of monsters. And the cops might be scared of *her*? Even worse, the only thing that might save her from suffering more terror at their hands was the fact she was *little*? Didn't they get it? She was the potential prey, not the predator.

It seemed like an eternity before Keri returned on her own. When I called the police back to let them know they no longer needed to look for her, the operator assured me that if Keri ran away again, I shouldn't hesitate to call. I hung up feeling conflicted. The police could have been the biggest danger of all.

> **Psych Nurse** says the appropriate entity to call when faced with a person experiencing a crisis due to a behavioral condition varies from city to city. Many cities have now implemented CIT (Crisis Intervention Training) for police officers.
>
> CIT programs enable trained emergency responders to handle such crises effectively and safely for all concerned and to take patients, without the use of excessive or deadly force, to hospitals rather than jails.
>
> Many cities, however, do not yet have personnel who've received this type of training. In this case, calling the sheriff's office, rather than the police, may be safer and less traumatic for all involved.

Chapter 22
Of Sisters and Spiders

Keri's constant, round-the-clock care took a physical and mental toll on both Greg and me. Though Greg tried to avoid job-related out-of-town trips, I found myself envying his nights away. At least he could fall asleep in a clean, orderly, peaceful hotel room. I worked mostly from home, doing much of my job at night and on weekends. I was determined to do whatever was required of me, at work and at home, but sometimes I wondered how much strain one person could take. Putting one foot in front of the other, I shrugged off my tiredness as best I could, but I desperately needed sleep.

In addition to taking care of Keri, Greg and I also made trips to a nearby city where our daughter Candace was going to college. Candace had gotten sick and needed our support. The girls enjoyed their visits when Keri went with us. Greg and I, on the other hand, were so exhausted it was all we could manage to do what needed to be done.

Keri continued to have fluctuating anxiety, irritability, frustration, negative thinking, inflexibility, extreme whininess, headaches, stomachaches, body pains, fatigue, and medication-induced hunger in addition to her hallucinations and terrifying nightmares. She was sleeping 10 to 11 hours each night and frequently emotionally needy, vulnerable, and just plain scared during the day. Gone was the independent, self-assured pre-teen of a few months before. When I sat at my desk, trying to meet the obligations of my job, she lay on the floor holding on to my ankle. It was as if she felt that letting go of me would plunge her once more into a roiling maelstrom of terror. When I had to leave the house, she remained behind with Greg, her woeful face peering at me through the storm door as I drove off. When I came back, sometimes hours later, she'd be sitting in the same spot, watching for my return.

Thank goodness for Sylvia, my stepmother. When I called her, which was often, she let me cry. Afterward, I knew she got support from talking to my dad. It was comforting, in a strange sort of way, to think our angst might become diluted by spreading it around, but what I needed most was real, live, tangible help at home.

In retrospect, expecting parents to be the sole caregivers of a child who requires round-the-clock care is ludicrous. In a hospital setting, such children have an entire support system, and help may be provided at home for some severely ill children discharged from a *medical* hospital. For other families, including some whose children have chronic medical needs, there is no such help. Many of these families have no insurance or battle with the insurance companies they have, finding respite care only by jumping through hoops—hoops they may not know exist, let alone have time to navigate. When a child has been diagnosed with a *mental* rather than a *medical* illness, the situation is even worse.

> **Respite-care** providers who are specifically trained to care for a scared child with hallucinations and paranoia still may be impossible to find in many areas. However, the increasing number of caregivers trained to give respite to families whose children suffer from autism or other developmental problems can be of assistance in some situations.

My mind pleaded for relief. From our earlier experiences, I knew there was no hospital within hundreds of miles appropriate for a little girl with a brain problem as opposed to a behavior problem, and I wanted to scream at the injustice of it all. Then, as now, children with broken limbs can go to hospitals with big, sunlit rooms and cheerful pictures on the walls, where an effort is made to include family and friends and plan happy events to make the child's stay as pleasant as possible. Children with broken brains aren't afforded this luxury. Organizations exist to support families of children with life-threatening medical illnesses, but they don't include children whose lives are threatened due to conditions considered mental. The bottom line was that we had no choice but to care for Keri ourselves.

After months of this, one night I succumbed to the exhaustion. The primal need for sleep came over me with an urgency I could not disobey. Keri still needed me, but I had nothing left to give. Through a thick haze, I heard her screaming in fear. She was achingly pleading for me to help her. I did not.

Candace came by that night, as she did occasionally when wanting the familiarity and comfort of home. On this occasion, she found no comfort in her sister's plight or in the fact that her father was away and her mother seemed absent as well. At the sight of me lying inertly in bed while her sister screamed in terror just meters away, Candace became furious.

"How can you just *lie* there while Keri is screaming for you?" I heard her ask accusingly.

Each word felt like a sharp jab, yet I couldn't muster enough energy to care. How could a mother be too tired to respond? I felt my actions were unforgivable, but still I couldn't move. "I just have nothing left to give," I mumbled. My need to sleep was more powerful than my will.

Through a strange, fuzzy veil of twilight between sleep and not-quite sleep, I heard Candace harrumph in disgust and leave my room to help her sister.

Keri was hallucinating big spiders. She was terrified of spiders, and there they were—great, hairy black creatures whose webs blocked the steps so she couldn't go down. They also blocked the way to her bedroom. With tears streaming down her cheeks, she was stuck on the staircase landing, terrified to move through the spiders she saw surrounding her.

Candace had learned from me to work with her sister's hallucinations rather than denying them. She explained to Keri that she was her "big bad sister," whose job was to kill the "big bad spiders." Down the stairs she went, destroying imaginary webs with her hands and arms. She squished spiders under her stomping feet. She went back to kill the spiders Keri pointed out she'd missed. Then she got the broom and swept them away, clearing a path to Keri's bedroom and making it safe for her sister to go downstairs.

Candace had saved Keri from her terrors. I went to sleep.

> **Psych Nurse Comment**: In some hospitals, personnel are *not allowed* to work with patients' hallucinations. They must always "reorient the patient to reality-based thinking," based on the idea that playing along with someone's hallucinations "only feeds into the psychosis." However, many times this reorientation method, when used on an acutely psychotic patient, merely serves to escalate the patient's fear, frustration, and agitation. Some hospital personnel, including doctors, will do what Candace did for her sister, even though it is against official policy.
>
> For example, a patient who believes there is a *real* monkey on her back pleads for hours for someone to remove the monkey so she can go to sleep. Nurses, expected to rigidly follow hospital protocol, talk themselves blue in the face and end up doing nothing except exacerbating her condition. A doctor, disregarding protocol and using a tactic frequently followed for patients with forms of dementia such as Alzheimer's, takes 10 seconds to comply with the patient's request by pretending to remove the monkey. Afterward, the patient proceeds to go to sleep.
>
> In Psych Nurse's experience, trying to reason with acutely psychotic patients only increases their fear and paranoia. It is best to leave the reasoning part until the acute psychosis is under control.

Darkness

Ages Twelve to Thirteen

Plea

Mother, Momma, please be accepting
Daddy, Papa, please just smile

Please, oh please . . . I need you now.

Mother, Momma, say it's all okay
Daddy, Papa, say you still love me

Say you'll be there for me, no matter what.

Mother, Momma, you still can trust in me
Daddy, Papa, you know I'm just like before

You've held my world together . . .
and now I need you more than ever.

— *Keri*

Chapter 23
On the Far Shores

Keri sat on the living room floor, mouth slightly ajar, with a school book open in front of her. Her glazed eyes stared vacantly into the distance. When I spoke to her gently, her unfocused gaze slowly shifted toward me.

After several agonizing months in the deepest bowels of Hell, Keri was no longer severely psychotic; the pharmaceutical cocktail was starting to make a difference. Shortly after she began taking Seroquel, the psychiatrist put her on Wellbutrin (buproprion), which moderately lessened her depression. She felt more awake and her concentration improved slightly, which alleviated some of the emotional meltdowns caused by her frustration with her brain for "not working." The Wellbutrin caused a side effect called akathisia, an "antsy" feeling that made her want to move, rock, or pace; she had a very difficult time staying still. Keri described it as anxiety of the body rather than anxiety of the mind. Fortunately, the condition was temporary and passed on its own.

The Seroquel enabled her to sleep better and alleviated some of her tics. It slightly decreased her wild mood swings, dampened her anxiety, and relieved *some* psychosis and hallucinations. She still had waking nightmares, but attempts to increase her Seroquel dosage resulted in glazed eyes, slowed movement, dulling of her cognitive abilities, and slurred speech. A lisp, which she'd corrected with speech therapy years earlier, was back. With permission from the psychiatrist, we experimented with splitting the dosage and giving it at different times of the day, which helped a little. Interestingly, Keri could tell me when she thought she needed the Seroquel dosage *increased*, but she had no idea when she seemed to have had too much. Her explanation for this discrepancy made perfect sense. "It's hard to tell when I'm feeling or acting doped up, or when my brain is running slowly," she said, "because, well, I *am* doped up and my brain *is* running slowly!"

Overall, it was a balancing act. Wellbutrin changed the balance slightly, but not enough. What was left of our daughter caused Greg and me our separate agonies. We felt spit out and stranded on Hell's desert shores.

Keri had quit doing all the things she loved. She no longer read for pleasure, complaining that reading was now too hard. Schoolwork was also difficult—she just couldn't concentrate. She was sleeping 11 hours a night, yet she was still profoundly tired during the day. She had frequent headaches and was often cold. But she *was* less anxious. Better able to tolerate the noise and commotion of school, she went to school for part of each day.

Math was especially difficult for her, although her ability fluctuated from day to day. Teachers asked what happened to her; she seemed so changed. We were evasive, glad she was not at a school where her impairments mattered. She was given math problems at a lower level, yet she still needed explanations before she could do them. Some days she felt as if her brain simply could not think, a state reflected by poor handwriting and disorganization. On other days, the setup of her math problems was neat and organized. Neatly done or not, however, she often tore up her homework in anger and frustration.

Figure 2: Good Day Math Sample

Figure 3: Bad Day Math Sample

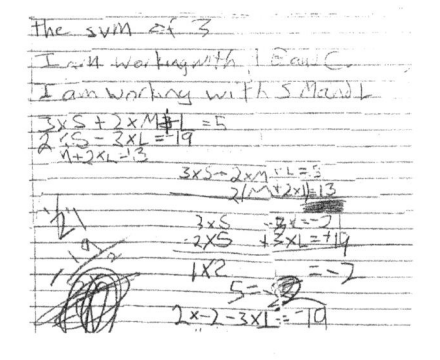

I was horrified at Keri's cognitive losses. It reminded me of Charlie, a character in the book *Flowers for Algernon*.[45] Charlie, a mentally challenged adult, receives an experimental treatment to enhance his intellect. Initially it works; in fact, it turns him into a genius. Eventually, however, the treatment loses its effectiveness. By the end of the book he's regressed to his original mental state.

At this point in her illness, Keri herself didn't care about her loss of cognitive ability. Soon enough, however, and for years afterward, she would remember that once school had been easy for her.

Previously, Keri had been open about her psychiatric diagnoses. Now she asked how to tell people about her psychotic disorder. "You don't," I told her flatly. "If you say you have a psychotic disorder, what people may *hear* is, 'I am psychotic.'" I worried her peers might disregard anything she said because she could have hallucinated it, or discount her still-impeccable logic because she was "nuts." Even kids who were friends *now* might someday use her illness against her.

Then Keri's psychiatrist did something for which we are eternally grateful. One of his young-adult patients with paranoid schizophrenia, now in graduate school and doing well, had allowed the local newspaper to do a feature story about her. Shannon, a beautiful, strong, intelligent young woman, was a superb choice to help destigmatize the label of *mentally ill*. The doctor arranged a time when his few adolescent patients with psychotic disorders, and their parents, could meet with Shannon. Keri was the youngest person there, and at first Shannon was hesitant to talk freely in front of a child. The psychiatrist, however, explained that regardless of her looks, Keri was mature enough to hear what Shannon had to say. As the group compared experiences and asked questions, Shannon told stories of stigma and advocacy. She also shared information about symptoms and medication side effects, as well as her strategies for managing both. The session was exhilarating. Greg and I came away with much greater hope and far less fear for Keri's future.

Keri's staring episodes, which initially looked like absence (petit mal) seizures, now developed a motor component mimicking com-

---

[45] Keyes, 1959.

plex-partial seizures. One day at school, she was holding a pen to a sheet of paper, going over and over it in a specific pattern. Suddenly, she became infuriated, asking who made those marks on her paper. When the other students said *she* had made them, she felt sure they were lying in order to mess with her mind. She knew she had *not* made those marks. One day, I saw her do the same thing at home. She was upset when she saw her paper was messed up. I explained what she had done and how it was possible for her not to have a memory of doing it. She then realized the children at school had been truthful.

Of much greater concern to me than her possible seizures was the increase in frequency and length of what the psychiatrist suggested were brief periods of catatonia, a state of motionless stupor in which a person does not react to external stimuli. Catatonia is a symptom of schizophrenia. Keri suddenly would freeze in place, even in the middle of talking, walking, standing, or reaching for something. Most episodes lasted from mere seconds to a couple of minutes; twice they lasted more than 10 minutes. When in this catatonic-like state, Keri was devoid of movement and unresponsive.

Toward the end of the school year, the school was taking some students on a trip to the ocean where they would be boating, swimming, and snorkeling (a skill Keri had learned at Ocean Camp the year before), and where their book learning would be put to use studying ocean biology and the surrounding fauna and flora.

Before the kids could snorkel, they had to pass a swim test. The test was given in a lagoon that looked like a scene from one of Keri's terrifying, recurring nightmares. Having a PTSD flashback, she refused to go near the area. She wasn't supposed to swim, anyway. An occurrence of one of her staring spells or rare catatonia-like episodes while swimming or snorkeling could be fatal. She didn't like having to stay on the boat while everyone else was in the water, but, still, she was glad she went.

The kids stayed in small cabins with bunk beds. When Keri woke during the night, the room had been transformed from a parsimonious square to a large, glamorous cabin. The meager windows had morphed into elegant bays. Rich velvet curtains and gilt moldings complemented the lush décor. The room was beautiful, but she knew she was hallucinating.

It felt strange, Keri said, to recognize she was hallucinating. She was not psychotic. She was just hallucinating. If her brain hadn't been able to tell her that what she was seeing wasn't real, her mind would have needed to supply a reason for how she came to be in a changed room. She might have decided she'd been abducted by creatures from another world and her classmates replaced by aliens. But Keri knew she was hallucinating. As she pondered these thoughts, she appreciated what she was seeing. Not all of her hallucinations were bad!

Within the hour, she snuggled under the covers and went back to sleep. When she awoke sometime later, the room was back to its small, drab reality.

At the end of the school year, students took the Comprehensive Test of Basic Skills (CTBS), which was given nationwide. Overall, Keri's scores were only slightly lower than the year before, even after suffering a major psychotic break and being on lithium, Seroquel, and Wellbutrin. Her largest drop was in math computation (see table 15).

During the summer, since we'd had no luck with the pediatric neurologist, Keri's psychiatrist asked a non-pediatric neurologist friend to check Keri for a possible seizure disorder. This doctor scheduled a sleep-deprived EEG[46] (electroencephalogram). The results were negative, but this alone did not rule out the possibility of seizures. The next step was a three-day EEG, during which time Keri would have to live with electrodes attached to her. She refused.

Keri had other plans for the summer besides dealing with her medical problems. She would be turning 13 in the fall, and her bat mitzvah was scheduled for Thanksgiving weekend. She didn't want anyone to make changes to the requirements to compensate for her problems, which she had avoided disclosing at the synagogue. She had

---

[46] A sleep-deprived EEG is brief, but it is done after the child has been awake for 24 hours. The theory behind the test is that seizures are more likely to occur during sleep. If the patient has been awake for 24 hours before the test, he or she is likely to doze off quickly after being allowed to lie down in a dark, quiet room.

the whole summer to study, and she felt confident she could learn the required material. She diligently studied the Hebrew texts and attended all the services she could, though her efforts were hampered by numerous side effects from her medications.

I also had summer plans. The house was a wreck. Keri's bedroom was worse than a wreck, and I wanted to have things in order when my family visited for the bat mitzvah. After Keri picked out paint colors for her bedroom, she and I began cleaning it up, repairing damaged plaster and painting as time permitted. We also converted what used to be the kids' playroom into an office for her, including a daybed so the space could double as a guest bedroom. Relying on Keri's good taste in decorating, we replaced the carpeting in this room with hardwood flooring, painted the walls a soft blue with white trim, and added a pretty wallpaper border.

Table 15: Comparison of Seventh- and Eighth-Grade CTBS Scores

	7th Grade Percentile	8th Grade Percentile	Difference
Total Reading	99	97	-2
Vocabulary	99	98	-1
Comprehension	99	93	-6
Total Language	97	98	+1
Mechanics	88	94	+6
Expression	99	99	0
Total Math	95	89	-6
Computation	90	80	-10
Concepts & Application	96	95	-1
Science	99	95	-4
Study Skills	98	99	+1
Social Studies	97	96	-1
Total Overall	99	97	-2

Note: A percentile of 99 on a national test means the student has scored at least as well, or better than, 99 percent of students across the nation in her grade taking that same test.

Chapter 24
The Roller Coaster through Darkness

When parents of children with still-unstable disorders affecting the brain get together, in person or online, they inevitably refer to the "roller coaster." In some ways, this ride is even more exhausting and emotionally damaging to the caregiver than the all-out Hell of a child's first acute psychotic break. Once on the roller coaster, parents never know what their child will be like from week to week, day to day, or even hour to hour. A happy mood can change for the worse in an instant. The parents end up watching for subtle clues that precede such a change. Is the child too happy, too loving, too loud, too quiet? Is the pitch of his voice just a little too high? Is a small lisp entering her speech?

Asking the child how he/she feels can trigger the very meltdown parents are trying to avoid, so they find themselves walking on eggshells, trying not to say the thing that triggers an episode of screaming, anger, wailing, or psychosis.

> **Keri's Comment**: A child can be aware parents are warily watching for changes in mood, and sometimes, this alone could be the last straw, plunging the child into the inevitable "switch."

Often this vigilance is of no use. The child almost seems to be waiting for something "wrong" to be said, just so he/she can fall apart. At least, to those on the roller coaster, this is what it feels like.

Sometimes I wondered if the interspersed good times in our lives made the inevitable bad times all the more painful. I'd read about experiments that measured the stress levels of various mammals when exposed to shocks or other stressors. Those receiving shocks at random, with no control over them and no warning, were horribly stressed. Animals receiving the same number of shocks predictably, or with advance warning, or with some control over the timing, fared much better. Given the unpredictability of Keri's symptoms and their effect on our daily lives, I felt like one of those lab animals exposed to random jolts.

Keri's vision changed with each change in medication, which meant we had to take her back to the eye clinic, get a new prescription, and order new lenses. She developed astigmatism. Then it went away. Then she got it again, but this time it was in another direction, so we couldn't use her previous lenses. The good thing was, we had vision insurance; the bad thing was, insurance paid for only one eyeglass prescription per year.

Keri made several trips to the dermatologist. Bumps on her face and arms were keratosis polaris, a benign side effect of the lithium. The dermatologist prescribed a lotion called Lac-Hydrin, which seemed to help. Later, a birthmark she had on her back mysteriously started to change color and shape. It was becoming cancerous and had to be removed.

Many things add to a parent's sensation of being on a roller coaster. Frequent trips to multiple doctors create a cycle of hope and despair. Then there is the trauma of numerous blood draws and the child's resulting fear, anxiety, and panic. There's the stress of more, fewer, or different symptoms, medication changes, side effects, good and bad and great and horrible days, screaming, canceled plans, worry, and lack of sleep. All the while, parents try to take care of everything else in their lives, including maintaining jobs to support their families and pay for this medical nightmare. This takes a toll on the parents' physical and mental health.

Most parents feel the roller coaster ride can't be truly understood by someone who hasn't lived it, which means most doctors haven't a clue. Parent and child speed over the tracks, gripping the safety bar as they hurtle through a long, dark tunnel. Although they keep watching for the light at the end of the tunnel, it's nowhere in sight. Perhaps, they begin to think, the tunnel *has* no end.

On our roller coaster ride, I kept a daily journal, logging the medications Keri was taking and how she was doing. Sometimes I recorded my feelings (see figure 4).

Figure 4: Sample of a Daily Journal

<new date>: Complaining of tiredness and feeling cold. Crying.

<new date>: Feeling cold and tired. Migraine in morning. Used ibuprofen. Felt better about 6 hours later. Crying at night.

<new date>: Warning signs: Loving. Repeatedly saying, "I love you, Mommy." I made her favorite food for dinner—pancakes. As I set her plate on the table, she suddenly turned on me, saying "BE NICE!" (another warning sign), accusing me of yelling, reprimanding her, and shoving the plate in her face (Psychotic?). I told her quietly, "You are not okay. I am going outside for a few minutes."

I felt abused.

She was talking in a higher-pitched voice. Begged me to "fix her." Took her Seroquel early. We went outside, and she again complained of feeling cold and tired. It was 80°F! Then she complained of headache and stomach pain. I gave her Tums (antacid) and Tylenol (acetaminophen). Became increasingly anxious and agitated. Had 0.25 mg of lorazepam.

Staying calm, loving, alert, and ready for anything makes me feel so old and beaten. I get the self-image of a fat old grey-haired peasant, stooped and frumpy, shuffling along a dusty road carrying a burden, looking like life has sucked her dry.

<new date>: Morning: Again saying, "I love you, Mommy," in a high-pitched soft voice that made us think she was not okay. Complained of being cold. Yelled "shut up" in the bathroom (voices?).

<new date>: Amazingly WELL!

Greg and I are stressed & tired. We feel like we are walking on eggshells. She criticizes & complains about everything. She is so often near tears. We try hard to help her so she isn't so frustrated—we never respond to her anger—and I am sure that helps, but she is unhappy. Life is unpleasant living with her. I am at a point where I hate my life.

From my journal entries, I prepared a summary of key points to take with us on visits to the psychiatrist, including Keri's current medications and dosages, usage frequency of as-needed medications since her last visit, and symptoms and/or side effects.

Figure 5: Typed Summary for Doctor

Name   Date

Current Meds:
- lithium   675 mg *b.i.d.* (just raised from 450)
- Seroquel   150 mg a.m.; 175 mg p.m.
- Wellbutrin   50 mg *b.i.d.*
- OmegaBrite   6 grams daily total, plus antioxidants
- lorazepam   *p.r.n.*: 0.5 mg – 3x, 1.0 mg – 2x
- analgesics   *p.r.n.*: ibuprofen – 2x;
                  Tylenol 2 reg. strength – 2x

Symptoms/Side Effects/How things are going:
- Blurred vision; change in eyesight—new lenses.
- Severe headaches; occasional migraines.
- Persistent nausea; abdominal pain.
- *Frequently* complains of feeling cold.
- Tired; easily fatigued.
- Low frustration and noise tolerance.
- Irritable. Critical of others. Whiny, clingy, insecure.
- Hard little bumps on face and arms.
- Depressed?
- Voice changes when "not okay"; prelude to distorting events.

Special Notes:
Keri feels strongly the lithium needs to be LOWERED and the Seroquel should be raised.

The psychiatrist ended each session with a plan, a set of printed instructions he gave to us each time we left his office. He also mailed a copy of the plan to Keri's therapist. These printouts were very helpful.

Figure 6: Plan from Doctor

> Date: _____
>
> - Continue current medications.
> - If she develops symptoms, adjust Seroquel upward.
> - If she develops side effects from the medications, lower the dose of lithium by 50 percent.
> - Bumps on face and arms could be from the lithium.
>   - Advise consulting a dermatologist.
> - Follow up: 1 month
>
> cc: _____ (therapist)

Chapter 25
Our Marriage, Our Depression

Objectively, Keri was making progress, but Greg and I were feeling no better. Unpredictability wears on a person. When Keri first became acutely psychotic, her psychiatrist impressed me with the fact that I had to accept Keri telling us about her symptoms as matter-of-factly as if she said she had a sore throat. "If Keri feels your distress or fear, she will close up to protect you as well as herself. This is an illness in which we can't use a thermometer to see if her fever is abating; we have to rely on her revelation of symptoms." The psychiatrist had given me a week to grieve and cry. "After that," he warned, "for Keri's sake you must pull yourself together and get over it."

Acting completely calm for the sake of the family only compounded the unbearable strain that threatened to break me. Only in the wee hours of the morning could I let down my guard and feel the emotional turmoil wash over me. I couldn't sleep, so in the middle of the night I shared stories, grief, knowledge, anxiety, and even joy with an Internet group from the Child and Adolescent Bipolar Foundation (CABF).[47] I felt as if I was drowning and my Internet group was a safety line. But I wasn't the only one walking on eggshells or grieving at the loss of what our child "could have been."

Greg and I had succumbed to the stress. Until the Internet support group suggested I was depressed, I didn't recognize symptoms of depression in either Greg or me. Ours was not a depression that made us lie in bed all day like characters in TV antidepressant commercials, nor did it cause us to wail in despair as Keri did. Greg's depression showed up as irritability. He was frustrated and intolerant. My distress

---

[47] http://www.bpkids.org.

was more internalized. I constantly felt stressed and anxious, and even though I was exhausted, I couldn't sleep.

Tension was beginning to build between Greg and me. To my husband, Keri seemed oppositional. I disagreed, and I felt his irritability was exacerbating an already bad situation. What sometimes seemed oppositional, I explained, was simply Keri being *incapable* of complying with what was requested of her. For example, one evening I was on the phone with a teacher at the same time Keri needed to go to bed. Keri no longer went upstairs alone at night and Greg knew this, but rather than go with her, he simply told her to go to bed. Of course, she did not. If he'd gone along, she would have complied willingly, but she could not go alone. Greg expressed disappointment in her, which made her cry. She sat on the floor, clinging to my legs until I was off the phone. Greg felt frustrated with Keri because she wouldn't do as she was told. I felt frustrated with Greg!

In my mind, what Greg did was selfish and immature. Not only had he not helped Keri, he'd further upset her, adding more for me to deal with. In his mind, it was a simple matter of a 12-year-old being told to get ready for bed. Such a request shouldn't have caused extra work for me, because Keri shouldn't have needed any help. In my mind, Greg was not accepting responsibility for helping a sick child. And in fact, the brunt of Keri's care *was* falling to me, as well as most of the family and household care. Greg was no longer doing his share.

In his defense, Greg says he didn't want to believe the extent of Keri's need. He was repressing anger about her bizarre behavior. He wanted his daughter back the way she was. He wanted his wife back. He wanted his family back. He felt as if he was at the center of an earthquake, his world collapsing around him. As a result, Greg's form of depression interfered with his ability to honor his responsibilities; mine did not.

Greg wanted Keri to be the responsible, independent child she used to be. She'd been his buddy, the mature, interesting kid he did things with on weekends. She used to contribute to the housework; now she wouldn't do so even when asked. It seemed like willfulness. If spoken to sternly, she acted fearful. Her fear frustrated Greg even more; to him it seemed as if she was putting on an act. Keri had no reason to fear her father, so to him her reaction felt like an insult.

Several times, Greg became so frustrated with Keri he slammed a door, which I'd never seen him do before. I, in turn, became irritable, impatient, and sarcastic with Greg. Feeling angry, I withdrew from him emotionally.

> **Comment from Psych Nurse**: Parents come to the hospital with a depressed, psychotic, or suicidal child. Sometimes interaction between the child and the parents has become dysfunctional, exacerbated by the way they respond to the child's psychosis and bizarre behaviors. The staff, observing this dysfunction and not realizing how stressed-out, anxious, anguished, and despairing the family has become, tends to think, "Well, no wonder the kid is a mess. Just look at the family!" It's easy for staff to forget that the severe, almost unbearable (for anybody) stress of caring for a deteriorating child with a mental diagnosis, coupled with the lack of support, sympathy, and proper care that is routinely afforded to a child with a medical diagnosis, is what is *causing* the family's distress and sometimes causing the observed dysfunction.
>
> Support for the entire family from the medical and therapeutic communities, along with support from extended family and friends, can go a long way toward preventing the oft-seen deterioration of a family under extreme duress.

At that time, Greg said, he simply didn't have the understanding and patience needed to provide long-term care for a psychotic child. His tolerance for Keri's whining, crying, and screaming was limited; he looked at her as a 12-year-old acting like a 2-year-old, and he wanted her to stop.

I viewed the situation differently. I was dealing with Keri's needs relative to her state of mind, not her chronological age. Greg tried to meet her at the level she *should* have been. I met her where she was. Both of us wanted to help our daughter regain her maturity and independence, but our ideas of how to do so were very different. Keri had the emotional neediness of a toddler for comfort, stability, and the security of a parent. I believed that pushing her to bathe by herself, do chores, or even sleep by herself, only worsened her turmoil. *Someday* she might regain confidence and become more independent. *Someday* there might be time for pushing. Now was not that time.

Keri began to sleep with me when Greg was away on business trips. Although she moaned, yelled, and thrashed about for hours, at least I could more easily calm her and sleep when I could. When Greg was home, Keri slept on our bedroom floor. This arrangement angered Greg. He wanted a good night's sleep, which he could not get with Keri moaning and crying out all night. He wanted her to sleep in her own room, in her own bed, *alone*. But she was terrified, and I was the one comforting her. Greg's insistence meant I spent hours in Keri's room in the middle of the night. I couldn't fall asleep in her softer, smaller bed, so my exhaustion grew even worse. Needless to say, I resented his resentment.

Keri's wailing also wore us down. Wailing is different from crying or sobbing. The wail, a loud, heart-wrenching sound of profound, unbearable grief, sounded like that emitted by mothers who have just lost their children or by a lover whose beloved has just perished. It drove us both to tears.

In times of trouble, traditional wisdom says we're supposed to get strength and comfort from our religious communities, but I felt more alone than ever before. As I watched other children play, sing, and talk together, flirt, even fight with each other, I grieved for the camaraderie Keri was missing. Our family felt invisible. Our pain and suffering were invisible, too.

This lack of support was largely a result of choices we made. We did not reach out to our friends, neighbors, or religious community— our social network—to help us through this horrible, emotionally stressful medical nightmare. Keri's was not a casserole illness, where people bring food and offer to help, and we were afraid of being stigmatized. For many people, the term *mental illness* conjures up words like evil, crazy, lunatic. *Mental* implies the illness is in the patient's head, that the patient and/or the family is to blame. *Mental* implies patients are responsible for their own symptoms and if they would simply choose to change their thoughts, they would no longer be sick.

Each week at the synagogue, the rabbi read the names of people who were sick so the congregation could pray for them. Keri's name was never mentioned. Even though it was obvious she was ill, only one person inquired about her well-being, and we kept the pain to ourselves. Each week, I felt sharp knives of despair rip through my chest, railing silently at the injustice of Keri not being recognized among those in need, of her being denied the prayers she would have received if her illness had been medical.

I felt silence was the only way I could protect my daughter, but in the process I isolated myself. I didn't let anybody know how badly we needed help and support. I didn't want the gossip that would be inevitable in our small, close-knit community. I'd been brought up in a society that believes such an illness brings shame to the entire family. I knew all too well that Keri and her illness would not be understood.

I hated my life.

"Be careful what you wish for; you might get it," says the old adage. Had I wished for patience and God was giving me the chance to practice it? *When things get really bad, I should thank God for giving me the opportunity to learn*, I thought. It was a wry twist of humor, but saying thanks to God was better than wallowing in pure despair.

Sometimes these thoughts made me laugh out loud, though if I forgot and laughed in front of Keri, she'd screamingly accuse me of laughing at *her*. Other times I cried, mostly in the middle of the night when I was supposed to be sleeping and gathering strength. When it got too bad to laugh or cry, I used fantasy as a coping mechanism. My fantasy of choice was to visualize, in detail, blowing my brains out with a gun. I understood that my fantasies were merely cathartic. I was *not* suicidal, but in some perverse way, contemplating escape through my own demise made me feel better.

Eventually I realized I had symptoms of major depressive disorder (MDD) and needed more help than just counseling.

Like bipolar disorder and epilepsy, MDD has an associated kindling theory. According to this theory, early episodes of situational depression may be triggered by events such as severe stress, trauma, or grief. Over time, however, someone with the disorder can become increasingly sensitive and thus more likely to suffer another depressive episode, even in response to minor events. Eventually, such a person may have depressive episodes without any triggers at all. Of course, underlying biology influences how sensitive each individual is to triggers to begin with, and thus how much kindling is needed to "light the fire."

Advocates of early and prolonged treatment of major depression cite this kindling theory as one reason why it's so important to stop the downward spiral. Another reason for prompt treatment, unrelated to kindling, is evidence indicating the longer depression remains untreated, the more atrophy (shrinkage) may occur in the hippocampus, that portion of the brain responsible for learning and memory.[48]

I wondered if MDD had been kindled in me. I thought perhaps it might have, except that it wasn't incapacitating. I was able to meet my obligations. I could still laugh and play. *Luck of the genetic roll of the dice*, I thought. And as for the brain shrinkage, *no wonder* my brain felt like mush!

Because of its benign side-effect profile when compared with pharmaceuticals, Greg and I first tried the herbal antidepressant, St. John's Wort (*hypericum perforatum*). I had no side effects, but I got no benefits, either. For Greg, it worked so well he stayed on it for years.

I then tried antidepressants prescribed by my family doctor. I started with Wellbutrin, the same drug Keri was taking. To my surprise, I got *worse*! I felt panicky. I'd wake up with my heart thumping, which quickly segued into extreme anxiety. Several other antidepressants produced their own terrible side effects. One caused me to gain a lot of weight, seemingly in a blink of an eye. On another I

---

[48] Sapolsky and Sheline, 2006.

lost motivation. The chemical effects of these drugs amazed me. Despite meticulously following the instructions for stopping two of these medications, I experienced severe withdrawal symptoms. Suddenly I had firsthand glimpses of how Keri must feel on her travels through the maze of pharmaceuticals prescribed to help her feel *better*!

The solution to my type of stress-induced depression ended up being rather simple; I shored myself up nutritionally. I guess my need was similar to that of an athlete who requires extra supplements for his much-used muscles. What I needed was extra nutrition for my brain. Using the well-researched protocol information from the nonprofit Life Extension Foundation,[49] I started cautiously on high-quality SAM-e,[50] along with vitamins B_6, B_9, and B_{12}, which were recommended for use with it. At night I added tryptophan, melatonin, and glycine, which helped me sleep. Greg began taking high-quality nutritional supplements as well. Later, we found a medical doctor knowledgeable in integrative medicine[51] to help ensure we were doing what we should to keep healthy.

In addition to dealing with our depression nutritionally, Greg and I sought counseling *together*, and I continued to see my therapist alone. I really enjoyed the just-for-me sessions.

Life with a severely ill child will test a marriage, and I now understand how such intense stress can either split couples apart or bring them closer together. Either way, I don't believe the marriage will remain unchanged. Greg and I were fortunate in that we had a strong foundation, a union based on love, respect, compatibility, and friendship. I had followed my grandmother's advice and chosen a man who respected and adored me. I respected him as well. It was a good beginning. As time went on, we grew to better understand each

---

[49] http://www.lef.org.
[50] SAM-e, or SAMe (pronounced "sam-ee") stands for S-adenosyl methionine. Shown to help with depression and osteoarthritis, it's sold in the United States as a nutritional supplement. It is used in a large mitochondrial energy production cycle along with choline, glycine, B_6 (pyroxidine), B_9 (folate), B_{12} (cobalamin), and other nutrients.
[51] Integrative medicine is considered to take the best from the fields of both traditional (pharmaceutical) medicine and alternative medicine.

other's abilities and limits and to work out mutually acceptable solutions to an extraordinarily difficult situation.

Although counseling and supplements helped to alleviate some of the stress, the most important aspect in Greg's acceptance and tolerance of Keri's behaviors and needs was *knowledge*. The psychiatrist helped by keeping us focused on Keri, the real person. Her behaviors were not her personality. They were the result of a biological problem affecting her brain. Labels such as mental, manipulative, spoiled, immature, and oppositional were not helpful. Only by refocusing on our daughter's needs of the moment could we accept and meet those needs with the patience required.

> **Family psychoeducation programs** teach families how to work together to help the patient. Programs are created and led by mental health professionals, usually as part of an overall clinical treatment plan. Groups are primarily diagnosis-specific and last anywhere from 12 months to 3 years. Some hospital treatment centers also provide family psychoeducation, but the majority of hospitals for children are geared toward behavior problems.
>
> Successful family psychoeducation programs generally teach family members to be patient with their ill loved ones by stressing that illnesses like bipolar disorder and schizophrenia are medical issues like cancer, diabetes, or hemophilia. Families are treated as partners in caring for the ill patient—part of the solution rather than part of the problem.

The National Alliance on Mental Illness (NAMI)[52] has free classes and support groups that help to educate patients and families and act as an emotional safety net. Greg and I signed up for a Family-To-Family class that met one night a week for 12 weeks. Here we met others dealing with loved ones who suffered from brain disorders. Learning about medications, grief, advocacy, and especially networking, was important to us. We hired an adult neighbor to be a babysitter for Keri while we were gone. We told the sitter that all she needed to do was sit downstairs while Keri was downstairs and sit

---
[52] http://www.nami.org.

upstairs with her when Keri wanted to go to bed. The neighbor complied with our request and asked no questions. Keri did not make a fuss about us leaving. She understood that the class doubled as a break for us. For Greg and me, it felt like a weekly date.

In the class we learned that a medical, biological, physiological problem was driving Keri's emotional state and current needs. This was a concept we could accept and work with. Greg and I, now on the same page, began to parent more effectively. By us *not* approaching her condition as a psychological/mental or behavioral problem that needed correcting with psychological and/or disciplinary techniques, Keri became more emotionally secure. Working together, we became stronger as individuals and as a family.

Table 16: Diagnoses: Ages 12 to 12½

Diagnoses
- Highly gifted-LD (learning disabled).
- Allergies.
- Migraines.
- Tourette syndrome.
- OCD (obsessive-compulsive disorder).
- ADHD (attention-deficit hyperactivity disorder).
- Constitutional delay.
- Major depressive disorder, re-diagnosed as bipolar disorder, then re-diagnosed as psychosis-NOS.

Table 17: Chronology of Symptoms and Drug Regimen: Ages 12 to 12½

- The month before her 12th birthday, while on **Adderall,** a stimulant for ADHD, and **Zoloft**, an SSRI antidepressant for depression, she became increasingly manic.
- She experienced several brief acute psychotic episodes immediately after turning 12. As a result, she was put on **Risperdal**, an atypical neuroleptic.
- Subsequently, she became anxious, paranoid, delusional, and psychotic. She experienced the following symptoms:
    - Auditory, visual, tactile, gustatory (taste-related), and olfactory hallucinations, as well as frequent hallucinations of pain.
    - Ultra-rapidly-cycling moods.
    - Voice changes preceding mood changes.
    - Extreme feelings of cold and intense sensitivity to pain.
    - Nightmares that wouldn't stop, even after waking.
- While almost completely off the Zoloft but taking a small amount of Risperdal and a tiny amount of Adderall, she became suicidal and psychotic and was hospitalized.
- Her life-long musical creativity ceased. She stopped playing musical instruments or even singing.
- Adderall and Zoloft were dropped and she was put on **lithium** plus a small amount of Risperdal. On Risperdal, she experienced EPS (extrapyramidal symptoms).
- A switch from Risperdal to **Zyprexa** resulted in weight gain and severe itching. A switch from Zyprexa to **clonazepam** resulted in escalating anxiety.
- She was put on **Seroquel**, which reduced psychosis and helped her sleep, but resulted in her acting "drugged"—spacey, with slowed movements and slowed, sometimes slurred, speech.
- A small amount of **Wellbutrin** was added. She had transient akathisia.
- An increase in the dosage of clonazepam resulted in agoraphobia. The drug was discontinued, after which her anxiety significantly decreased.
- She additionally had an increase in the following symptoms:
    - Migraines.
    - Brief catatonic, seizure-like episodes, sometimes with a motor component.

Table 18: Medication History Chart: Ages 12 to 12½

Medication	Age	Purpose	Unexpected Results
Zoloft	9.5–12	Depression	Minor color vision loss in left eye & worsened close-up vision.
			Required increasing dosage.
			Episodes of hypersomnia started.
			Decreased parasomnias & sensory hypersensitivity.
			Frequent illnesses.
			Increased "spacing out" / brief catatonias.
			Anxiety & anxiety attacks.
			Worsened OCD.
			Hypomania & psychosis (after Adderall added).
Adderall (+ Zoloft)	11.5–12	ADHD (misdiagnosis)	Increasing hypomania.
			Decreasing sleep.
			Major, prolonged psychotic break: Hallucinations involving multiple senses including pain.
			Decreased cognition after psychotic break.
Risperdal (1mg)	12y 0m– 12y 2.5m	Hallucinations & mood	EPS - Dystonia & severe pain in muscles and joints.
Zyprexa (12 mg)	12y 2.5m– 12y 4m	Hallucinations & mood	Weight gain; intense hunger.
			Appearance of hypoglycemia.
			Severe itching.
			Increased anxiety.
OmegaBrite + antioxidants	12y 3m– Present	Mood instability; EFA deficiency?	None.
Lithium	12 y 4m– 13y 4m	Mood instability	Headaches, nausea, diarrhea, stomachaches.
			Increased sleep.
			Temporary vision changes (astigmatism in one axis, changed to different axis, etc.).
			Keratosis polaris (used Lac-Hydrin).
Clonazepam	12y,4m– 12y 5m	Anxiety	Worsened anxiety. Agoraphobia.
Seroquel	12y 4.5m	Hallucinations & mood	"Overdosed" at necessary dosage—spacey, glazed eyes, slowed movements, sometimes slurred speech.
			Increased hunger.
			Gingivitis.
			Skin photosensitivity.
			Frequent illnesses continued. Neutropenia.
Wellbutrin	12y 5m– 22	Depression	Transient akathisia.
			Improved alertness.

The Long Tunnel

Ages Thirteen to Sixteen

Some days I can smile through the pain
Some days I go on, ignoring all my fears
Some days the sun feels good shining on my face
And some days, I have no choice.

Some days the pain reduces me to tears
Some days all the fear becomes too overwhelming
Some days I sink down so low the sun is darkened out.

And so maybe I'm not strong enough
Maybe I'm not brave enough
Maybe I give up too easily
When the light begins to fade.

Or maybe I'm already bowed, with weight that you don't know
Maybe I've been a long time, fighting battles you couldn't imagine
And maybe even in the darkness, I'm dreaming of the sunlight on my face.

– Keri

Chapter 26
Determination

I was awed by Keri's determination to continue studying for her bat mitzvah. All the other children at her religious school were doing this, and she desperately wanted to do it, too.

Despite her constantly changing vision, days lost to incapacitating migraines and fatigue, passing out (causing a concussion), stumbling over her feet, bumping into things (thus injuring a shoulder), and falling down stairs, Keri studied. She continued, as often as she could, attending classes and going to the synagogue. I talked to her about not having a bat mitzvah, but she was adamant she could to do it.

To help her prepare, she was assigned a mentor. Keri could have learned to chant the long Hebrew portion for her bat mitzvah much more easily by listening to the tune. But her mentor—explaining that since the object was for her to be able to take part in the adult religious community by acquiring the knowledge to chant *any* text—firmly insisted she learn without listening to the melody in advance. Keri must learn to fluently chant haftarah and master her portion by reading the trope (cantillation marks that accompany Hebrew text).

Keri was not learning things as swiftly as she used to, but no one at the synagogue except the rabbi knew about her problems, not even her mentor. And I couldn't help; I don't know how to chant haftarah trope.

One afternoon, as I was catching up on work in my home office, I half-listened as Keri studied her haftarah portion in the living room. For 45 minutes or so she worked steadily, repeating the beautiful melody of the passages until she could chant them smoothly. Suddenly I was startled into full awareness by the agitation and anger in her voice. When I heard her stomp with frustration, I ran out of my office to see why.

Keri was slumped on the couch with the Hebrew text clutched in her hand. After asking me to read some of it to her, she looked up at me, stricken. "Mommy . . . I was *hallucinating* the text on the page. What you just read is not what I was *seeing*. I just spent all this time practicing *hallucinated* words and trope!" Needless to say, her practice ended for the day. Later, she again rejected my suggestion that she give up. My daughter was determined.

Keri often felt so fatigued when standing during services at the synagogue that she leaned against me for support. When sitting, she struggled to stay awake. Sometimes we had to leave early because her head hurt too much or she was hallucinating and felt scared. Once she described what she was seeing as if looking through pieces of different-colored cellophane or painted glass. We couldn't know whether some of these visual phenomena were migraine auras or hallucinations. One day while standing and singing, Keri looked at me with a stricken expression. She explained she'd just seen me turn my head, say something nasty to her, and then return to singing. She felt a weird split with reality. She knew I would never say to her what she'd just heard. Yet she'd seen and heard me do so. The hallucinating part of her brain registered the incident as reality, while the logical, analytical part knew it couldn't be true.

On another occasion, Keri asked me on the way home where we were. She knew she was hallucinating, but she felt neither panic nor confusion. Her brain was simply registering two contradicting "facts," and she serenely asked me for clarification so she would know which fact was real. She'd read a sign indicating she was on a road 100 miles from home. At the same time she expected to be close to home. Which was real—the sign or where she thought she should be? It was the wording on the sign that was not real. The visual part of her brain seemed to be providing the thinking portion with incorrect information.

We often drove on a road close to our home that meandered through a large park with fields, green bushes, and robust trees. On one of these excursions, Keri again knew she was hallucinating, since she was clearly seeing slow-moving, three-toed sloths hanging from branches high in trees much taller than trees native to our area. She asked if I saw the animals, which, of course, I did not. She then described the park as looking like a tropical rain forest, with dense vegetation, thick vines, and hanging mosses one would expect to see in the bayous and marshes of the southern United States.

Usually Keri got upset, angry, frustrated, and sometimes even scared by her hallucinations, and I had learned the hard way that asking how she felt or what was going on while she was hallucinating only increased her agitation. More often than not, if I listened in a non-reactive way, she would tell me about them. Fortunately, this hallucination made Keri feel giddy with laughter. I was glad she wanted to share it with me, and I was glad to have the memory of being able, at least this once, to laugh along with her.

We designed and printed the bat mitzvah invitations ourselves, using a picture Keri had made in class the year before that illustrated the haftarah text she was to read. Family members would be traveling long distances at considerable expense to attend the ceremony. I let them know that because of Keri's health issues, there was no guarantee she could do anything until she actually did it. Everyone said they would come anyway. They assured Keri they supported and loved her and would celebrate with her regardless. The bat mitzvah was scheduled for Thanksgiving weekend. If nothing else, we would share a wonderful Thanksgiving together.

One day after Hebrew class, Keri said, "You know the bumper stickers that say, 'You're just jealous because the voices are talking to *ME?*'"

"Yes," I questioned, tensely.

"Well," Keri continued, "in class Ben said that to me, and I thought, *Ben, if you only* knew . . . *if you only* **knew**!" I asked Keri if she actually said anything back to Ben, and she said she hadn't.

Somehow, this interchange led to a discussion of drug use. I had shared with Keri the research that for some people predisposed to psychotic illness, cannabis (marijuana) might actually cause psychosis. The controversial part of this research is the theory that for these individuals, the psychosis is not transitory and the episode can actually trigger a full-blown, life-long psychotic illness. We talked about people who use hallucinogens. She found it odd they would want to take drugs to *cause* the very symptoms she took drugs to *stop*. If she wanted to do what they did, she laughed, all she'd have to do was *not* take her drugs!

The medications were helping, but improvement was slow. I admired my daughter's ingenuity in dealing with chronic hallucinations. On one occasion I watched as she grabbed the yappy little poodle, Mugsy, took him upstairs, and held him in front of a closed bedroom door. She waited a moment, then cracked opened the door, shoved Mugsy into the room, and closed the door behind him. She waited a few more moments, opened the door, and went into the room. When I asked her why, she explained that since Mugsy barked at *everything*, if he was not barking at something she was seeing or hearing, then whatever she was seeing or hearing was not really there and she could ignore it. She'd heard voices in the bedroom and was scared to enter in case there were burglars or other sinister characters inside, but since Mugsy didn't bark, she knew no one was really there.

We didn't schedule a party for after the bat mitzvah, as many people do. Just having so much family around for days was wonderful. Cat, my friend from my time as a college undergraduate, came to stay with us. She cooked most of the Thanksgiving meal, leaving me to socialize with family. Keri was so happy to have her cousins visiting; she was in heaven.

The bat mitzvah itself went smoothly. We knew that leading the service Friday night and staying up late, followed by rising early the next day for Saturday morning services, would be impossible for Keri in her current state. So the rabbi scheduled Friday services to begin extra early, and we had a simple dinner right at the synagogue. Keri got a nosebleed during the Friday services, and her hand bled out of nowhere during the Saturday services, but she took it in stride and everything was wonderful. At home, all her aunts, uncles, grandparents, and cousins understood when Keri holed up in her bedroom, needing dark and quiet for a few hours. I can only wish all children with disorders affecting brain function might have such supportive, loving, extended families.

Despite continued medications in the years to come, Keri still heard sounds and saw movement in her peripheral vision. At first she was hyper-vigilant, always feeling paranoid that someone was around or that there might be spiders or other bugs. In time she adapted, figuring out ways to be alone in her bedroom and get her schoolwork done without constantly being distracted by hallucinations. She hung bells by her bedroom door so when the door was opened, they would chime. She knew the bells would also set off the "Mugsy alarm"—an extra bonus.

One day Keri was hallucinating the doorbell ringing. After repeated interruptions to "answer" the front door, she thought of another adaptation. She kept Mugsy on her lap while she did homework, training herself to ignore sounds and movements by knowing she could rely on the dog's senses. Perhaps once again she was doing cognitive behavioral therapy (CBT) for herself.

Sometimes, however, Keri's migraines and her inability to cope with noise made it difficult to be with the yappy little poodle. When she wasn't feeling well, I had to take the dog and the bird into my office and close the door, doing my best to keep them quiet. I thought how much more help a dog might be if he was as attuned to the environment as Mugsy but trained *not* to bark. Such an animal could alert Keri to movement and sound in much the same way hearing dogs do for deaf people, allowing her to distinguish real sounds from hallucinatory sounds. I read a book called *Lend Me an Ear* by Martha Hoffman that detailed the temperament, selection, and training of hearing-ear dogs. Inspired, I thought about how a service dog could help Keri. Maybe we could make that idea a reality, even if only to help her at home. In the meantime, Mugsy was the best substitute for a service dog we had.

Chapter 27
The Boo-Boo Mobile

One Friday afternoon we took Mugsy to the veterinarian for what turned out to be a spontaneous disc rupture. Due to a genetic problem that had caused calcified "pebbles" in several of Mugsy's discs, his back had been an accident waiting to happen, but this was not the first of his medical issues. In fact, we'd already nicknamed him Boo-Boo due to his history of physical problems and traumatic life events, among them a congenital, inoperable liver shunt.

There was still sensation in Mugsy's hind legs, so the vet sent us home with strong anti-inflammatory pills, but by Monday morning, the back half of the dog's body was completely paralyzed. Without immediate surgery, the paralysis would get worse, and the closest vet who could perform the needed procedure was two hours away.

Without hesitation, Greg and I took the day off from work and drove to the veterinary spinal specialist. Keri sat in the backseat with the carefully secured Mugsy next to her, ensuring his calmness and safety, full of confidence that he would be all right.

The veterinary surgeon found no deep pain sensation in either back leg. Even with surgery, he explained, Mugsy had less than a five percent chance of being able to walk again. In fact, he'd only known of one dog with such severe paralysis that regained its ability to walk, and that animal's owner had been a veterinarian. The surgery cost thousands of dollars, and the recovery would be long. We were not rich. To spend thousands on a dog with virtually no chance of recovery is a difficult decision, especially when the animal is already living on borrowed time. Because of his liver problems, Mugsy had only been expected to live until age four; he was now five. To humanely euthanize him seemed the only sane thing to do.

I looked at Keri. Then Greg and I left the room to discuss what to do next. Keri loved Mugsy. She *needed* Mugsy. Having him with her allowed her to walk around the house without me by her side, because she could rely on *him* to let her know if things she heard or saw were real. The dog was her reality-check, helping her deal with the confusing world of her hallucinations, plus his playful zest for life cheered her up. Losing him now, in her already fragile state of mind, would be harsh.

Next we discussed what would be best for the dog. He loved to run and play, but the vet held no hope that he would ever walk again. He would have no bowel or bladder control. Even without considering the money issue, it would not be right to make him live like this, especially since he was already a year beyond his life expectancy.

On the other hand, what message would we be sending to our ill daughter if we did nothing? Not many months before, Keri had wanted us to let her die because of an illness that was causing her great suffering and for which she felt there could be no positive outcome. There was more at stake here than just throwing away money. By making the choice to treat Mugsy, would we be helping Keri believe that life was worth the fight?

It was a difficult decision, but we elected to go ahead with the surgery. We also accepted the responsibility of catheterizing the dog and doing physical therapy on him indefinitely. Many people would not have understood our choice, but to us it was a message of life, hope, and commitment.

A week later we returned to the surgeon's office to bring Mugsy home. He had no sensation in his hind quarters, and the vet had not changed his prognosis. Mugsy would not walk again. Our only ray of hope was that he might regain bowel and bladder control. I could look forward to that!

When we got Mugsy home, he seemed depressed. The once feisty, active little dog was now paraplegic. When I catheterized him, he detested it. *He must have some sensation*, I thought, *since the process seems to cause him discomfort*. Because the catheter tube was an issue, we ended up choosing another option. As the vet had shown us, we expressed urine from Mugsy's bladder by pressing on the sides of his abdomen. Greg and I had trouble mastering this procedure, but Keri's small hands were just the right size, plus she had the technique we lacked. Thus, expressing the dog's bladder several times a day became her job.

We also had to be Mugsy's physical therapists. Each morning and evening, I held him while Greg stretched and worked the dog's stiff legs. In the afternoons, Keri took over. With a heavy heart, I began looking into custom-made doggie wheelchairs. It didn't seem like one would work well in our small, cluttered house or even in our sloping yard. Mugsy had so loved to play—fetching balls, playing tug, and jumping into the shallow creek that ran between the houses at the back of our property.

Now his eyes remained dull with depression.

Then Keri got an idea. She rummaged through the attic and found her old Waffle Blocks. With them, she built a flat cart with wheels, to which she fastened a sturdy cardboard box she'd decorated. She now had a cart in which she could pull Mugsy around. Dubbing it the Boo-Boo Mobile, she added a plate on the back declaring it such and took the dog for a walk around the neighborhood.

When they returned, Mugsy looked alert and alive. The sparkle was back in his eyes. Keri explained what she'd done. "What do male dogs live for?" she asked. "To sniff and to pee. Sniffing around posts and brush is their equivalent of receiving messages. Peeing is their equivalent of sending messages. So I stopped at every lamppost and fire hydrant, took Mugsy out of the cart, let him sniff, and expressed his bladder."

At home, we continued doggie physical therapy. We bought a plastic kiddie wading pool and encouraged Mugsy to walk in it using his front legs. He tried the same procedure in the house, though sometimes he tried so hard that he actually lifted himself onto his front legs, the doggy equivalent of a handstand!

One day, Keri had Mugsy in the Boo-Boo Mobile when she stopped to talk with friends. Mugsy started rocking from side to side in his little box, hopping up and down on his front legs and acting agitated. When Keri took him out of the box and put him on the grass, he pooped. He had felt the need! Some sensation was returning.

Keri became a familiar sight around the neighborhood, pulling the dog in his homemade cart. People came up to me to say what a great kid she was. They didn't know the half of it. What they were witnessing was a little girl helping her dog to heal, which, in turn, was helping the little girl heal. Keri and Mugsy were dealing with depression and despair together, both moving on with their lives, both overcoming severe obstacles. At one point, each had lost the will to live. Now each had grown stronger and was fighting back.

Mugsy beat the odds. Soon there was no need to express his bladder. And despite diminished nerve impulses to his rear legs and diminished sensation, he *did* learn to walk again.

Mugsy couldn't read the veterinary manuals, so he had no way of knowing his prognosis was bleak. Today he's more than 15 years old, with no sign of deterioration from his inoperable liver problem. His hind legs are withered, but they carry him; his gait is stilted, but he walks. He also runs. At first, each time he tried, his body twisted and he flipped head over heels. But he kept trying. Eventually he learned to run with both hind legs moving together, like a rabbit. He runs fast!

Chapter 28
Medications and Food Supplements

Would the hallucinations, psychotic episodes, brief catatonia, hypersomnia, depression, mood swings, and anxiety ever stop?

Keri was on fish oil—two grams of essential fatty acids (EFAs) in the form of OmegaBrite plus antioxidants. Fish oil had been shown to alleviate inflammation, as well as depression and mood swings. It could help protect brain cells (gray matter) from damage, as well as help them to grow back. Later, a study showed that just 1.5 grams per day could help temper the escalation of symptoms in children who experience brief psychotic episodes.[53]

My psychiatric nurse friend told me that vitamin E was prescribed for some of the patients in the state hospital, but none were given fish oil. From talking to other parents, it seemed as if *some* doctors instructed their patients to be on vitamin E, but not all. And *some* said to be on fish oil, but not all.

Keri's doctors didn't know the appropriate amount of vitamin E for a child taking both fish oil and a neuroleptic. I contacted two major manufacturers of this vitamin, who in turn put me in touch with their research departments. I also talked with two nutritionists, after which I came to the conclusion that I should put Keri on a total of 400 IU of vitamin E per day. When I discussed this with the pediatrician, she agreed. As we learned more, we switched to a mixed tocopherol and tocotrienol vitamin E supplement rich in gamma tocopherol.

I was intrigued when several parents of children with mood and psychotic symptoms told me their children's symptoms were effectively treated, with *no* side effects, using nothing but nutritional supplements. I wished I had known this before Keri started on

---

[53] "Daily Dose of Fish Oil May Keep Schizophrenia at Bay," 2007.

psychotropic medications. At least I would have been able to say I'd tried the benign and found it didn't work before moving to heavy-duty pharmaceuticals with their severe health consequences. And what if Keri were one of those children who *could* have been helped by food supplements alone?

Next I read about a multi-nutritional supplement marketed by a Canadian firm called Truehope.[54] I took the ingredient list from the product, which at the time was called Synergy, to Keri's pediatrician, who thought it was a good, benign formulation for Keri to be on. Having everything in pills from one bottle was easier for me than doling out different supplements from multiple bottles. (Later, the Synergy product was reformulated into a more concentrated form and renamed EMPowerPlus, but it would be another decade—while research accumulated about the effectiveness of *micronutrients*, as the product would be generalized and referred to in the scientific literature—before the Truehope product was better accepted.)

The folks at Truehope suggested I stop Keri's Seroquel. Greg and I would have done this if we'd just started treating Keri's ailments, or if she had not been helped by any pharmaceutical medications. But now we were unwilling to stop a medication that was clearly helping her, at the risk of throwing her back into a psychotic hell.

Keri, not yet 13, had been on the combination of Seroquel and Wellbutrin for several months. Things were somewhat better, but she was still desperately impaired. Her Seroquel dosage was already fluctuating up and down, a constant balancing act between symptoms and side effects, but she often looked overdosed (glassy-eyed, with slowed speech and movements) from the amount necessary to combat her symptoms. Thus, although we weren't willing to stop altogether, we were more than ready to lower the dosage if at all possible. If the food supplement could help us to do so, great, but I was not hopeful.

On the Truehope supplement, Keri's symptoms improved. Her hallucinations, irritability, and mood instability lessened. As a result,

---

[54] Truehope's Web site is http://www.truehope.com. There are good supplements from other sources, the biggest differences among them being the specific ingredients in each.

we were able to lower the Seroquel enough so she no longer acted overdosed. Her mental fog lessened. Some of her motivation and spunk returned. But if I lowered the Seroquel too much, her mood and psychotic symptoms worsened.

I still didn't believe it was the supplement that was helping. At the time, most professionals believed it was quackery, and her psychiatrist did not believe in it. *She must be just getting better*, I thought, *because she's been on the Seroquel long enough for it to help.* After she'd been on the Truehope supplement for a year, I decided not to buy any more.

Big mistake!

Within a month, she was going nuts. Her moods started to fluctuate rapidly. She became irritable, whiny, anxious, and paranoid. She cried within minutes after being happy. In short, she was reverting to an anxious, scared little girl and we were walking on eggshells once again. Was our life turning back into the Hell we thought we'd left behind? We raised her Seroquel dosage and she again developed extrapyramidal symptoms (EPS) along with an overdosed, doped look.

I put Keri back on the Truehope supplement. Each day I carefully logged how she was doing (see Appendix C: Charting Symptoms). At her next appointment, Keri's psychiatrist was surprised to see her doing so well within a month of what had appeared to be another major psychotic break. When he asked what had changed, we told him we'd put Keri back on the Truehope supplement. The psychiatrist blew us off. "What *really* changed?" he asked, explaining that he meant changes in environmental factors—psychological or emotional—in school or at home. But there hadn't *been* any other changes; adding the supplement had been the only difference in her routine. The psychiatrist did not believe in food supplements that had not been proven to work on a mental illness through a double-blind, placebo-controlled clinical trial, such as the one conducted on OmegaBrite. Nevertheless, I knew from the irrefutable evidence of Keri's behavior that something in that bottle was helping her.

Keri asked me to promise I would never again take her off the Truehope supplement.

Later, I asked Keri's pediatrician about the supplement. She opined, "It might be just a single ingredient in the supplement that she needs. It might be a synergistic combination of ingredients. To find which specific ingredient or ingredients her body needs could take years of trial and error. In the meantime, she would continue to suffer. So you may as well continue to give her the mix of ingredients contained in the supplement."

I couldn't have agreed more. We continued the Truehope, but we missed a major signpost. Somehow, Keri's mental illness was inextricably intertwined with her nutritional needs. Did this mean that at least some of her symptoms weren't just "in her head"? And if so, then at least part of her problems weren't *mental* at all.

Our daughter was once again semi-functional. But she still was very ill.

Chapter 29
High School

Keri greeted me excitedly. "They're like *me*, Mommy!" Playing outside with her schoolmates, she'd found that many of them, like her, were clumsy or uncoordinated. For others, visual-spatial and kinetic skills were their strengths—but enough were uncoordinated to make an impression on her. She soon found other things in common with her new classmates.

Keri loved her freshman year at a small school for bright students with special educational needs (dyslexia, auditory processing disorder, attention problems, etc.). The classes were mixed age. Some kids in high school did reading with the elementary school kids, while some kids in elementary school did math with the high school kids. There was no stigma attached either way, and she was pleased to find the other students were polite.

"The kids are so accepting of everyone's weaknesses," she related happily. I reminded her that the children at the Montessori school were also accepting. Keri explained the difference. "At Montessori, acceptance came from the top down. At this school, acceptance comes from the kids themselves, without anyone telling them it has to be this way." She told me about a time when the kids were at a table working together. One was being funny, saying, "I'm *special*," in a funny voice. Everyone at the table cracked up, because *all* of them were special. Keri said if someone had said the same thing at another school, it would have been derogatory.

Keri's reaction to her new school made me think about the big push to mainstream kids. I had no idea she would be so happy with this group of bright kids, all of whom had special educational needs.

Most of the children at this school were on one or more medications. Many also had experienced hallucinations or even brief periods of psychosis as side effects of these meds. Others, just as sweet and wonderful as Keri, suffered from the same symptoms and diagnoses of depression, bipolar disorder, and schizoaffective disorder.

As the school year progressed, I was amazed how quickly several of Keri's learning-related problems vanished. The first improvement I noticed was in writing. Suddenly she could write incredible book reports—better than I ever could! "How?" I asked. Keri explained. Her teacher taught them how to write a book report for each type of book (fiction, nonfiction, science fiction, biography) and then provided an instruction sheet and a template they could use for any book of that type. Up to this point in her educational career, I realized, she'd been asked to write book reports without ever having been formally taught how to do so.

In middle school Keri had a problem with organization, which caused her to lose and redo many assignments. At this school she never lost anything. Once again, the children were taught a formal method to use. In addition to a loose-leaf binder, each student was given a multi-pocketed accordion folder with labels for each subject. All homework papers and all completed homework went immediately into the correct slot in that accordion folder. As long as the student diligently followed this method, which Keri did, nothing was lost or overlooked. In addition, teachers wrote all assignments on the board, and students recorded them in their assignment books. Each day, every student's assignment book was checked before he or she left the school, and each evening, parents initialed the books to acknowledge they knew what assignments their children had been given. I didn't need to know what Keri's assignments were—she did them independently—but this formal method of communication between school and home helped keep everyone working toward a common goal.

Another skill taught at her new school was outlining. Because many of the students had problems with attention, organizing, processing, and retaining information, they outlined almost everything they read. It was a tremendous amount of work, but Keri actually appreciated doing it. She felt it improved her writing ability as well as her ability to retain information. Outlining was a skill that helped immensely after she got to college.

Keri's biggest remaining school problem was that she was often unable to get there. Her sleep remained extremely disturbed. She thrashed about, moaned, and talked most of the night, and in the morning she was almost always tired. One day a week at random, she slept all day.

For much of her 13th year, Keri was congested. Although on an antihistamine and decongestant, she still had allergy problems. She got more than her share of colds, ear infections, and other respiratory infections, and when the school called to tell me she was coughing up blood, I knew she had pneumonia. This wouldn't be her only bout of pneumonia during high school. When she was actively sick, blood tests showed barely elevated white cell counts, indicative of minor infection, but we had no explanation for why she kept *getting* sick. Her immune system just seemed compromised. As I listened to her struggled breathing one night, I wondered if she had sleep apnea. I mentioned this to her primary-care doctor as a possible reason for her daytime tiredness, but this suspected cause was not investigated.

Keri had repeated bouts of viral illnesses that caused fever and vomiting. The first time this happened while she was on psychotropic medications, I tried to keep up her normal medication schedule, despite her excessive sleeping and vomiting. She seemed to get over "the bug," but afterward she remained in bed, in a stupor, for three days. I took her to the pediatrician, who determined she was dehydrated and had acidosis. At this point, the doctor surmised, the meds were so concentrated in Keri's bloodstream she was essentially overdosed. Never again did I worry about her taking psychotropic medications on schedule when she was ill and slept or vomited through dosage times. Apparently, if she was that sick, her body wasn't processing the medications effectively, anyway.

During the next few years of Keri's imperceptibly gradual growth, she gained no weight and thus slowly slimmed down. She was very careful about her diet, not accepting soft drinks or processed, refined, or junk foods, in spite of *not* having her mother as a good role model. She was on various nutritional supplements, including the Truehope and OmegaBrite, and I was buying some healthier foods at a time when going organic was not in vogue and the safety of chemical food additives was mostly unquestioned. Still, Keri seemed sickly. She continued to have the same aches and pains in her muscles, back, ankles, and knees she'd had for years. The shoulder she'd injured when she bumped into a post never healed. And she had intermittent, burning pains in her extremities she could hardly bear.

Between the days lost to sleeping and the days she was sick, suffering from migraines, and/or experiencing hallucinatory symptoms and anxiety, this girl was missing way too much school. At first, she was able to make up her schoolwork without incurring more stress and had at least a little time to socialize and indulge in hobbies. By the end of her senior year, however, her body and her energy level had deteriorated to the point that completing schoolwork became an all-consuming task.

It wasn't just in-class times that Keri missed. The students were learning about caves and were going on a spelunking expedition to caves in the area. They commemorated the occasion with specially imprinted T-shirts, for which Keri's cave-related artwork had been selected. She excitedly prepared for the trip. We splurged on sturdy, waterproof boots.

When the big morning came, however, things did not look good. We reached the school bright and early, but Keri was too quiet. She looked tense and refused to get out of the car. When she finally spoke, it was to ask me to describe what I saw. I was puzzled. "What do I *see*?" I asked quizzically. "I see the school, and the grass, and trees." Keri decided she must be hallucinating because I would not be so calm if I were seeing what she was seeing. She saw a tall tree on fire. A small white dog was running across the field away from the burning tree, which was now spreading flames to surrounding trees.

When people read that stress exacerbates psychosis, migraines, and epilepsy, they sometimes think of physical or emotional abuse, sexual abuse, severe bullying at school, neglect, or deprivation. But stress is merely a biological response to environmental stimuli, and such stimuli are not always negative. Stressors also can be things such as a party, receiving a gift, or, in this case, the excitement of getting to go spelunking.

Keri just wanted to go home. And so we did. Instead of going on the field trip, she went to bed. Her body and brain had simply shut down. She needed to sleep.

~~~~~~~~~~~

On Sundays and Tuesdays (when she was awake and able to go), Keri worked as an aide for religious school. Since I taught on Tuesdays and for a short time on Sundays, it was no extra work for me to take her, and while she worked for two hours on Sundays, I had a chance to walk in the surrounding neighborhood. I liked this time to myself.

On breaks and vacations, and a few times after school, Keri had another enjoyable job. When people around the neighborhood were out of town, they paid her to take care of their pets and plants.

Keri squirreled away the money she received from her jobs, her allowance, and her birthday and holiday gifts. Her life was full and busy . . . when she was awake.

The summer after her freshman year, her school relocated. For years, they'd rented space from a local church, but now the church needed the rooms, so the school moved to a commercial building, sharing the facility with administrative personnel from a nearby clinic. Unfortunately, in this new building Keri had an allergy and migraine problem.

Staff and clients of the clinic smoked indoors in their part of the building, which triggered Keri's migraines and worsened her allergies. I do not like confrontation, but I swallowed my fear and explained to a clinic manager that I had a special needs child across the hall who could not tolerate the smoke. They agreed to limit smoking to outdoors, but the problem was still not resolved. People now smoked immediately outside a side door that was left open. Just inside the door was an air intake vent that pulled smoke into the children's classroom. So now we had to convince the clinic folks to smoke outside but in a different location, or at the very least to remember to close the door. This was the beginning of a struggle that would last for years—a battle to keep Keri away from the smoke that triggered the migraines, which then caused her to lose more precious days of her life.

Meanwhile, I was contacted by NAMI to become a co-facilitator for a class called Visions for Tomorrow being started for families of children diagnosed with mental illnesses. I declined the training session, since I already felt overextended. I was working full-time, teaching Hebrew twice a week, volunteering at the Child and Adolescent Bipolar Foundation (CABF), and preparing to teach an introductory Spanish class at Keri's school. CABF had also requested I do a Web page with information about medications, but I didn't even have the time for that. I handed over all the information I had, leaving it to someone else to take over the task. Later I quit my volunteer position at CABF altogether for the sole reason that I was overextended. Years later, I would be able to volunteer again, becoming a trained educator and support group leader for NAMI.

My experiences as a volunteer in these organizations leads me to wholeheartedly recommend joining, and, if possible, volunteering in such groups. Volunteering helps focus grief into action and turn anxiety into advocacy. In my case, I was able to help myself while giving back to others, and networking with other parents was sometimes the best way to get information about doctors, programs, and available resources.

Migraine Misery

We were not sure if lithium was helping Keri, plus we suspected her almost unbearable migraines, fatigue, and need for sleep might be side effects from it. Yet I was afraid to take her off the drug. Working as a volunteer on a drug committee with CABF, I was familiar with reports that lithium lessened the chances for suicide. I had read books written by Danielle Steel[55] and Trudy Carlson,[56] each the mother of a bipolar child who had committed suicide. Carlson's son was being taken off lithium at the time he killed himself.

People write books so others can learn from their experiences, and learn I did. I was terrified. Still, I knew we needed to remove the lithium, which we proceeded to do, very slowly and cautiously, over the course of many months.

We had hoped Keri's migraines would diminish once off this drug. No such luck. In fact, they got worse, plus they became more frequent, sometimes occurring more than once a week. Some were so bad they incapacitated her for days at a time. Often they were accompanied by odd prodromes or auras before the actual head pain hit. Sometimes she experienced severe depressive symptoms as part of the prodrome. Other times she experienced visual phenomena, such as seeing the world through static on a TV. To alleviate her symptoms, we tried various over-the-counter (OTC) migraine medications, to no avail. About all we could do was put cold compresses on her head to help ease the pain.

We could not differentiate between a migraine prodrome and when Keri was about to have another psychotic-like fit. Before a psychotic episode, just like before many of her migraines, she could feel "off," unwell, cold, fragile, and/or like her brain was fuzzy. Some people with epileptic seizures describe the same phenomena. We usually could tell it was a bad day as soon as we saw Keri in the morning. She would soon be in agony once again, either from a migraine or from one of her fits that started out looking like a

---

[55] Steel, 1998.
[56] Carlson, 1999.

migraine, or she would be in one of her odd sleep days. We began to believe Keri's migraines, psychotic-like fits, pain, mood swings, hypersensitivities, and sleep disorders—although each would be labeled with a separate diagnosis—stemmed from the same underlying problem.

The absolute worst kind of migraines (fortunately, Keri had only a few of these) were the infamous cluster type, also known as suicide headaches. When she started bashing her head against a wall, screaming in pain, I thought she'd gone nuts. It made no sense to me that someone would deliberately hit herself in the head when she hurt so much already. Once again, the Internet came in handy. When I read about cluster migraines, I learned they are so painful some sufferers do exactly as Keri had, that somehow head-banging serves as a coping mechanism for bearing the unbearable!

We knew of no pediatric neurologist in town other than the one at the hospital medical center who had been such a huge disappointment. Because of an exodus of specialists from our city due to a problem with a physician management company, we were limited in our choices.

Since we had to look elsewhere for a pediatric neurologist, I decided to find the best one I could. I started with Larry Robbins, M.D., the author of a book about migraines. His name was also associated with papers about the increased incidence of mood disorders in migraine patients. He directed me to three other doctors. Through them, I was put in contact with a pediatric neurologist in Baltimore who specializes in treating adolescents. He was passionate about the topic of pediatric migraines; the fact Keri had so many other health issues didn't bother him in the least. He was happy to work with her local doctors and to act as a consultant with her psychiatrist via teleconferencing. As a migraine prophylactic (a medication to prevent the migraines), he put Keri on an antiseizure medication called Topamax (topiramate). For acute episodes, he prescribed Imitrex (sumatriptan succinate).

When this doctor first suggested Topamax, I was concerned because of its notoriety for causing cognitive side effects. In some circles on the Internet, it had been dubbed "Dope–a–max" because it made people "stupid." Keri already had cognitive problems. She didn't need more! The neurologist explained we could try to minimize the chance of cognitive side effects by starting the drug at a very low dose and raising it very slowly. I liked that idea.

We ever-so-slowly increased the dosage. When we finally reached a level that helped Keri's migraines, she still had no noticeable side effects. This may have been because she was already so impaired, or because we'd raised the dose so gradually we didn't notice the slow decrease in cognition. Later the dosage was raised even more, and then we did notice the decrease in her verbal skills. Still, Keri felt the benefit to her overall quality of life was worth the trade-off.

The Topamax lessened the frequency of Keri's migraines to between four and six per month. It also reduced their severity. The Imitrex did nothing. Once again, the psychiatrist asked the neurologist who had done her last EEG to please accept her as a patient, even though this doctor's practice was normally limited to adults. The neurologist agreed, following Keri over the next few years, raising her Topamax dosage, discarding the Imitrex in favor of Zomig (zolmitriptan), then trying Axert (almotriptan malate) when Zomig caused side effects worse than the migraines themselves.

Most surprisingly, when Keri's Topamax dosage was increased, her strange staring spells and episodes of brief catatonia stopped completely. Her strange psychotic-like episodes, during which she suddenly reacted to her environment through a filter of terror with no apparent trigger, also nearly disappeared. Keri's psychiatrist had wondered if these episodes could be neurological, saying they might be the result of migraines, sleep disorders, or seizures (complex partial seizures in the temporal lobe region of the brain, called temporal lobe epilepsy or TLE). Since we had no concrete evidence the episodes were due to seizure activity,[57] however, there had been no reason to put her on antiseizure medication until it was prescribed to help control her migraines.

Gingivitis and Metal Allergy

The orthodontist announced Keri had gingivitis (severe inflammation of the gums with bleeding), which he thought might be exacerbated by her congested, open-mouthed breathing at night.

Keri brushed her teeth three times each day. Each night she spent 40 minutes carefully flossing each tooth and brushing both manually and with an electronic toothbrush. Then she used an oral irrigation device, called Hydro Floss, which used water pressure to clean between her teeth and around the gum line. When the gingivitis didn't abate, the orthodontist admonished her for not flossing enough.

In addition to gingivitis, she also had an awful-looking rash inside her mouth where her lips brushed against her metal braces. I mentioned to the orthodontist that Keri had a contact allergy to metals. He explained that although having a contact allergy on the epidermis (outer skin) is common, we do not react to metals—especially not the surgical-grade stainless steel of which the braces were made—inside the body, as this skin is different. "Inside the body" included inside the mouth.

One day the other orthodontist in the practice was talking with us about the sad shape of my daughter's gums. Keri burst into tears. After I explained her meticulous brushing and flossing routine, the orthodontist said the only other thing that might cause this type of gingivitis were medications like neuroleptics or antiseizure drugs, and

---

[57] Wellbutrin, which Keri continued to take for depression, was not supposed to be given to a person with seizures. However, given Keri's history and how well she was doing on it, the doctor continued to prescribe it.

he sincerely doubted she was on such medications. "But she *is!*" I gasped at the same time Keri exclaimed, "But I *am!*"

Her braces were removed, replaced by a small metal retainer behind her bottom teeth and a plastic retainer for her top teeth. The gingivitis around the top teeth healed completely, but the area around her lower teeth, plus the inside of her lower lip near the metal retainer, remained inflamed. Keri believed the inflammation was due to the metal.

Discussing her symptoms with colleagues at a professional meeting, the orthodontist confirmed that dermis inside the mouth could not react to the metal. To prove his point, he removed her lower retainer. To his surprise, the rash went away. He put the retainer back. The rash returned. Keri could not have metal in her mouth.

How much metal had she been exposed to during her life? All her vaccinations and yearly flu shots contained thimerosal as a preservative. Thimerosal has a heavy metal in it—mercury—which can accumulate in the body.

I know people can be allergic to thimerosal without knowing it. I'm allergic to it, which I learned only because I had reactions to eyedrops and nose sprays with thimerosal (once a common preservative in such medications but later eliminated because so many people suffered adverse reactions). I had never had a noticeable allergic reaction to the thimerosal in flu shots, yet, clearly, I was sensitive to it. Could Keri be also? Added to the metal allergy inside her body, could thimerosal sensitivity have been another source of stress to her physiology?

I wondered then, as have many parents, about the effects of multiple vaccinations and/or thimerosal on a child like my daughter, a child who has allergies and a weakened immune system. At the time, there were no answers to these questions. Years later, research elucidated the potential for thimerosal in vaccinations to adversely affect a subset of children, as studies showed a connection between mitochondria, thimerosal, and neuronal death.[58]

---

[58] Yel, L., et al., 2005.

~~~~~~~~~~~~

The psychiatrist never formally announced he was changing Keri's diagnosis to schizoaffective disorder. It was just there, in something he handed us one day. Her diagnosis was changed based on the length of time her symptoms persisted. He had to wait until he had no doubt the symptoms were not due to the Adderall or Zoloft, or withdrawal from them. And the symptoms had to persist for at least six months. He also needed time to verify that the mood symptoms were separate from the psychosis, and the psychosis was separate from the mood symptoms.

Chapter 30
Dashed Dreams

Keri had just turned 14. A sophomore at her small high school, she was physically immature for her age. Mentally and emotionally, she vacillated. Some days she seemed like a normal teen, usurping the phone with her bedroom door closed, music blaring. Other days her emotional needs for parental love and protection were those of a young child. Heartbreakingly, her wisdom and insight were always those of someone much older, someone who had already experienced too much suffering in life. I knew she sometimes felt old, jaded, and impatient with the superficiality and lighthearted concerns of "normal" 14-year-olds.

On this day, Keri was extra-quiet in the car on the way home. Her eyes were watery, which meant she was *extremely* upset. For all the wailing and sobbing she did when "not okay," Keri rarely cried as a result of self-pity, hurt feelings, or disappointments. In other words, she cried from the pain of her illness, but rarely from sadness in her real life. I had learned not to pressure her for information about what was wrong, so I waited for her to start talking.

"I wish you had *told* me," she said, speaking softly and carefully. There was no tone of anger or accusation in her voice. No whininess. She just sounded old. Old and resigned.

"All these years," she continued, "I've been envisioning myself as a mother and a doctor. These have been my life's goals. They've always been what I saw myself becoming. But you *knew* I couldn't be either. I wish you had *told* me rather than let me go on thinking I could."

My mind couldn't think fast enough to reply. *I should have been ready for this conversation*, I growled to myself, but I wasn't. Sitting erect in the front seat, holding back tears, Keri looked like a little girl, but she sounded decades older.

She is too young for this! I screamed to myself. My mind wanted to retreat into denial. I sidestepped with a question, tackling what I hoped would be the less emotionally laden topic. "Why do you say you can't be a doctor?"

"There is no way I can go through medical school and residency, for several reasons. My illness dictates that I can't stay awake for a couple days at a time like the residents do. I can't have an erratic sleep schedule. And you know medical school is very stressful. I couldn't handle the stress, either. It would just make me sicker. I'd become psychotic. I wish you had pointed this out to me instead of just letting me go along thinking I really *could* be a doctor."

Every point she enumerated reflected a concern I'd had for years. I thought I'd been doing the right thing by encouraging her to be and do anything she wanted. Now I wasn't so sure. Should I have warned her that health might factor into her life's goals? Yet how could I have said anything? I couldn't know the future as a fact, so how could I dash her hopes and dreams. I sidestepped again. "Why do you say you can't be a mother?"

"I can't get pregnant while I'm on these medications. That would be harmful to the baby's life. But I can't get off the medications or it would be harmful to *my* life."

I could not completely dispute that, but I offered her this hope, "Honey, even 10 years from now you will only be 24 years old. A lot can change in 10 years. You may be on different medications by then, ones that wouldn't harm a baby."

"Oh, there are more reasons," Keri continued. "Even if I could get pregnant, it still wouldn't be fair for me to pass on my genes. I would not want to bring a child with this same illness into the world. And there is another problem. If the baby turned out to be like me, I don't think I could handle it. What if she cried like me? I couldn't handle the noise. I couldn't handle the stress!"

I reminded her, "Keri, there is always adoption." But my daughter, always realistic, had thought of this as well. "Mommy, think of it!" She was admonishing me for my lack of insight! "Any baby I adopted would also have the possibility of being like me. The probability of the child coming from parents who have similar genetic problems, or who abused alcohol and drugs, may be higher. I couldn't handle a child with special needs like me. *You* can. *I* could not!"

I suggested we bring this topic up with her psychiatrist. He might have some insight that neither of us had.

I also decided to talk with another expert—my older brother—who had a special needs son. He reminded me that everyone has dreams and goals, and that most people have a handicap in some form or another that gets in their way. If this handicap makes their first dreams impossible, they simply modify their goals and move on. His son had the same hopes and dreams as any other person, he explained. So when my nephew wanted to drive a car, my brother didn't tell him he couldn't, nor did he say this goal was unrealistic. He simply said that to drive he would have to learn signs, rules, and about the vehicle. My brother began to teach him. It was very difficult for my nephew, and he eventually lost interest.

I relaxed. A lifetime is a lifetime. Goals are great guidelines, but they are also fluid. If they have to change, that's okay as well.

I also had to be honest with myself. I felt a twinge of grief for the grandchild I might not have, along with guilt and embarrassment at having such a selfish grief. I also grieved the loss of my daughter's dreams, but I didn't feel as bad as I would have just a few years before. If nothing else, having a special needs child makes the parents grow up. Separating your own goals from your child's is a big part of this growth. I had learned to let go.

Keri and I were both pleased when Martha Hellander of CABF wrote an article for the CABF newsletter[59] that brought up special concerns about girls with bipolar disorder, concerns that are just as relevant for girls with schizoaffective disorder. A drawing of an elfin lady suffering from depression, which Keri had done a few years earlier, was solicited for the article. Keri wrote about the elf, ". . . she

---

[59] "Girls With Bipolar Disorder: Special Concerns," by Martha Hellander, CABF e-bulletin, September 29, 2004.

didn't even bother to remove her heavy cloak. Instead, she lies still in the water and drifts away. Perhaps she just cannot find it in her to care anymore."

Unfortunately, although the article addressed girls' feelings about their illness, the effects of treatment on fertility, and the risk of premenstrual symptoms, there were no hard and fast answers. Are there ever? Still, the information was interesting, including the statistics on the large percentage of teenage girls with bipolar disorder who suffer from anovulation—the absence of menstrual periods. Years later, this article would come back to haunt us when Keri experienced anovulation (amenorrhea) and again when she had abnormal uterine bleeding including both infrequent and too frequent menstrual periods, and dysmenorrhea (severe pain during menstruation).

Chapter 31
The Endocrinologist Who Could Have (But Didn't)

Later in Keri's sophomore year, she had another three-week-long sleep episode. When she was awake, she was unable to walk without assistance, bumped into things, and fell down, but, mostly, she slept. This time there was no doubt—she was *not* depressed. The pediatrician thought she had mononucleosis. Keri did not understand how she could get mono; she was OCD-ish about not sharing germs. Because Keri was so phobic about blood draws, the doctor tested for the illness with a less accurate, but also less traumatic, finger prick test. The results were negative. "Still," said the pediatrician, "it appears she has some type of viral infection, so we may as well call it mono." This diagnosis seemed to placate the director at the school as an explanation for Keri's three-week absence.

Because Keri had so many inexplicable symptoms, the pediatrician decided it was time to send her back to a pediatric endocrinologist. Perhaps a thorough workup by a specialist in this discipline would provide some answers for her extreme fatigue, sleep days, sleep weeks, short stature, delayed puberty, migraines, hallucinations, mood swings, anxiety, depression, frequent infections, muscle and joint pains, the need for food supplements to maintain her sanity, and severe sleep disturbances. (In addition, she still had dry skin; dry, thin, brittle hair and fingernails; feelings of cold; and frequent abdominal distress common with low thyroid.)

Keri had begun to get striae (stretch marks) on her body, even though her weight hadn't changed. She bruised easily, and intermittently she developed small, localized patches of tiny red pinpoint spots called petechiae. The petechiae, caused by leaky blood vessels, appeared where articles of clothing, folds in bedding, backpacks, etc., pressed against her pallid skin. Although they looked cosmetically strange, we were assured the spots were benign. Meanwhile, Keri's friends teased her affectionately about having fairy-tale-princess syndrome, saying she was a combination of Sleeping Beauty (with her sleep episodes), Snow White (with her pale, ivory skin) and The Princess and the Pea (because of her bruising and skin petechiae).

Both the pediatrician and psychiatrist wanted blood tests to be run, but they believed an endocrinologist could: (1) best determine exactly which tests were needed, and (2) order all needed tests at one time, eliminating the necessity for multiple blood draws. The pediatrician set up an appointment with a pediatric endocrinologist at the local hospital medical center. In preparation, I carefully typed a short report listing Keri's current medications and all our concerns. The psychiatrist and pediatrician looked it over and made some modifications. When it was finished, we agreed this one-page paper provided a clear and succinct summary of Keri's case. She was looking forward to having just one blood draw instead of several. She was also looking forward to finding out what was *really* wrong with her.

Unfortunately, the meeting with the pediatric endocrinologist was a fiasco. When I handed him the sheet with the list of symptoms that concerned us, explaining that both Keri's pediatrician and her psychiatrist had contributed to the write-up, he gave me a disdainful look. As he began to talk, it was obvious he thought of me as an hysterical mother who thought things were wrong when everything was fine. Keri was seething inside at his arrogant attitude. The doctor dismissed our concerns with a wave of his hand. "She looks fine to *me*," he said "*If* anything is wrong with her, it's due to the medications she's taking, so it's not my responsibility to order tests. It is the responsibility of the prescribing physician to do so."

He refused to order a single test.

I wished Greg had come with us. I doubted this male doctor would have acted the same way if Keri's father had been in the room.

Keri was very upset by this encounter. She didn't appreciate what she described as being treated like an idiot. "He doesn't *care!*" she said irately. I agreed. He had arrogantly dismissed our concerns. "And how can he say I *look fine*!? How can I be *fine* when I feel sick all the time and sleep half my life away? How can I be *fine* when I always feel cold and tired? I hallucinate! I have migraines! I am *not fine*!

"No more!" she cried angrily. "I'm done with doctors. I don't *ever* want to be treated like that again. He didn't even listen. Doctors don't know *anything*; they don't care; and I don't want to go through such humiliation ever again!"

The pediatric endocrinologist dutifully sent a hard-copy report of the visit, reporting only on Keri's short stature and "constitutional delay in growth and development." Based on my statement that I had entered menarche just after turning 14 (thin, quite athletic, and younger than Keri was now) he wrote "family history of delayed menarche." (This was incorrect; other family members had begun menstruating at 12.) The section of the report for lab work listed "none obtained." The report also said "Multiple other medical concerns: I have encouraged Keri's mother to contact Dr. B. [the pediatrician] to address these individually."

Obviously, if the pediatrician had felt qualified to "address these individually," she would not have sent Keri to *him*. I was bewildered. How could an endocrinologist not investigate the possible endocrinological contribution to a child's hallucinations, fatigue, pain, and host of other problems? How could he have such a cavalier attitude?

When Keri turned 15, she was more physically developed but was still not menstruating. The psychiatrist asked how the follow-up appointment went with the endocrinologist. Of course, there had been no such appointment, since the endocrinologist had said it wasn't his responsibility to run blood tests on Keri. I gave the psychiatrist a copy of the letter from the endocrinologist's office, from which it was obvious he had wiped his hands of the case.

Still, I had a mother's gut instinct something was wrong. Not menstruating was simply one more symptom. Yes, it could be normal for a girl to start later than average, especially if she was highly athletic (but Keri was not athletic). A diagnosis of primary amenorrhea (never having started menstruating) is not made until after a girl turns 16, however, so the doctors felt it was useless to take her to a gynecologist before then.

To my deep regret, my desire not to be seen as a parent who inflicted her own worries on her child overrode my instinctive concerns. I dropped the issue.

Chapter 32
Surviving School

One of Keri's major struggles during her last two years of high school was to stay awake. At the age of 15, she had yet another three-week-long sleep episode. This time we knew the drill. It wasn't depression, and it wasn't mononucleosis. What it *was*, we had no idea. She slept 22 hours of each 24-hour period, rising once or twice a day to eat, use the bathroom, and—sometimes with my help—bathe. Each time she got out of bed, she was dizzy, her thinking felt fuzzy, and she stumbled when she walked. It was very difficult to wake her at all, and when I had to take her to the doctor, it took hours to get her up, dressed, and out of the house as she cried and staggered about.

When the sleep episode was finally over, it took another week before the sparkle was back in her eyes. Now she faced the task of catching up on a month of schoolwork while simultaneously trying to keep up with new assignments.

Then she began to have numerous shorter sleeping attacks, each lasting one or two days. During them, she could barely walk without assistance and she kept falling down. She definitely would have failed a sobriety test. For a day or so following each of these occasions her thinking was still fuzzy and she couldn't concentrate.

Due to her sleep episodes, Keri missed at least one day of school every week. When she was awake, almost all her time was spent catching up on numerous writing assignments or doing new schoolwork. Is it any wonder she was getting precious little time for fun, exercise, play, or just relaxation? When I took her to the pediatrician with complaints of tightness in her chest and difficulty breathing outdoors, the doctor assumed it was anxiety. It didn't feel like anxiety, Keri insisted, but she complied with the doctor's instruction to breathe into a paper bag the next time the tightness occurred. It did no good whatsoever. Further investigation showed she had asthma, for which she was prescribed still more medication. In addition, she now had to carry around an inhaler.

Then came the hives. She could feel them develop as a stinging sensation before they became visible. Then they felt stingy/itchy. They would come and go, mostly covering the back of her neck and spreading to her arms. The allergist diagnosed them as cholinergic urticaria, a fancy name for hives that appear as a result of a rise in body temperature or from excitement, exercise, or stress—probably related to the functioning of the hypothalamus.

I found this interesting. For some time we'd been saying Keri seemed to have a problem with her hypothalamus, which, as mentioned earlier, contributes to the regulation of body temperature, sleep, dreams, anxiety, stress, hormones, and more. Her hives appeared from going outside when it was hot. They also appeared when she was excited or feeling strong emotions. One day I bought her some expensive colored pencils for her artwork. This made her so happy she broke out in a *miserable* case of hives. I guess she really liked the gift!

She was now on two different once-per-day antihistamines (double the normal dose), plus an antileukotriene to keep her hives, allergies, and asthma under partial control.

Near the end of her senior year, one of her teachers began assigning much more written work than usual. In the past, the school had granted an accommodation regarding the amount of written work Keri had to turn in. She had been graded on the quality rather than the quantity of her work. In this case, the accommodation was not forthcoming.

The additional work became a nightmare. I suggested she give up. Stop. Take an extra year to graduate or be homeschooled. My suggestion was met with near-hysteria. She was determined to complete her work and graduate with her peers, in spite of the stress.

She'd been involved with Greg and me as we worked to put supports in place for college, and she had tremendous hope for the future. In the meantime, she just had to survive.

But she was so very, very tired.

Table 19: Diagnoses: Ages 12½ to 16

Diagnoses
- Highly gifted-learning-disabled.
- Immune/autoimmune issues: allergies, asthma, cholinergic urticaria.
- Migraines.
- Tourette syndrome.
- OCD.
- ADHD, inattentive (diagnosis didn't persist).
- PTSD (from her nightmares and hallucinations; slowly diminished over time).
- Vision-related issues: acquired dyschromatopsia, convergence disorder, and farsightedness.
- Delayed puberty.
- Psychosis-NOS, re-diagnosed as **schizoaffective disorder**.

Table 20: Characteristics, Problems, and Chronology: Ages 12½ to 16

- Allergic rhinitis and occasional allergic hives.
- Seizure-like episodes and brief catatonias.
- Some cognitive impairment.
- Tics diminished on Seroquel.
- Use of Truehope's EMPowerPlus lessened symptoms while reducing the amount of Seroquel required, which alleviated side effects.
- Delayed and erratic growth and physical development.
- Test for Turner's Mosaic at age 12 was negative. Thyroid was normal as well.
- Fatigue, lethargy, cold, tired; frequent bouts of dizziness and falling.
- Removed from lithium. No difference in mood symptoms noticed (but migraines increased).
- Due to increasing migraines, added Topamax.
- After adding supplements and increasing Topamax, seizure-like spacing out and brief catatonias stopped.
- Remained stable on the combination of Seroquel, Wellbutrin, Topamax, and supplements.
- Three bouts of pneumonia.
- Found metal allergy caused contact dermatitis inside mouth.
- Three-week sleep episodes, then increasingly frequent, shorter bouts of hypersomnia (sleep days), each 2–3 days long plus recovery time.
- Back and neck pain. Chronic pain in joints and muscles. Intermittent burning pain on the surface of muscles in arms and legs. Overly sensitive to touch, bumps, and pain.
- Mini-megacolon continued.
- Dry, thin, brittle hair and fingernails. Dry skin.
- Sensitive to heat and cold; mild hyperthermia during school field trip.
- Developed striae (stretch marks). Intermittent bruising and skin petechiae.
- Difficult to tell the difference between migraine prodromes, sleep days, psychosis, and medication side effects!
- Stopped use of Truehope supplement for brief period, which resulted in recurrence/exacerbation of mood and psychotic symptoms, lowered frustration tolerance, and more disturbed sleep.
- Asthma.
- Cholinergic urticaria (hives from minor rise in body temperature).

Light at Tunnel's End

Ages Sixteen to Nineteen and a Half

Waking

Been there . . .
  Been there sleeping, far too long now?
Where . . .
  Where did all the time go?
and When . . .
  When did life start passing me by?
Don't know . . .
  Don't know whose skin I'm living in;
but I swear . . .
  I swear it isn't mine.
Why . . .
  Why now are these thoughts so muddled?
Before . . .
   Before, I remember thoughts as clear.
Unsure . . .
  Unsure why things are the way they are.
Holding on . . .
  Holding on to my last tangible memories;
I'm waking . . .
  Waking to a life I do not know.

– Keri

Chapter 33
Looking To the Future

Keri, now a senior in high school, was talking to a friend, catching up on what she'd missed at school. As I looked at my 16-year-old daughter sprawled on the couch, book open in one hand, phone glued to her ear with the other, I thought of my mother.

She, too, had been sweet, intelligent, and loving. She, too, had been sick. And, sadly, she had died young. In the intervening decades, there was no question society had moved forward. We now had a diversity of medications, supplements, therapies, accommodations at work and school, and even service dogs to help people with disabilities live fuller lives. The availability of medical tests had also improved, even if sometimes these tests were not used to their full advantage.

Nevertheless, my sweet, intelligent, loving daughter was still sick.

Keri had matured. She'd adjusted to her limited energy and environmental restrictions (having to be careful about heat, cold, and smoke), and to her feelings of pain, fatigue, depression, tics, and the hallucinations that waxed and waned. "We should all be this mentally healthy," I thought ruefully, watching her cope with a diagnosis society still stigmatizes and considers a *mental* illness—as opposed to simply an illness—as if it was the result of something psychological or simply bad behavior.

With her typical resolve, and with what I now understand was resilience on a deeper scale than most people could know, Keri persevered with altered goals for herself. Gone was her dream of going to medical school. Her new goal was to somehow get through high school, and then to attend college while exploring satisfying career options that fit her abilities and limitations.

On her bad days, Keri still felt irritable. It was hard not to have meltdowns when she felt so bad and was constantly making up for lost time at school.

"Keri! We need to get going to your new GP."

Keri, who had already heard many positive things about this doctor, was almost looking forward to the appointment. We'd found him by word of mouth—family friends urging me to try him when I was looking for a GP for myself.

"He's like a young version of an old-fashioned family doctor," my friends said enthusiastically. "He takes your history himself. He takes as much time with each patient as needed, and he's willing to order as many tests as he thinks may be useful."

When we arrived at Dr. David Marwil's small practice, we were the only ones in the cozy, unpretentious waiting room. Paintings and drawings from his artistic family members adorned the walls, and fresh-cut flowers from his wife's garden brightened the gently lit office. Dr. Marwil didn't over-schedule his patients, so he had plenty of time for each of them. If he was late, we knew it was because the patient before us simply required more time. We also knew he would do the same for us.

The doctor walked in unhurriedly, shook our hands, and sat down next to us. As he looked at Keri, he said, "I hear you've had a hard time of things. I don't know how much I can help, but we'll work together and do our best, okay?" With such unassuming simplicity, my daughter's defenses relaxed. Rather than having a nurse ask questions, summarize answers, and hand her notes to the doctor for review, Dr. Marwil himself asked the questions. Compassion was written across his face as he intently listened to Keri's tale, taking notes. He had already read the medical file we'd brought in advance from the pediatrician's office, along with a 10-page summary of Keri's medical history that I'd prepared.

We didn't know it yet, but this day marked a turning point in Keri's life.

Without medical care that went beyond psychiatric medication, Greg and I doubted Keri would have the strength, or be awake enough, to go to college. We had not shared this opinion with our daughter. Instead, we'd been working for several years on ways to help her attain the best life possible, but in our heart of hearts, we weren't sure such an outcome would include either higher education or even the most simple job.

The year before, we had worked on getting Keri accommodations for taking the College Board entrance examination (SAT), the results of which would follow her to college. We'd also worked on having a service dog trained to assist her in being more independent.

Since Keri was already familiar with the SAT, having taken the test in the seventh grade, we decided she would take it again as an actual entrance exam for college. The plan was for her to do so while still a junior in high school. If needed, she could retake the exam as a senior.

From the College Board online Web site,[60] we obtained a brochure describing "Services for Students with Disabilities (SSD)," which lists all the forms and documentation needed to apply for accommodations as applied to the testing process.

First of all, the testing, labeling, and establishment of required accommodations Keri had gone through at the end of sixth grade had to be updated. We needed new test results, doctors' letters, and other documentation dated within two years of when we requested accommodations for the exam.

To complete these requirements, Keri went to a psychologist specializing in the administration of tests for learning disabilities. She took double the time the psychologist allotted, so she had to return for a second three-hour session.

Although the psychologist gives a multi-page write-up of observations, explanation of test results, conclusions, and recommendations, the College Board requires the raw data as well. The raw data showed that although Keri's overall grade equivalency was greater than 18.0,[61]

---

[60] http://www.collegeboard.com/ssd.
[61] Grade equivalency of 18 means at the level of a master's degree (high school graduate [12 years] plus 6 years of college).

her actual scores ranged from higher than the 99.9th percentile in her writing content to 1st percentile in her ability to spell sounds, even though at this point she could spell words (at the 70th percentile). Her math scores varied greatly as well, from math reasoning in the 81st percentile to math fluency in the 4th percentile. Some of the psychologist's observations were:

- *Difficulty with fluency or the speed at which she can access cognitive skills.*
- *Did not appear to be over-processing or obsessing over her answers, but instead had difficulty retrieving the information she needed.*
- *May be due to innate cognitive style, side effects of medication, or processing deficits.*

Then came her conclusions:

- *Meets the criteria for learning disability in math calculation.*
- *Significant delays in her ability to write short sentences quickly.*
- *Deficits in spelling.*
- *The stress of intense intervention should be weighed against the stress of managing her clinical diagnoses.*

Finally, there was the all-important recommendation of:

- *Should be allowed accommodations when taking college entrance exams. Because of her diagnoses, along with her slower processing speed, extra time and testing in a room with a proxy is warranted.*

Keri's psychiatrist wrote an extensive letter "Regarding Special Accommodations." He listed pertinent diagnoses and medications and his review of her last psychoeducational testing, along with a discussion of her problems and how he arrived at her diagnoses. Lastly, he wrote his recommendations for special accommodations while taking the tests, followed by his credentials.

The director of Keri's school, a former special education instructor in the public school system, gave us a simple IEP (individualized education program) form stating what the school essentially had been implementing for years. Areas of need included "Expressive written language" and "Paper/pencil tasks in mathematics." The "Goal" was stated simply as "Relieve anxiety and teach strategies that will allow her output to be at her 'gifted' level." Academic objectives included easing hand fatigue (because of her Tourette syndrome). The IEP included a list of recommendations.

After the paperwork was mailed in, Keri received notice from the College Board allowing her to take the SAT with extended time for the math portion, which was *already* about four hours long. The psychiatrist suggested multi-day testing, but the board rejected that recommendation.

Keri took the test at her own school in a familiar, non-stressful setting. The test administrator was the school's director. She did very well, scoring high enough on one portion of the test to qualify her for college honors classes in non-mathematical courses.

Once accepted to community college, getting further accommodations was easy. We made an appointment with the college's Disability Support Services (DSS) department, to which we brought the supporting documentation we had used for the SAT. We included additional medical information accumulated in the intervening year, a letter from a doctor listing some newly found diagnoses and their possible effects, and a short new letter from Keri's psychiatrist that included a list of diagnoses plus recommendations for special testing accommodations as follows:

- *Extended time due to being slowed down by the conditions themselves as well as by the medications to control the symptoms.*
- *A different location or time, if necessary, to avoid odors and noises.*

As for all the days Keri would miss, we were informed it was ultimately up to the individual teacher whether to accept absences. Although there could be excused absences with letters from doctors, there was no rule requiring teachers to *accept* them. This made perfect sense, since, for some courses, class interaction and participation were part of the grade.

Luckily, our determination to support Keri paid off. Not only did it enable her to receive accommodations for college, it also led us to her service dog, without which she could not have started her college career.

Chapter 34
A Service Dog for Keri

Based on Keri's experience of using our yappy little poodle, Mugsy, as a reality checker, I knew that a specially trained service dog could be even more helpful. Obtaining such a dog proved more difficult and expensive than I had imagined, but I remained determined to find a solution. Perhaps we could at least find a professionally trained, really good companion dog to assist Keri at home.

I envisioned a dog able to quietly alert Keri to sounds important to her, allowing her to ignore extraneous distractions while she worked. The dog would need to be as vigilant to the environment as Mugsy, so Keri could rely on it for reality checks, but be able to react with body language, nudges, etc., instead of barking.

I imagined a service dog checking rooms for Keri and being able to get me when she indicated a need, such as during a migraine. Maybe the animal could even be trained to a support harness to help on the many days Keri could hardly walk. With the right dog, she could get to the bathroom independently, without falling, and climb up and down stairs safely.

Keri's psychiatrist agreed that a service dog was a great idea. He told me to do Internet searches on service dogs, anxiety, and psychosis. From there, I discovered a write-up on the International Association of Assistance Dog Partners (IAADP)'s Web site, listing "tasks to mitigate certain disabling illnesses classified as mental impairments under the Americans with Disabilities Act."[62] The write-up outlined approximately 30 physical tasks a service dog could be trained to do for a person with a psychiatric disability. I learned that disabilities which are not always obvious, such as epilepsy, hallucina-

---

[62] "Service Dog Tasks for Psychiatric Disabilities," Joan Froling, http://www.iaadp.org/psd_tasks.html.

tions, anxiety attacks, Ménière's disease, and many others, are referred to as "invisible disabilities." A person with an observable disability is abbreviated as a PWD, while someone with an invisible disability is described as a PWID.

Investigating further, I found that for a fraction of the cost of a service dog from a large organization (and in years less time), we could train a dog ourselves with the help of a professional service dog trainer. Of course, the dog needed to have the right temperament. I knew we ran the risk of investing a year in raising a dog, only to have it turn out not to have the proper temperament for use in public. Nonetheless, I was willing to give it a try. Even if we ended up with a dog Keri could use only in the house, it still would be a helpful companion for her.

> Even a well-behaved companion dog—one that is not certified as a service dog with public access—can help a child with mood and hallucinatory problems at home. However, it is imperative that the child is not violent toward the pet.

Joan Froling from the IAADP recommended we look into obtaining a smooth-coat collie. This breed is innately sensitive and intelligent, and its shorter fur makes grooming easier. Word-of-mouth (or maybe fate) united us with a breeder who had set aside a young female collie as a possible service dog due to the pup's exceptional sensitivity, intelligence, and temperament. Keri named the puppy Kira.

The professional trainer we chose was Janece Rollet of Shepherd's Crossing Dogs for the Disabled, about an hour's drive from us. Janece, an animal behaviorist with several degrees, had disabilities of her own, making her an ideal choice. Kira would have to learn how to behave appropriately in public, mastering tasks such as lying quietly under the table or next to Keri's chair in a restaurant, not jumping on people, ignoring other people and animals in public, going on escalators, not whining or barking in public, not stealing food, and more. The dog also would need to learn tasks specific to Keri's needs.

Our first job was to raise the puppy as a well-trained, well-behaved companion dog, while at the same time trying to prevent her from acquiring bad behaviors that would later have to be unlearned. During the day, we kept her on a leash attached to me or Keri so she was constantly supervised. We taught her the usual good manners: come, sit, down, stay, stand, up, off, heel (with me), leave it, drop it, give it, and bring it, as well as how to do things like walking calmly on a leash. The more difficult behaviors we left to the trainer. We also gave Kira words for natural behaviors, such as "go potty," so the dog would do them on command. We took training classes together. We took her everywhere we could and socialized her daily. The director of my daughter's school, aware of what we were trying to do with Kira, allowed the puppy to wait in the school foyer with me for the children to be dismissed. Kira practiced sitting, lying down, and staying while being petted by hoards of children.

We encouraged wanted behaviors, such as whining, nuzzling, and giving Keri "kisses" when she moaned and cried. Soon, Keri could tell the affectionate canine to give her a "kiss kiss," for licks on her face.

We reinforced Kira's innate desire to find a parent when Keri was distressed and not responding to the dog's overtures. These instances occurred most often in the middle of the night when Keri was thrashing and crying in her sleep. Kira became distressed when Keri had severe nightmares—ones that continued indefinitely, sometimes even after she awakened.

Each time the dog came to us, we said, "Show me," as we walked to Keri's room. Spectacularly attuned to the humans in the household, Kira quickly understood she was to take us to the area of concern.

Being a herding breed made Kira a natural at trying to herd and mother Keri. Watching the two of them, I thought how wonderful this dog would be for a child with a tendency to wander off. One Saturday morning when we were at Keri's school for a meeting, Keri took Kira for a walk in the field next door. When Kira thought Keri had gone far enough, she started herding her back to the building!

Kira quickly learned our names and the words for several objects. Everything was a game to her. When we asked her to fetch or deliver an object, we always rewarded her for bringing the correct item. I would give her a small bottle and instruct her to "Take it to [whomever]." Upon successful delivery to the correct person, she was given a treat and sent on to a new destination. In this way, the dog learned to obey commands from Keri to "Take [something] to Mommy" or even to "Get Mommy." I liked the idea of being able to send Kira to give Keri her medications. Because it was less of an intrusion, it made Keri less annoyed that she had to take pills and less frustrated when she had to stop what she was doing. She did, however, complain about the container getting slobbery.

One important game we played with Kira was "find and take me to." Each of us would take turns hiding. The others would tell Kira to find the hidden person. "Find Mommy!" Keri would say excitedly, and Kira would take off through the house looking for me. When she succeeded, I would greet her excitedly and give her a treat. "Go to Keri!" I'd say, sending the dog back. "Take me to Mommy!" Keri would command, as Kira led her back to me. We had Kira find objects, other people, even Mugsy.

One night, Greg and I could not find Keri. We looked everywhere we could think of, with no luck. When we called, there was no answer. Suddenly, Kira appeared. "Show me. *Find Keri. Take me to Keri!*" I urged. Kira led me up the stairs and through Keri's room. She kept looking back to ensure I was following. She stood before the closet doors, but when I looked inside, I saw no one. Still, Kira stood her ground, insistent that her charge was in the closet. I looked more carefully. Finally I saw her, hidden behind all the clothes on the side farthest from the door. If the dog had not insisted Keri was there, I wouldn't have found her and Keri would have been awake and terrified, hiding through the night. As it was, I gave her emergency medication and got her to bed, and she was able to go to school the next morning.

We also discovered that, just by being herself, Kira could stop anxiety attacks. Keri had a phobia of certain bugs. Seeing these bugs triggered attacks of escalating anxiety that often became a downward spiral, necessitating emergency meds followed by her going to sleep. The first time this happened with Kira around, I watched as Keri started panicking. The dog jumped up on her and Keri toppled over, entangled with the puppy, as Kira tried to lick her face. My daughter wasn't sure whether to laugh, cry, or be angry. It seemed as if she was trying to do all three at the same time, but the anxiety stopped. This reaction, which Kira provoked instinctively and which doctors refer to as "responding to an anxiety attack with tactile stimulation," meant Keri did not require pharmaceutical intervention and was able to go to school that day. Later, the trainer taught the dog to respond as effectively without actually jumping on Keri.

Remember how Keri used Mugsy to check out a bedroom before she entered it? With Kira, the trainer went one step further, teaching the dog to enter the room and turn on the light. Kira's body language announced clearly whether someone was in the room, without the incessant barking that made Mugsy a liability. From watching the dog, Keri also knew if a person or animal she was seeing was real or a hallucination. "Who is it, Kira?" we would ask in an excited tone. If it was a living being, she would sinuously wiggle her slender collie body in delight and be rewarded with a treat. If nobody was there, she would look at us as if to ask what in the world we were talking about.

The dog's responsiveness to the environment dramatically increased Keri's independence by allowing her to focus on the task at hand. She no longer needed to be hyper-vigilant. She could ignore superfluous sounds. If the doorbell *really* rang, Kira stood up and nudged her. An added "Show me" resulted in Kira leading the way to the location she felt needed attention. Now Keri could do her schoolwork without interruption and go to bed independently.

Later, Kira gave Keri the same kind of independence outside the home, as the trainer taught the dog how to help Keri walk using a sturdy support harness with a strong handle. Although Kira always wore a type of harness when working in public, Keri switched to the support harness on those days when she could walk only with assistance. Even without the special harness, however, Kira learned to brace herself, lending support when Keri suddenly became dizzy or needed help standing up.

In crowded places, the dog provided another unforeseen benefit. Kira's harnesses each had a small tag with a medical emblem, indicating her status as a service dog. When people saw Keri and Kira together, they seemed less likely to jostle her and cause her pain. Although no one would think Keri was delicate merely by looking at her (hence the term PWID), she suffered from fibromyalgia-like pain and was easily hurt.

During Keri's senior year, while Kira was still in training, we published a solicited article titled, "How a Psychiatric Service Dog Changed Our Lives," for an IAADP newsletter.[63] I was glad Keri and I were able to add to the list of tasks psychiatric service dogs can provide. Although we had to use the term "psychiatric service dog" for the article, in real life I saw no benefit in distinguishing between psychiatric and medical disorders, especially since, based on our family's experience, many severe psychiatric disorders *are* medical. A better term for these animals would be "medical-assist service dogs."

Also during that year, the director of Keri's school invited Janece and her co-workers to bring several service dogs to the classroom. The trainers explained to the students what went into training the dogs, the requirements for a career of training service dogs, and the different types of training for various disabilities. They also taught the kids the differences between a therapy dog and a service dog, along with the rules of service-dog etiquette. Some of these rules were not to pet a service dog, especially without permission, and never to ask the owner what his or her disability is (that's rude, and nobody's business). The trainers also discussed the ADA (Americans with Disabilities Act) and the concept of public access.

---

[63] Wolfson, 2004.

Soon Kira began accompanying Keri to school three mornings a week, and Janece came to the school intermittently to continue Kira's training in a school environment. Once again, we were lucky that the school director supported this endeavor. Since Kira was not yet a fully trained service dog, the director could have refused to allow her to accompany Keri or to be trained in the school at all.

It took several years from the time I first had the idea until Keri had a trained service dog, but the wait and the effort were worth it. We'd started out to find a steadfast companion who could hear and see reality for her, but the result was so much more. We had no idea Kira would be so skilled at sensing something amiss—perceiving migraines in their prodromal stage and alerting Keri to drops in blood pressure, as well as once to high blood pressure (in this case, a teacher's—not Keri's). I'd have been content if the dog had been able to do nothing more than help Keri at home with her hallucinations and anxiety, and possibly with her walking and balance on bad days. But Kira far exceeded my expectations, including eventually helping Keri walk to college classes when she otherwise would not have been able to go.

Individuals differ in how much they want to tell people at school, work, and elsewhere about their disabilities. They differ in how they interact with the curious public. Through reading stories and participating in discussions online in a listserv group (e-list) for people with service dogs trained to assist those with invisible disabilities,[64] I learned about problems Keri might encounter and how to deal with them. Eventually, she developed a support network of her own.

Working with a service dog gave Keri coping strategies that proved invaluable as an adjunct to pharmacological interventions. Although the dog was trained to help with many tasks, the interaction between the two created a synergistic effect far beyond the scope of those tasks. Keri gained confidence, which alleviated some of her generalized stress and anxiety. She knew auditory or visual

---

[64] This group was led by Joan Esnayra, Ph.D., who later founded the Psychiatric Service Dog Society—http://www.psychdog.org.

disturbances, embarrassing phobic reactions, or a migraine prodrome phase could occur suddenly, at any time. Having the dog to help deal with these phenomena steered her toward a degree of independence we never thought possible.

Table 21: How a Well-Trained Dog Can Help at Home

- **Go into a room and check for occupant**: Keri realized that if she put Mugsy, the yappy little family dog, into a room before she entered and the dog did not bark, nobody was there, regardless of what or whom she was hearing. Kira, the service dog, served this purpose and more by learning to turn on a light in the room as well.
- **Provide a reality check**: This is important and complex. The child becomes hypervigilant due to the bombardment of auditory and visual hallucinations. Knowing he/she can rely on the dog to react to noises (such as doorbells, footsteps, cars, etc.) and movements (Keri was plagued by seeing distracting movements in her peripheral vision) allows the child to relax and focus on homework and other tasks. Kira, responded to "Who's that?" either with delight, if someone was really there, or with a puzzled expression if nobody was there.
- **"Go get" a parent:** Without any training, and while still a puppy, Kira would try to get us to come to Keri's aid when she was in distress, whether awake or asleep. With a little training, the pup quickly learned our names and to go to the person named. She was also taught to "go get" an object, as well as to "bring." Keri could count on her dog to "go get" me when told.
- **"Find" someone**: We made a game of "finding" different family members. That paid off when I told the dog, "Find Keri," and she took me to my terrified, hiding child.
- **"Take" meds to my daughter:** Giving the dog a packet of pills and saying, "Take it to Keri," caused less resentment than me nagging her to take her medicine.
- **Provide necessary support, balance, and steadiness**: Keri had low blood pressure and as a result was often clumsy. Kira steadied her and helped her get up from the floor. As needed, a special harness allowed Keri to use the dog for support when walking.
- **Stop anxiety attacks**: Regardless of whether a person in the midst of an anxiety attack gets annoyed with, becomes angry at, or laughs at a dog licking her face, the effect is the same—the anxiety attack stops.

Chapter 35
Finding Answers

Keri was still small in her senior year of high school, and her list of problems seemed endless. I desperately wanted someone to take a look at the whole puzzle of her medical issue, but we seemed to find doctors who looked at only one piece at a time.

One of these doctors was a gynecologist. Since Keri had passed the magical age of 16 without starting to menstruate, she could be evaluated for primary amenorrhea. It is possible for neuroleptic medications, particularly the older (typical) neuroleptics and the atypical neuroleptic, Risperdal (risperidone), to prevent menstruation. These drugs can cause hormone imbalances—galactorrhea (lactation), gynecomastia (breast growth), amenorrhea (lack of menstruation), and anovulation (lack of ovulation)—similar to a post-pregnancy state. But Keri was not on any of these medications.

Another problem that can cause delayed menarche is Turner syndrome, a genetic condition also characterized by short stature. But Keri's DNA test for Turner had been negative. Numerous other possibilities, including disorders of the pituitary, thyroid, or adrenals, could be checked with blood tests.

Since amenorrhea can be a symptom of hypothyroidism, I discussed this possibility with the gynecologist. Table 22 lists some symptoms of low levels of thyroid hormone.

The gynecologist ordered a blood test to check Keri's female hormone levels. The doctor reported that the results looked normal for a girl who was just too young to start menstruation, even if she *was* 16. With normal levels for a girl in the process of undergoing puberty, the protocol would be to do nothing further. "Just wait," we were told.

Table 22: Possible Signs of Hypothyroidism

- **Cold intolerance**
- Bradycardia (slow heartbeat)
- **Fatigue, lethargy**
- **Hypersomnia (excessive sleeping)**
- Anemia
- **Decreased metabolism, weight gain**
- **Constipation**
- **Brittle nails, dry skin**
- **Thin, brittle hair**
- **Amenorrhea** (not menstruating)
- Menstrual irregularities
- Galactorrhea (lactation)
- Hypercholesterolemia (high cholesterol)
- **Depression**
- **Slowed Achilles reflex**
- Apathy
- **Cognitive or mental deterioration**
- **Attentional problems**
- **Myalgia** (muscle pain)
- **Arthralgia** (joint pain)
- **Psychosis**
- **Mood instability**
- **Anxiety**

Symptoms Keri experienced are marked in bold.

After starting on some hormones, Keri finally started menstruating when she was 17, but her newfound womanhood was accompanied by terrible menstrual-related depression and migraines. Worse yet, she was unable to tolerate the medications that might have been able to help her.

An osteopathic doctor had helped a friend's son with facial tics. In hopes of easing Keri's body pains, migraines, and tics, we took her to this doctor for a few sessions of osteo-cranial manipulation. It made her feel worse. For a few days after each session, she felt foggy, slept more, and had increased pain. Surprisingly, an X-ray of Keri's neck showed she already had degenerative changes. Chiropractic treatment and physical therapy (PT) helped to address her limited mobility, as well as the pain in her back and neck and in the shoulder she'd injured years before, which had never completely healed. Although, unfortunately, medical insurance paid for a very limited number of PT sessions, she found further relief from daily yoga, which helped keep the pain at bay.

The Sleep Study

The first thing Keri's new GP, Dr. Marwil, did was schedule a sleep study. He felt she was long overdue for an evaluation by a neurologist at a sleep disorders clinic to determine the reason for her frequent sleep episodes. He believed such a study might also shed light on past and ongoing symptoms, including nightmares, hallucinations, paranoia, insomnia, hypersomnia, body pain, anxiety, fatigue, moodiness, irritability, low frustration tolerance, sensory overload, and/or attentional and cognitive problems, symptoms that until now had been labeled as schizoaffective or attributed to medication side effects.

Keri's diagnoses after the sleep study were narcolepsy, idiopathic hypersomnia (sleeping excessively due to an unknown medical reason), and obstructive sleep apnea. Day or night, the study showed, Keri fell straight into REM (rapid eye movement) sleep, a state during which people dream. We were told that this immediate fall into REM sleep (day or night), along with numerous brief arousals disturbing her sleep at night, indicated a form of narcolepsy. The diagnosis of sleep apnea was borderline.

> **Narcolepsy** symptoms can include REM-sleep intrusion hallucinations during the day. Some patients can have such frequent hallucinatory intrusions that they appear delusional.
>
> Narcolepsy can begin in infancy and can profoundly affect the circadian rhythm of growth hormone release.[a] More may be released in the daytime, and less at night, than would normally be seen in those without this disorder.[b]
>
> Narcolepsy can be misdiagnosed as a psychotic disorder, such as schizophrenia, with symptoms of thought disorder, delusions, and bizarre and agitated behavior.[c]
>
> Some people with narcolepsy may not have the most obvious symptom of falling down (cataplexy). However, they may feel fatigued, not do well in school, have frightening visual disturbances, and experience social difficulties. Narcolepsy symptoms can be confused with medication side effects, attentional difficulties, or depression.
>
> **Microsleeps**, which are so brief people may not be aware they've occurred, can happen to someone with narcolepsy or to anyone severely sleep deprived. These microsleeps can cause memory lapses that result in the person bumping into things, misplacing things, or writing nonsense. In this respect, microsleeps can mimic absence seizures.
>
> A person with narcolepsy can also develop **insomnia**.
>
> [a] Witmans, M. B., and Kirk, V. G., 2002.
> [b] Overeem, et al., 2003.
> [c] Bhat, S. K., and Galang, R., 2002.

Previously, the psychiatrist had not allowed Keri to try melatonin for her disturbed sleep—waking during the night and too early in the morning. After the sleep study, he gave his approval. Melatonin, a hormone that helps regulate sleep, is produced by the pineal gland, which works in harmony with the hypothalamus. Although she still woke at night and too early in the morning, now she sometimes could fall back to sleep quickly.

Keri also started to take narcolepsy medication, a central-nervous system stimulant called Provigil (modafinil).[65] Unlike traditional

---

[65] Cephalon, the manufacturer of Provigil, developed a longer-acting version called Nuvigil (armodafinil), approved by the FDA in 2007, to which Keri later switched.

amphetamine-like stimulants (those commonly used for ADHD), we were told Provigil selectively targets the brain's sleep center in the hypothalamus, mostly leaving the rest of the brain alone. Although there are risks associated with any medication, we were assured this drug was less likely to trigger the potential agitation, mood, and psychotic side effects, or have the withdrawal symptoms sometimes associated with traditional stimulants.

Initially, the GP cautiously suggested Keri take a 100 mg dose of Provigil only when she started one of her sleep-day episodes. Unfortunately, a dose this low, taken only at the start of a sleep episode, had no effect at all.

A New Endocrinologist

A three-word response to a query I made on an Internet discussion board changed our lives. I had described Keri's puzzling long sleep episodes and countless shorter ones. The response suggested the name of a disorder I had never heard of—Kleine-Levin syndrome (KLS).

The information I read about this disorder, described on many Web pages, said it occurred predominantly in males and was accompanied by hyperphagia (overeating) and hypersexuality. This description did not fit Keri, but as I read further, I learned that about 40 percent of those with the disorder are female. Additionally, just as the rare coprolalia (swearing) tic of Tourette syndrome gets a lot of publicity because of its social impact, so, too, do the hyperphagia and hypersexuality of KLS, even though in either illness these more sensational symptoms are far from ubiquitous.

The importance of those three words—Kleine-Levin syndrome—lay not in giving us a diagnosis for our daughter, although, like the label for Keri's tics years earlier, it did provide some solace. But researching the disorder led us to Dr. Robert Fredericks, a Nevada-based endocrinologist who had helped others with sleep symptoms similar to Keri's. One of his patients put me in touch with other patients, people who, in some cases, had traveled from countries around the world to consult with him. Dr. Fredericks looks at the person's entire endocrinological picture, I was told, takes a complete history, and performs numerous tests, including what is called a "structural ecology workup." This comprehensive approach was exactly what we'd been trying to find for so many years—someone to look at Keri as a whole person in order to figure out what was out of whack.

Dr. Marwil was relieved we'd found an endocrinologist who would run a broad range of tests. I was bolstered by his affirmation that we were doing the right thing by not giving up and by doing whatever it took to get Keri definitive medical testing and care.

We planned to take the trip to Nevada right after high school graduation. In the meantime, we prepared a write-up of Keri's history and diagnoses and a list of symptoms—details of the mystery we wanted solved. The list was fairly extensive, but it didn't include everything (see table 23). We didn't think to mention such things as burning pain in her extremities when hot and fatigued, abdominal pain, grey hairs, etc. At the time, we failed to see these indicators as significant.

Table 23: Some of the Puzzle Pieces at Age 16½

- Migraines (dilated blood vessels).
- Sleep days/sleep episodes.
- Major depression.
- Hallucinatory phenomena and psychotic disorder.
- Need for both neuroleptics and food supplements to stave off psychosis.
- Intermittent dizziness/low blood pressure.
- Oversensitivity to heat, cold, sound, and smell.
- Nightmares that don't stop when waking.
- Intermittent days of body pain and fatigue.
- Cholinergic urticaria (hives from excitement, stress, happiness, exercise, and heat).
- Delayed menstruation.
- Striae (stretch marks) without weight gain or weight loss.

The tests, conducted in Dr. Fredericks' clinic, took two and a half days. During this time, the doctor popped in and out energetically, saying "hi" with a friendly smile and checking on how things were going. The patient who had helped us with information and travel arrangements came in to meet us. He and Keri had a lot to talk about. It was the first time Keri had met someone with a host of symptoms similar to hers. The two of them talked about the problems affecting their bodies and brains, the pain, the fatigue, sleep episodes, depression, dizziness, trouble walking, and the fluctuating nature of their symptoms. They even discussed the sensitive topic of sometimes feeling like giving up and ending their suffering through suicide. I could not help but think that the opportunity for Keri to talk to this other patient was, in itself, worth the trip.

Even before all test results were complete, Dr. Fredericks met with us to discuss the findings. Sitting across from us at his massive wooden desk, he had Keri's medical papers spread in front of him. But before he said anything, he wanted to hear what *she* had to say about her problems. He leaned forward, listening attentively, sometimes having her pause while he checked a lab value or jotted a note. When she was finished, he offered me the same opportunity, giving the impression that what we had to say was as important as the clinical test results.

When we finished, there was a moment of silence. "Keri's symptoms," he began, holding up his hands and splaying his fingers, "and her myriad of diagnoses, are like the branches of a tree." Moving his right hand, he demonstrated with his left, fingers still spread apart to simulate branches, forearm propped vertically on the desk. "The real problem, however, is in the trunk."

Dr. Fredericks went on to explain that Keri's blood chemistry and history were so odd he suspected the origin of her problems was systemic—something happening at a cellular level that was affecting her body-wide. The definition of this "something" was still a mystery, and he was not offering a cure. But he did come up with the beginnings of a treatment plan to help her feel better.

To begin with, even though her daytime testing still showed no deficiency, he started her on a low dose of human growth hormone. He based this controversial decision on experience, looking at the whole picture and formulating a scientific theory supported by current research. When he documented his reasoning for the medical insurance company, they agreed with his decision and paid for the hormone, which is incredibly expensive.

This kind and creative endocrinologist was thinking outside the box, and his approach was based on treating Keri the person, not Keri the diagnosis. He was also right. The treatment didn't cure her, but it had a profoundly positive impact on her health and her life. And once she started to feel a lot better, she began to wake up.

Another test showed she had an unusual acid/base balance, a low white cell count (neutropenia), and imbalances in hormone levels, along with a vitamin B_{12} (cobalamin) utilization problem (called a functional or metabolic deficiency), which the doctor said he'd seen in a subset of patients with symptoms similar to hers. Possible symptoms of a B_{12} deficiency include fatigue, abdominal pain, burning pain in the mouth or extremities, difficulty walking, depression, and dementia-like symptoms. Later, Dr. Marwil tested her folate (vitamin B_9) levels and found the same oddity. A metabolic problem with folate also can affect vitamin B_{12} metabolism. These B vitamins work synergistically with a host of other nutrients such as choline, glycine, fatty acids, carnitine, and more, affecting mitochondrial function and thus, every cell in the body, especially cells with high energy needs such as those in muscles and the brain. I wondered if this was one reason the multivitamin supplement EMPowerPlus helped Keri so much.

Her blood calcium was extremely high; her parathyroid hormone level was suppressed and very low. Such blood values could be indicative of an autoimmune disorder called neurosarcoidosis, but further tests showed a different reason. Instead of building bone, Keri's bones were leaching out calcium, elevating the levels in her blood. Furthermore, she could not effectively absorb calcium even with added vitamin D, a vitamin needed for calcium absorption. Keri had intestinal malabsorption syndrome.

A bone scan revealed her bones had become thin; she had mild osteoporosis. I was stunned! (Oddly, although medical insurance paid for subsequent scans, they would not pay for this first bone density scan, saying there was no prior diagnosis warranting it. Yet how *can* there be a diagnosis warranting it until one has a test with which to make such a diagnosis?)

After we returned from Nevada, Dr. Marwil scheduled additional tests to verify and further investigate Keri's hormonal woes and thinning bones. The tests confirmed what Dr. Fredericks had found. He then ordered an MRI of her pituitary and arranged an appointment for her with a bone metabolism specialist. The MRI revealed no visible lesion or tumor, but other than being told to put her on a few supplements, we were given neither follow-up recommendations for finding the cause of her malabsorption nor information on how to correct it.

Tests run by Dr. Fredericks—confirmed by more tests in the coming years—also revealed Keri had low levels of a host of hormones. Among them were multiple thyroid hormones (free T_3, free T_4, and reverse T_3), Angiotensin II (which, we were told, is sometimes associated with fibromyalgia), testosterone (which females also need in small amounts), progesterone and other reproductive hormones, endothelin (which is used by cells all over the body and acts as a neurotransmitter in the hypothalamus), cortisol, and ACTH (adrenocorticotropic hormone). In addition, her cholesterol, a necessary precursor to the synthesis of many hormones, was slightly low. This deficiency could have occurred because of her sleep problems, intestinal malabsorption, or nutritional insufficiencies and low-functioning mitochondria, since each of these problems can affect other bodily functions.

In addition to diagnoses of Tourette syndrome, gifted-LD, schizoaffective disorder, and migraines, Keri now met the criteria for Kleine-Levin syndrome, narcolepsy, fibromyalgia, chronic fatigue syndrome, osteoporosis, intestinal malabsorption, possible endothelin insufficiency, and central hypothyroidism. The next challenge was to figure out what all of this meant and then to come up with a meaningful plan to help my daughter feel better and give her a decent quality of life.

Dr. Marwil cautiously prescribed T4 thyroid replacement in minute doses, afraid of her becoming hyperthyroid. Working together, Dr. Fredericks and Dr. Marwil also decided she should take a full-strength dose of narcolepsy medication on a regular, twice-per-day schedule, even doubling her morning dose on sleep days.

Finally, we were moving beyond the stagnant, tunnel-vision diagnosis of mental illness into the world of biomedical tests and treatments designed to address Keri's underlying biology. We still had a long way to go, however, and while we worked on what really ailed her, she would need all the determination and spunk she could muster to succeed in college.

If she gave up now, all would be lost.

Chapter 36
College

Keri was ecstatic to graduate from high school and start at the local community college while living at home. Before classes began, she went to the school's disability office to establish accommodations for her writing disability and medical-related absences. Of course, she went with Kira.

Accommodations are provided by a school to even the playing field—an attempt to give each student an equal opportunity for success. Using a service dog is not an accommodation, any more than allowing the use of crutches, a wheelchair, or eyeglasses, so we were not required to explain Keri's need to have Kira by her side. However, having been forewarned by people on the listserv for PWID's with service dogs that it would be a good idea, Keri gave the director of Disability Services two sheets—one with information about her medical issues (see table 24) and one about the dog (see table 25). Fortunately, with greater emphasis on the acceptance of the disability laws and service dogs in general, such documentation may not be needed, especially in larger university environments.

Kira's presence also helped Keri socially. It drew faculty, staff, and students to her and was a great icebreaker as she got to know other students, with and without disabilities. She was happy in this socially, culturally, and academically diverse group. She made friends, went places with them, dated, and had fun. Fortunately, Keri's friends understood her frequent need to cancel because of not feeling well.

The regular use of Provigil, along with the growth hormone, seemed to decrease the severity of Keri's Kleine-Levin syndrome sleep episodes and shorten the time afterward when she was cognitively impaired. Whenever possible, she scheduled her classes later in the day so she could take extra narcolepsy medication on sleep days and go back to bed for an hour while the drug started working. This way, even though her brain might be in a fog, she could make it to school more often, using Kira to help her walk as she stumbled into the classroom. (Sometimes "just being there" was what a teacher most cared about.)

Keri functioned better than she had in her last year of high school, but her first year at the local community college was still a nightmare of sleep days and feeling bad. Without a local endocrinologist to treat her, adjustments to hormone dosages were slow. She couldn't take a full load of classes, since so much of her time was lost to migraines, sleep days, and hormonal fatigue and depression. Stress was also a killer, and if she'd tried to carry a full load, making up all the work from days absent or sick would have made the situation worse.

Occasionally she used a small amount of Xanax, a preventative emergency medication that allowed her to battle stress and anxiety while remaining able to function mentally and physically. Taking this drug before certain medical procedures and during final exam week avoided the stress cascade that could result in an escalation of anxiety and hallucinatory symptoms. There was little danger in her becoming addicted, since she used it so infrequently and sparingly.

Another emergency medication she kept on hand was Atarax (hydroxyzine). Prescribed by her allergist, it was to be used in the event of a severe outbreak of cholinergic urticaria (hives), which could happen if her body became overheated from physical activity or fever. (I found it interesting that some doctors also prescribe Atarax as an emergency medication for anxiety.)[66]

At age 18, after finishing her second year of taking a few classes each semester, an increase in growth hormone lessened the frequency of her sleep days and a thyroid hormone adjustment gave her increased energy. Once she felt better physically, she experienced a slight reduction of her anxious feelings and a slight increase in tolerance to stress.

---

[66] Atarax (hydroxyzine) is a piperazine derivative used as an antihistamine (especially for hives or itchiness). It is also used for nausea and as an anxiolytic (anxiety-reducing) drug.

Table 24: Summary of Medical Issues (for college)

Some Current Pertinent Diagnoses:
- Severe migraines with prodromes consisting of confusion, ataxia, aphasia, mood changes, and vision changes.
- Mild Tourette syndrome.
- Schizoaffective disorder.
- Sleep disorders—Kleine-Levin syndrome, narcoleptic disorder.
- Cholinergic urticaria.
- Calcium malabsorption/thinning bones.
- Fibromyalgia/chronic fatigue syndrome.
- Learning disability in written communication (requires "double time" for math and writing).
- Allergies.
- Asthma.

Some Pertinent Daytime Medical Issues:
- Migraines—have been lessened by antiseizure medication. Medication must be taken at initial onset, but that onset is not easily recognized, as it can include mood change or confusion.
- Allergies.
- Mild temperature dysregulation—sensitive to cold and heat; prone to hypothermia and hyperthermia.
- Cholinergic urticaria—hives from small increases in core body temperature, which can result from stress, excitement, exercise, or exposure to heat.
- Overly sensitive to sounds, smells, and pain.
- Easily injured (physically).
- Residual, mild, chronic auditory and visual hallucinatory phenomena.
- Narcoleptic-type symptoms/Kleine-Levin-like sleep symptoms—can appear confused, be physically and mentally sluggish with slowed speech, and lack the ability to walk without assistance. This can be a dangerous state, as accidents and falls are likely.
- PTSD-like anxiety attacks can be precipitated by exposure to phobia.

Table 25: Summary of Service Dog's Public Tasks (for college)

Kira is a multipurpose service dog, very different in nature and behavior from the more familiar guide dogs for the blind. Guide dogs are trained to ignore sounds and other environmental stimuli, Kira has been trained—much like dogs that help the hearing-impaired in public situations—to quietly but enthusiastically respond to environmental cues.

Additionally, Kira is a medical-alert dog, much like the well-known seizure-alert dogs. She can detect and alert to migraine prodromes and dangerous changes in blood pressure.

She is also trained as a physical-support dog for the occasional instances when her handler is dizzy or unable to walk without assistance due to medication side effects, migraines, and/or a narcoleptic condition and to perform tasks that help mitigate multiple other disabilities.

- **Alert to migraines** at an early stage (prodrome) so the medication has a better chance to be effective, which will lower school absences and in turn lessen overall stress.

- **Help handler walk** to safety when a migraine has hit and during a Kleine-Levin syndrome sleep episode.

- **Provide necessary support, balance, and steadiness**, preventing falls when dizziness occurs from low blood pressure and/or medication side effects, as well as when narcoleptic/Kleine-Levin-type episodes occur.

- **Respond to anxiety attack or stress with tactile stimulation:** Lessen residual symptoms by responding to stress and anxiety signals with tactile stimulation techniques, which empowers handler to cope with phobic reactions in a more socially acceptable and effective way and decreases school absences.

- **Mitigate hallucinations by providing a "reality check":** Provide a quiet response to the environment, which mitigates the effects of residual hallucinatory phenomena by allowing handler to ignore them.

One spring day, with Kira by her side, Keri and I walked in the nearby arboretum as we talked of her plans for the weekend. It was a chilly afternoon, but my daughter was no longer as intolerant of the cold. After our walk, she had enough energy to return to class, come home, do some homework, and chat with friends. This was a good day.

There were also bad days. At school the very next morning, the dog alerted her that something was wrong. Keri wasn't sure if the warning meant she was about to pass out or a migraine was imminent. She assessed her condition and realized her thinking was slowed and her mood dull. She decided she'd better take her migraine medication and call home. Within a half hour, the migraine hit, but because of early intervention, it was not severe and subsided within hours.

For now, progress meant there were more good days than bad. Instead of hearing Keri sobbing and seeing her holed-up in her room, I was more apt to find her sitting on the couch preening her bird, reading, doing art, or knitting a new sweater for Mugsy. Or, I might not see her at all because she was at school, studying, at the park, or out with friends.

Keri continued to grow, eventually reaching a height of 5 feet, 2 inches (157.5 cm), 4 inches (10.2 cm) greater than the 4 feet, 10 inches (147.3 cm), predicted. She still had sleep problems, fluctuating energy levels, occasional bouts of pain, and times of emotional fragility that fluctuated along with her hormone levels, but at least those levels were now being monitored. She had a healthier glow about her, and while her health and well-being remained precarious, things were definitely improving.

Keri had lost years of her life being ill, years she should have spent learning life skills. Going into a bank, using a check card, filling out forms—things we take in stride—can seem daunting to a person who missed out on so many aspects of teen development. Now, with the help of friends and family and with Kira by her side, she was gaining confidence by mastering these useful life skills. Although it took her an extra year to get her first college degree (an Associates of Science), she was growing up and enjoying life. She even took classes beyond those needed for her degree because she wanted to explore areas of interest to her.

~~~~~~~~~~~

Young adults need insight, stability, and cognitive ability in order to pursue and implement available options pertaining to their health, and these traits are dependent on a certain degree of wellness. Some people whose brains are adversely affected also suffer from anosognosia, which means they are unaware their brain is so compromised. Many of these individuals have difficulty seeking or accepting help for problems they do not understand or sometimes even acknowledge.[67] Our family was lucky. Keri was one of the 75 percent of people with the diagnosis of schizoaffective disorder with insight.[68]

Even so, a small incident brought home to me the dangers we faced now that Keri was 18. A new allergist had her try a twice-a-day inhaler for her asthma, in hopes it would improve her lung function. Keri reacted with escalating anxiety, agitation, and paranoia. It looked like acute psychosis was imminent. And this time, if Keri became too paranoid, or frankly psychotic, the outcome could be dire. She was legally an adult, and if she chose to do something irrational, such as discontinuing all medications, there would be nothing I could do. The only way I'd be able to force treatment would be to obtain a court order and commit her to the state psychiatric hospital—not an appropriate place for a person like Keri.

Luckily, in this case Keri's GP immediately recognized the problem as a reaction to the asthma medication. Side effects of two of its ingredients—corticosteroids and salmeterol—could cause a reaction that looked like mental illness. When Keri stopped using the inhaler, her anxiety was reduced and her paranoia abated.

This incident motivated us to look into what could be done under the laws of our state to help Keri in the event she became acutely psychotic in the future. If she was ill, she wanted to be treated. Even if she stated this wish while healthy, if later she said she *didn't* want

---

[67] To understand the nightmarish difficulties of trying to get help for adults suffering from anosognosia, read *Crazy: A Father's Search Through America's Mental Health Madness* by Pete Earley and *I Am Not Sick I Don't Need Help!* by Xavier Amador.
[68] Amador, 2007, p. 6.

treatment, even if she was acutely ill when making this statement, the law would be on the side of her being *denied* treatment.

One complicating factor in this legal morass is the Health Insurance Portability and Accountability Act (HIPAA). While meant to protect the privacy of patients against discrimination or persecution if their conditions were known, this law can have tragically damaging repercussions. One such repercussion adversely affects the most vulnerable patients—those with severe brain disorders—by excluding from the circle of treatment the only people who truly love and care about them. Family members no longer have access to what is being done for, or *not* being done for, their loved ones behind the closed doors of psychiatric hospitals.

Keri wanted something that would ensure treatment in the event she didn't even know she needed it. We found she could complete a psychiatric advance directive as well as grant me a *durable* medical power of attorney. Both are revocable, but together they could ensure she would receive *some* treatment, if only in the time it took for them to be contested and revoked. This small window might buy Keri the time she needed to become aware she was becoming paranoid or psychotic again.

Templates for psychiatric advance directives (PADs) can be found on the Internet, printed, and completed without needing an attorney—just a notary—but state laws differ as to whether hospitals are legally bound to honor such directives. PADs outline some general aspects of care, list types of treatment a person does or does not want to have, and include the designation of a person authorized to make treatment decisions in the event the patient becomes mentally incapacitated.

The durable medical power of attorney gave me permission to carry out Keri's wishes as if I were her personal attorney. It covered what I was already doing for her—talking with doctors and staff, making and rescheduling appointments, and dealing with medical bills and insurance claims. Because of HIPAA, many doctors' offices will not even talk to a parent about the bills of an adult patient, even if the parent is paying them. Unless the patient signs a release form with each medical entity, even to admit the patient *has* a bill goes against HIPAA privacy laws. Once I had Keri's medical power of attorney, I was legally allowed to have two-way conversations with doctors, handle bills, deal with insurance claims, and reschedule appointments.

With this safety net in place, Keri could focus on moving forward. Following the path laid out by her GP, Dr. Marwil, and the endocrinologist, Dr. Fredericks, we continued with biological testing and biomedical treatments. The results far exceeded our expectations.

Table 26: Diagnoses: Ages 16 to 20

- Gifted-LD.
- Migraines (symptoms eliminated by age 20).
- Tourette syndrome (very mild).
- Schizoaffective disorder (symptoms eliminated by age 20).
- Immune: cholinergic urticaria (disappeared by age 20), neutropenia, allergies, asthma (mild).
- Vision problems: Acquired unilateral dyschromatopsia (left eye), convergence disorder (left eye) and farsightedness (both eyes).
- Primary amenorrhea changed to erratic, infrequent menstruation (age 17 on thyroid hormone).
- Sleep disorders: Kleine-Levin syndrome (diminished symptoms by age 21); narcolepsy & idiopathic hypersomnia (better control of symptoms by age 20); borderline sleep apnea (not sure if still exists).
- Central hypothyroidism (treated; substantially better at age 21); idiopathic hypopituitarism.
- Intestinal malabsorption, celiac/gluten & other food intolerances (dietary changes in full effect at age 20).
- Osteoporosis (slowly improving but still present).
- Chronic fatigue syndrome & fibromyalgia (symptoms reduced by age 21, although still does not have the energy level of her peers).
- Vitamin B metabolic problem/functional insufficiency (adequately treated by age 21).

Sunshine

Ages Nineteen to Twenty-one

I Am
(Remember . . .)

Remember the little one
The one with the questioning eyes
Who played by herself
Who cried all the time
And questioned the meaning of love eternal?

I was that little one.

Remember the child
The one with the bright eyes
Who never smiled
Who still cried often (just not when she was sad)
And never ever knew just what she'd done so wrong?

I was that child.

Remember the girl
The one with the defiant stare
Who painted her face and went out with friends
Who bit her lip, hid her tears
And prayed for reality to fade away, into the light of the strobe?

I was that girl.

Remember the adolescent
The one with the vacant gaze
Who sat apart from everyone else
Who was swallowed in dreams and pain
And all the while fought to stay above it all?

I was that adolescent.

Remember the woman
The one with wonder in her eyes
Who laughs when she's happy, cries when she's sad,
      and smiles in-between
Who stands afraid yet ever looking towards the future
And is not quite certain how she ever made it this far?

I am that woman.

– Keri

Chapter 37
Endocrine Treatments

"They're gone," Keri solemnly informed me. "The last of the voices and even the background noises are gone."

Growth hormone therapy, followed by the partial correction of her thyroid levels, had diminished the intensity of Keri's audio hallucinations. Her physical malaise, along with her psychiatric symptoms of anxiety, stress intolerance, and frustration intolerance, lessened along with them. As her body grew healthier, so did her brain functions. She was able to decrease the dosage of her antipsychotic medication.

Keri's eyes sparkled in wonder. She was 19 years old. Her reproductive hormone levels had been as low as an old woman's. During normal fluctuations of her menstrual cycle, the levels dipped even lower, incapacitating her with depression and migraines, so the doctor added one more hormone: progesterone. As promised, the progesterone helped her mood and menstrual-related migraines, but it did so much more.

The voices and the hallucinations, including visual hallucinations where she saw movement in her peripheral vision, simply *stopped*. Keri had lived with voices and/or hallucinations to one degree or another for nearly her entire life. And now, with the replacement of a deficient hormone, the last of her hallucinatory symptoms vanished. We were stunned! We hadn't been trying to rid her of schizoaffective symptoms, or even to help her with hallucinations. We'd only been trying to improve her *physical* health. We had no idea progesterone could help a symptom considered a severe *mental* illness.

We were not so naïve as to believe this one hormone was the cause of, or the complete answer to, Keri's schizoaffective disorder. After all, she'd already been improving on other hormones and we were addressing her sleep problems and other medical issues. Years later, Keri temporarily stopped the progesterone to see if it was still needed. Although her level was still low, the hallucinations did not return.

We knew Keri was far from well, but even before the addition of the progesterone, she was already taking less neuroleptic medication than before. Now, progesterone, added to the changes we'd already made, seemed to tip the balance.

After adding a supplement recommended by a consulting doctor to help mitochondrial function, followed by dietary changes and treatment to heal her gut, Keri found her migraines disappeared as well. At this point, the psychiatrist stated that all the symptoms of our daughter's schizoaffective disorder—her *mental* illness—could have been caused by the biological problems we'd uncovered. "In fact," the doctor mused, "it could have been caused by any of these [biological] issues. Low hormones of hypopituitarism *alone* can cause symptoms of schizoaffective." Laughingly, he compared Keri's story to *Lorenzo's Oil*, in which the parents relentlessly searched for a solution to their son's incurable neurological problem. The psychiatrist said we'd found *Keri's Oil*—a magic elixir made just for her.

And she did feel better. That she suffered fewer psychiatric symptoms was like winning the door prize after being given free tickets to a concert. But she was far from cured. I read more about Lorenzo. He was never cured, either. For him, it was too little, too late.

The difference, of course, is that Lorenzo's parents had been searching for a cure. We were not.

~~~~~~~~~~~~

Keri had long ago adjusted to being in the life-long recovery stage of mental illness—*acceptance*. She'd been building her life, adhering to regimens for medication and therapy, and using supports and accommodations to minimize the impact of her ongoing residual hallucinations, anxiety, occasional fits, and medication side effects. She just wanted not to feel sick all the time, and we helped in every way we could. In this respect, we were succeeding on all fronts—in part because of Keri's determination, attitude, and what I can only call *mental health* in the midst of her biological *mental illness*.

Keri's problems were incredibly complex. Putting the puzzle pieces together, and then tailoring treatment accordingly, was far more involved than diagnosing an infection and prescribing an antibiotic.

Diagnosing and treating Keri's endocrine problems had not been within her doctor's abilities as a psychiatrist. However, perhaps psychiatrists, as medical doctors, may need special training regarding diagnosis and treatment of problems related to the hypothalamic-pituitary-adrenal axis. Hormones produced by this system profoundly affect brain function, sleep and arousal, anxiety, and mood; they have been documented for decades as being intertwined with cases of depression, bipolar disorder, schizophrenia, schizoaffective disorder, and, more recently, autism spectrum disorder.

We soon discovered that resolving pituitary-related endocrine problems completely was not within the capabilities of current endocrinological medical knowledge. To do so would require a treatment that reproduces the human body's precise responsiveness to immediate needs—in other words, a treatment that could mimic Mother Nature exactly. Still, Keri's hormonal issues were finally diagnosed.

Even as a young child, we knew she was very sensitive to endocrine-system disruptions, so perhaps I should not have been so surprised that part of the solution to her chronic hallucinations was endocrinological. I had read that some women with symptoms of schizophrenia and low estrogen had had their symptoms alleviated with estrogen-hormone-replacement therapy.[69] Other studies implicated cortisol, another hormone, as playing a role in some cases of teen schizophrenia.[70] I read about clinics and treatment centers for fibromyalgia and chronic fatigue—once considered mental illnesses—where doctors now focus on achieving optimal hormone levels as part of a treatment strategy.

---

[69] Busko & Lie, 2008.
[70] Emory University press release, 2008.

While I was searching for information that might help Keri, one psychiatric medical researcher sent me articles about women whose mood and psychotic disorders in women that were improved by increasing their thyroid-hormone levels.[71] Some of these studies were more than 30 years old, some recent, yet I hadn't seen this type of research reflected in practice by either endocrinologists or psychiatrists.

Over the years, family and friends had suggested Keri might benefit from treatment normally thought of as anti-aging, because some of her symptoms overlapped those normally observed in older women. Even as she was growing up, it seemed as if she was advancing in age like an old person rather than developing into a voluptuous young woman with obvious signs of fertility and health. When we learned about her hormone deficiencies, as identified by Dr. Fredericks, this connection made sense.

DHEA (dehydroepiandrosterone), testosterone, progesterone, estrogen, melatonin, thyroid hormones, and somatotropin (growth hormone) all have an impact on brain function and other organs. All are hormones that decline with age. Neurotransmitters in the brain, such as dopamine, acetylcholine, norepinephrine, GABA, and serotonin, also decline as we grow older. As a result, our immunity decreases and our inflammatory processes increase.

These hormones and others affect biological processes such as growth, reproduction, sleep, hunger, digestion, metabolism, cognition, and mood. And science continues to discover new hormones and to learn about their complex interaction with body, brain, and mind.

Between the growth hormone shots and partial alleviation of her low thyroid levels, Keri continued to feel stronger, more energetic, and less fatigued.

Telling friends about the effects of these hormones, I felt like an announcer for an infomercial: "But wait! There's more!" Her hair grew. Before, it was dull, thin, graying, and brittle. With the new medica-

---

[71] Bauer, Heinz, Whybrow, 2002, and Bauer, et al., 2005.

tions, it got thicker, longer, stronger, and shinier. Her nails grew stronger, too, and she enjoyed doing the usual girlie things with them—letting them grow longer and making them look pretty. The skin on her hands was no longer dry and cracked. A year after starting medications to address some of her medical issues, she didn't have as many sleep days, days when she couldn't walk, or days when she could barely think. She was no longer constantly dizzy, and she didn't fall or bump into things as often.

By 19-1/2, three years after starting on the growth hormone and thyroid medication, Keri had grown nearly three inches (7.6 cm), and her bone density was closer to normal. She was no longer in constant pain. She no longer felt physically sick most of the time. Her immune system was improving.

Sometimes we see best how much something helps when it is removed and then restored. Keri once missed her growth hormone shots for a week. She again felt dizzy, fatigued, achy—in her word, "yucky." She said it felt as if she was coming down with the flu, that this was how she used to feel *all* the time. She became depressed and unable to think well. Even trying to decide which of two foods to eat felt too stressful. Stress is involved in mental illness, but we could see clearly that stress was not the cause of Keri's illness. Indeed, the reverse was true; her illness caused everyday living to be too stressful.

We knew growth hormone wasn't the whole solution. We had to correct multiple hormone problems. In the meantime, we continued to work on improving her thyroid hormone levels, which turned out to be a challenge in itself.

The Thyroid Connection

When Keri was first tested by Dr. Fredericks at the age of 16-1/2, we had been amazed to discover she had low levels of thyroid hormone. Because previous tests had shown no abnormality, doctors had dismissed this possibility for years. None of these medical professionals had tested *all* her thyroid-related hormone levels, nor had they done a complete thyroid panel (see Appendix A: The Thyroid Connection). So nobody caught *her* form of hypothyroidism. When I later asked, "Why not?" one doctor answered, "Because it's rare." But can we really know how rare it is if we aren't even checking for it?

I felt betrayed. Fortunately, some newer books now mention rarer forms of thyroid malfunction, and more doctors are writing articles about testing multiple factors before ruling out a thyroid hormone problem. In addition, if a doctor doesn't do a thorough job, families today have access to information allowing them to follow up with testing on their own, or to search for a doctor who *will* order the full battery of tests.

Some studies suggest that even low-but-normal thyroid hormone levels in a female with a cyclical mood disorder might clinically worsen the illness, adding to the effects of bipolar mood disorder.[72] However, many doctors (including clinical endocrinologists with little expertise in complex cases involving psychiatric symptoms) will not treat thyroid levels until they drop below normal.

The protocol for treating Keri's type of hypothyroidism indicated that she needed to reach the *upper third* of the normal range. But for years, doctors couldn't maintain her levels at even the *lower third* of normal. Dr. Marwil found nothing in his medical textbooks to help, yet the few times Keri's thyroid levels measured in the low-normal range, she felt significantly less fatigue.

Each time the GP increased her thyroid dose, her levels would go up temporarily. Then her TSH would drop further, and with it her thyroid levels. To assess the results of each increase took months, waiting for blood levels to adjust, getting a blood test, waiting for the results, and then getting a new prescription. Another four months were wasted when the mail-order pharmacy sent a different generic. *Thyroid hormones are not interchangeable.* Now we ensure "dispense as written" (DAW) gets put on Keri's prescriptions.

---

[72] Bierkowska and Rybakowski, 1994; and Papadimitriou, Calabrese, Dikeos, and Christodoulou, 2005.

Dr. Marwil turned to the endocrinologist for advice. Dr. Fredericks had no definitive answer regarding Keri's dropping hormone levels, either, but he did have a suggestion. He recommended the GP switch her to a thyroid hormone that could be dissolved under her tongue. It would be processed differently by her body, bypassing any intestinal absorption problems that might be interfering with her treatment.

The suggestion sounded promising, but the results were the same. Her levels dropped again.

The GP was baffled, so he referred Keri to a local thyroid specialist—a doctor at the same hospital medical center as the pediatric endocrinologist who had cavalierly dismissed her all those years ago. This local endocrinologist stated dismissively that Keri's medications were probably interfering with her thyroid levels and she should therefore "discontinue some of them." "Oh?" I queried, "Which ones would you have her stop?" The endocrinologist immediately proceeded to list three: Seroquel, Wellbutrin, and food supplements. "Someone so young should not be on these meds."

My daughter and I gaped at the specialist in disbelief, as I half-asked, half-stated, "So you would have her be psychotic instead?"

Keri chimed in with, "That's literal. I would be *literally* psychotic."

(The day eventually came when Keri was able to slowly taper off Seroquel, but only *after* her hormone levels were being corrected, and only *because* of nutritional supplements.)

In defeat, we returned to the GP, who just shook his head. With a sad smile, he said of the medical center endocrinologist, "She must be young." Keri's take was different. Since the same problem had occurred earlier with another endocrinologist, she felt the problem must lie within the curricula of at least some medical schools.

Dr. Marwil, taking up the slack for local endocrinologists who seemed loath to treat anyone on psychotropic medications, attended continuing medical education seminars in an attempt to help his patient. He learned that hormones produced by the adrenal glands, as well as other hormones and even nutrients, are intertwined with levels of thyroid hormone. Until this point, none of these issues had been addressed in my daughter's case. Since Keri's T3 level was even lower than her T4, an indicator she was insufficiently converting T4 into the useable T3 form, perhaps she needed a T3 supplement as well. But Dr. Marwil did not feel he had sufficient training to prescribe T3 replacement. Instead, he prescribed a natural desiccated thyroid hormone replacement containing both T4 and T3, along with minute amounts of T1 & T2. His research indicated the natural thyroid replacement worked better for some people. But when this failed as well, the GP felt he was in over his head.[73]

He then sent Keri to another local endocrinologist, this one in private practice. He carefully prepared a half-inch (1.3 cm) thick medical report he felt the new doctor needed to have, plus a cover letter with a short summary. Since he suspected the previous endocrinologist may not have received all the information he'd submitted by fax, he advised me to hand-carry the report to the doctor's office. He also faxed a "heads-up" to the new endocrinologist. We were desperate for help, and he didn't want anything to go wrong.

Still, the visit nearly ended in disaster.

The endocrinologist sat across the desk from us in confusion, obviously not understanding why we were there. Looking at Keri's low TSH levels as reported in the head's-up fax from Dr. Marwil's office, he assumed her thyroid levels were too high. I grew increasingly alarmed. Where were the report and cover letter from the GP I'd given to the receptionist, which the doctor was to have reviewed?

With growing alarm, I explained what was missing. When he insisted he had everything he should, I jumped up and began agitatedly rustling through papers on the doctor's desk. This really got his attention! He left the office to search for the records I allegedly had handed over to the front desk. It took some time, but he found them. They'd accidentally been thrown in the trash.

Keri and I sat quietly while this new endocrinologist read her extensive medical history. He occasionally uttered a surprised, "Oh!" and "Now I understand!" then put the papers down to talk to us. He

---

[73] T1 and T2 are lesser thyroid hormones scientists don't know much about. T2 is theorized as playing a role in the use of some types of fat cells for energy production.

recognized she had idiopathic hypopituitarism (low functioning of the pituitary from an unknown cause). A low-functioning pituitary does not release enough TSH to stimulate adequate production of T4 and T3, even if the person needs more thyroid hormone. In Keri's case, we needed to get her T4 and T3 levels up to a normal level—all the way up—however much it took. By administering T4 and T3 separately, each was independently adjustable. The endocrinologist prescribed a high dose of each. After we knew the levels of each that were required to help her, she would be able to switch back to the appropriate amount of desiccated thyroid hormone.

If Keri started to feel bad, we were told, it could indicate an overdose, which might in turn cause temporary hyperthyroidism. She did, in fact, develop hyperthyroidism for a short time, but she felt so bad already it made little difference. Another adjustment was made. And then another. Finally, her thyroid levels were correct. By then, she was 21 years old. *It had taken over four years!*

> Following is a simplified version of how the thyroid works. The hypothalamus sends TRH (thyrotropin-releasing hormone) to the pituitary, telling it to send TSH (thyroid-stimulating hormone) to the thyroid. TSH tells the thyroid to create thyroid hormones, including a lot of thyroxine (T4) and a little bit of triiodothyroxine (T3).
>
> T3 is the thyroid hormone actively used by cells throughout the body. T4 gets converted to the active T3 form mostly in the liver and kidneys, but some gets converted in the brain itself. The hypothalamus is supposed to sense the body's thyroid hormone level and release more TRH when the level drops. This sensing mechanism is called a feedback loop.
>
> The hypothalamus acts much like the thermostat in a building, sensing when the temperature drops and signaling a mechanism in the heating system that causes heat to be generated. If the thermostat is set too low, it doesn't give this signal often enough and not enough heat is produced.
>
> In Keri's case, her hypothalamic-pituitary-adrenal axis did not send out messages strong enough to maintain a sufficient level of hormones. The "thermostat" controlling her thyroid level was set too low.

Figure 7: Hypothalamic-Pituitary-Thyroid Axis

Hypothalamic-Pituitary-Thyroid Axis

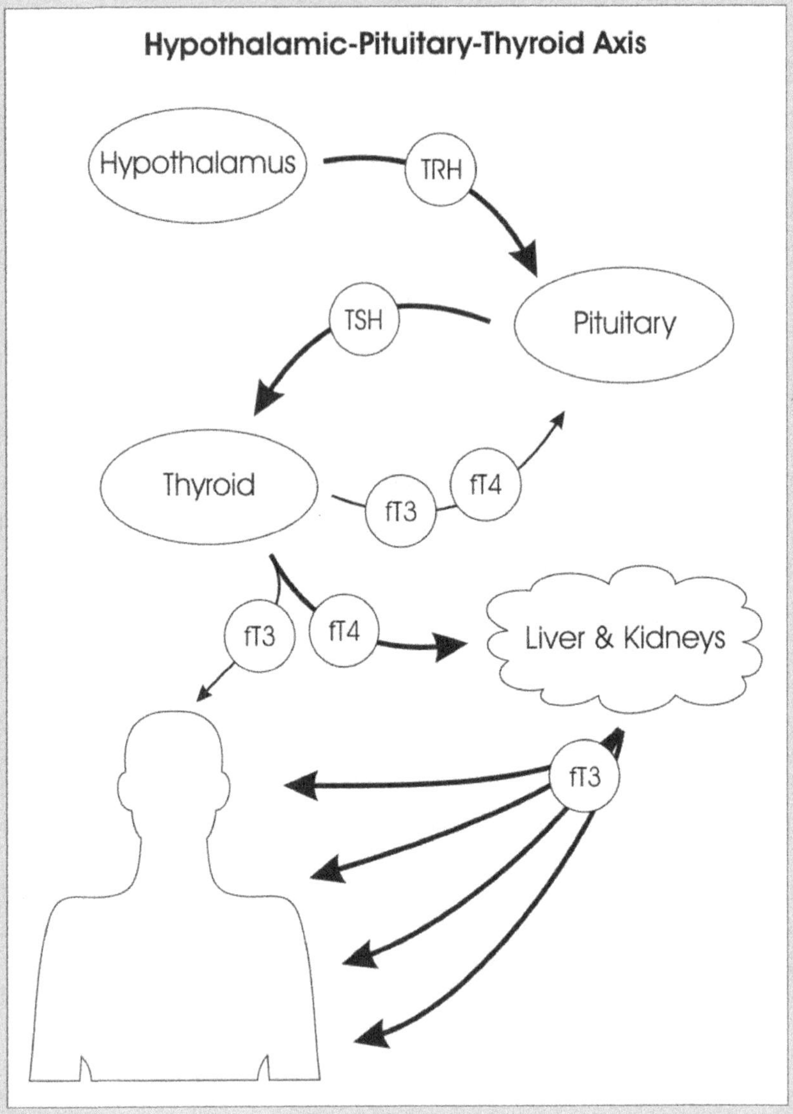

Many doctors measure TSH only, instead of measuring the levels of T4 and T3, the actual thyroid hormones available for the body to use. Plus, there are other hormones and nutrients connected to the functioning of thyroid hormones (see Appendix A: The Thyroid Connection).

The Adrenal Connection

Hormone tests showed Keri had low adrenal function. Adrenal function can be impaired from medications; nutrition problems in the hypothalamus, pituitary, or the adrenals themselves; tumors; or autoimmune response. And either low or high adrenal function can produce symptoms affecting mood, anxiety, pain, sleep, immune function, startle response, energy, stress response, and blood pressure.

Before receiving integrative biomedical treatments, Keri had been easily overwhelmed by stress. Whether caused by illness, fatigue, migraines, frustration, allergies, medication side effects, or lack of sleep, stress had led to anxiety, crying, paranoia, and an increase in hallucinations. The severe stress of hallucinations and nightmares when she was younger had spiraled into symptoms of phobia, pain, and even, temporarily, PTSD. She'd often been dizzy, clumsily bumping into things and falling, and she'd had emotional meltdowns as a result of these sudden feelings of malaise—falling to the floor, whining, and crying. I wondered if she'd had low blood sugar.

Since adrenal hormones influence the conversion of T4 into T3, there is a connection between thyroid hormone function and adrenal function. Some reproductive hormones, such as testosterone and progesterone, are produced or partially produced by the adrenals as well. We knew Keri was deficient in reproductive hormones, thus the spectacular results yielded by the addition of progesterone to her drug regimen. Her testosterone levels, however, fluctuated so much that replacement therapy was ruled out for fear of making her levels too high.

Cortisol is also affected by adrenal gland malfunction, and Keri had a low cortisol level. Cortisol protects the cells of the body from the effects of oxidative stress and inflammation. Low levels can mimic symptoms of psychiatric disorders, inducing feelings of depression and moodiness. They also can cause fatigue, dizziness, weakness, nausea, low blood sugar, low blood pressure, muscle and joint pain, and stress intolerance. In the extreme, insufficient cortisol is life-threatening. Thus, in order to protect itself from excess inflammation and other deleterious effects, the body naturally increases cortisol levels when it is under stress.

On the one hand, low cortisol reduced Keri's ability to deal with stress, both physical and emotional; on the other hand, the stress of prolonged illness—whatever was going on with her neuro-endocrine system—could cause further deterioration of her adrenals and a corresponding dip in cortisol levels—a condition referred to as adrenal fatigue or partial adrenal insufficiency.

Although low cortisol levels can cause or be interconnected with psychiatric symptoms, many people diagnosed with bipolar disorder and schizophrenia tend to have *elevated* levels of this stress hormone, and some neuroleptic agents (antipsychotics) tend to lower the levels, thus normalizing them. Seroquel, the atypical neuroleptic Keri was taking, is one of these drugs. In a study where Seroquel was given to healthy people with normal cortisol levels, subjects showed a drop in this hormone while on the drug.[74] In cases where the medication itself is the cause of low cortisol, but switching medications is not advised, a small amount of cortisol replacement hormone may be needed.[75] Obviously, adrenal function should be periodically checked in people under stress or on psychotropic medications, but no one had checked Keri's cortisol levels until she went to Dr. Fredericks. (Note: Even after Keri was no longer taking Seroquel, her cortisol was still low—just not *as* low.)

There was yet another connection. Both thyroid hormones and cortisol are involved in the functioning of mitochondria—the powerhouses of our cells, whose dysfunction is correlated with cases of autism, bipolar disorder, and schizophrenia.

In addition to some of the reproductive hormones and cortisol, adrenals produce hormones that regulate salt and fluid balance. Before Keri's visit to the endocrinologist who prescribed T3 replacement hormone, Dr. Marwil had looked at the supplements she was taking and said she needed even more, including vitamin B_5

---

[74] Cohrs, et al., 2006.
[75] Anderson, 2007.

(pantothenic acid) and antioxidants like vitamin C. He wanted to shore up her adrenal glands and get her cortisol levels to go up and to stay up. With additional support, he hoped her adrenals would produce more reproductive hormones and more cortisol, which in turn would help with her low T3 levels.

We knew there were precautions to take—and problems to rule out—before increasing some nutritional supplements. For example, hemochromatosis is a common genetic disease that causes the excessive retention of iron. Excessive iron can cause a hypofunctioning of the pituitary that gets mislabeled as idiopathic hypopituitarism, which in turn can result in psychiatric symptoms misdiagnosed as mental illness. Since Keri had a diagnosis of idiopathic hypopituitarism, and since Vitamin C increases the absorption of iron, she was screened for hemochromatosis before increasing her vitamin C supplementation.

Nutritional therapies sometimes help to protect adrenal function under stress. Unfortunately, in Keri's case these therapies did not improve her low hormone levels. Later we learned some doctors use specific herbal supplements to help stimulate the hypothalamic-pituitary-adrenal axis, resulting in a more natural increase in adrenal hormones. If we had known about these supplements before starting hormone replacement therapy, we would have tried this approach first, because hormone replacement therapy causes additional stresses on the body and does not completely mimic Mother Nature. An integrative medical specialist put Keri on a supplement that did normalize her cortisol levels, as well as her testosterone levels.

When dealing with adrenal function abnormalities, other strategies, such as therapeutic hormone replacement, may be needed, even if the problem is not at the level of the adrenal gland itself but rather the result of medications, the hypothalamus, or the pituitary.

Some people opt to supplement these replacement hormones with precursors (such as DHEA and pregnenolone), but we did not, simply because blood tests did not show a deficiency in the precursors—only in the hormones themselves.

Keri's brain function turned out to be very sensitive to hormonal fluctuations. As her hormone levels improved and her nutritional needs and sleep issues were addressed, her psychiatric symptoms of mood instability, depression, anxiety, and hallucinations were reduced, along with her fatigue and pain.

It was with growing horror that Greg and I, and Keri herself, began to understand the import of what we'd learned. In short, if all of her *physical* issues had been addressed first, she may never have had any *psychiatric* issues to treat.

We now had a deeper understanding that Keri's remaining *mental* problems (stress intolerance and moods that fluctuated with her hormone levels) were due to biological/medical issues not yet sufficiently addressed—limited either by our understanding or by lack of sufficient advances in medical knowledge. *Acceptance* of Keri's status was no longer an appropriate state of mind for her or for us. To the contrary, there was still much hope for continuing improvement.

Chapter 38
Integrated Treatment

"Dinner's ready!" A delectable mix of aromas permeated the house. As usual, Keri and her boyfriend were serving an enticing array of healthful, colorful foods lightly cooked in olive oil and seasoned with spices, cloves of garlic, and home-grown herbs.

Keri talked excitedly about the classes she was taking as part of her program to be a dietitian. She loved the courses in nutrition and biology. Chemistry was hard, but doable. The conversation drifted to plans for vacation, doctors' appointments, how family and friends were doing, what was going on in our lives, and Keri and her boyfriend's dreams for the future.

~~~~~~~~~~~

When Keri was 12, we had missed a major "Aha!" moment. We had seen that the multi-nutritional Truehope supplement, EMPowerPlus, partially alleviated her schizoaffective symptoms, thus allowing us to lower her Seroquel dosage. We understood the concept of nutritional deficiencies. However, since Keri was being fed a good diet, we had no reason to suspect she might be nutritionally deficient. No doctor had mentioned the words "gluten" or "celiac" to us, and we had not heard of *functional* nutritional deficiencies, in which a person can ingest food containing sufficient nutrients but not be able to utilize them effectively. We also didn't know of genetic problems—problems more common in those diagnosed with autism and associated conditions such as bipolar disorder and schizophrenia—in which an individual may not be able to adequately metabolize or synthesize nutrients such as folate (vitamin B_9), cobalamin (vitamin B_{12}), or even cholesterol, all of which are required for the proper functioning of brain connections and the production of many hormones.

Keri had been caught in a perfect storm of genetic and environmental factors, an unfortunate alignment that created a complex pathological condition. Real-life biology is complicated, a fact borne out by studies implicating a multitude of genes that play a role in conditions we call bipolar disorder and schizophrenia, and underscoring the importance of focusing on individualized treatment. Ultimately, it was this focus on the unique needs of Keri the individual, as opposed to her diagnosis of schizoaffective disorder, which led to treatments that ameliorated her symptoms.

The Gluten Connection

When Keri was in her early teens, my father began talking about celiac disease (also called sprue), because some of its possible symptoms matched Keri's. Specific issues that concerned him included hard stools (the opposite is also a symptom), depression, chronic fatigue, bone pain, neurological symptoms, headaches, irritability, and osteoporosis and osteopenia. As he pointed out, there is evidence, some dating back decades, of a higher incidence of celiac diagnosis (and, as we know now, gluten sensitivity) in people diagnosed with schizophrenia than in the general population.[76]

Yet it was not until after Dr. Fredericks ran tests that identified Keri's intestinal malabsorption issues that Greg, I, or Keri herself took this idea seriously. We took it upon ourselves to have her tested for immune-system reactions against gluten and other common sources of food allergies. She also had nutritional DNA testing and DNA testing for celiac and gluten-sensitivity genes.

Genetic and nutrigenomic (genetics relating to the absorption and metabolizing of vitamins and minerals) tests revealed she had two

---

[76] Dohan, 1973; Horrobin, 1981; Johns Hopkins University Bloomberg School of Public Health News Center, 2004; and Ludvigsson, Osby, Ekbom, and Montgomery, 2007.

copies of the genes involved in gluten sensitivity, three genetic variants that would hinder the absorption of calcium, and gene variants (including the MTHFR variant) that hindered her processing (methylation) of a number of critical B vitamins. These results shed some light on problems doctors had already found through other testing.

Additional tests revealed Keri was indeed reacting to gluten, but also to dairy (specifically, to casein—the milk protein in dairy products), soy, and eggs. For her, consuming these foods generated an immune response by increasing the inflammatory proteins in her gut. This inflammation could have contributed to her feeling bad for so much of her life. Once she eliminated the offending foods from her diet, she found great relief. Her inexplicable mini-megacolon and abdominal pain, along with the bloated belly she'd had since toddlerhood, simply dissipated.

True, we had tried food-elimination trials back when she was still a toddler, but we hadn't continued them long enough. Also, at the time she was reacting to so many things and feeling so bad, it was difficult to identify what was causing what.

Keri handled news of her food sensitivities with the same passion and determination with which she faced everything else in her life. Finding a plethora of information about celiac, gluten sensitivity, and other food sensitivities in books and on Internet Web sites, she learned about eating healthfully without the offending foods. A local dietitian[77] helped her choose foods that complied with her restrictions yet ensured diversity and sufficient nutrients. Now her diet consists primarily of minimally processed or unprocessed whole foods—fresh fruits and vegetables and whole grains such as brown and wild rice and quinoa—cooked in a multitude of new ways. As a result, rather than being boring or feeling restrictive, her meals are more creative and diverse than ever before.

If we'd been aware earlier that simply eliminating gluten alleviates symptoms of a psychotic disorder in a subset of patients diagnosed

---

[77] Loiselle, Beth, R.D., author of *The Healing Power of Whole Foods*.

with schizophrenia,[78] or that nearly one-quarter of those diagnosed with schizophrenia (as opposed to a scant three percent of the general population) may have significantly elevated levels of gliadin (antibodies to gluten proteins),[79] we would have tried such a diet even without the testing—or we would have looked into testing sooner.

The plan was for Keri to continue taking supplements while her intestines healed—or perhaps for life, since celiac is correlated with an impaired metabolism of some nutrients. Given her specific biology, coupled with the stress and trauma she'd already experienced from her symptoms, she might need more palliative supplements than someone without such a history. However, to some degree, obtaining the nutrients needed to maintain optimal health is an issue for all of us. Due to modern methods of crop production, transport, and storage, the quality of our food is often compromised, resulting in the loss of many micronutrients. In short, many foods today are simply not packed with the same diversity of vitamins and minerals as in our great-grandparents' day.

Thyroid, Nutrition, and Vitamin D

Since her initial bone density scan at the age of 16-1/2, Keri had visited a bone metabolism specialist yearly for a follow-up scan and a checkup. At 18, the scan showed she was gaining bone mass, and her blood test results prompted only one suggestion from the specialist—tweak her food supplements to contain a little less magnesium. We did. Unfortunately, subsequent scans and blood tests did not always show improvement.

The bone metabolism specialist kept talking about the necessity of Keri achieving better thyroid levels, something we'd worked on for years. Other doctors were concerned about how her thyroid hormones actually functioned in her body. As we learned more, we

---

[78] Kalaydjian, Eaton, Cascella, and Fasano, 2006.
[79] Cascella, et al., 2009.

discovered that the synthesis, conversion, reception, and utilization of even one thyroid hormone is an integrative dance between biology and nutrition. Adequate amounts of nutritives such as selenium, iodine, and tyrosine are needed to produce the thyroid hormone T_4 and convert it into the usable T_3 form. But even when there *is* enough T_3, progesterone, omega-3 fatty acids, and adequate vitamin D are needed for our cells to use it. Keri had been deficient in progesterone and vitamin D, as well as in the thyroid hormones themselves.

Vitamin D, known as the sunshine vitamin, is involved in much more than the functioning of thyroid hormones on a cellular level. It also affects mitochondrial function, and it works in conjunction with calcium to maintain strong bones. Low vitamin D levels are implicated in a multitude of ailments, from autoimmune problems to an increased risk of cancer. In our modern environment, where many of us spend much of our day indoors, people often do not get sufficient vitamin D from the sun. Keri, with her sensitive skin and one skin cancer scare already, was particularly careful not to expose her skin to excess sunlight.

On the other hand, her low vitamin D level was cause for concern. Initially, the GP prescribed 2000iu per day of vitamin D_3. When this dosage failed to raise the levels of this vitamin in her blood, he had her take it in a more easily absorbable gelcap. This didn't alter her levels, either. Another specialist increased the dose fivefold, to 10,000iu per day, but even this megadose failed to substantially impact her blood levels. Finally, she started on a liquid, more highly absorbable form of the vitamin, which quickly worked, allowing her to reduce the dosage.

Implementing dietary changes and adjusting her supplements helped Keri to become less reactive. She no longer had cholinergic urticaria (hives), which gave her increased freedom to be active in the summer heat. Her allergies improved, and she outgrew her extreme allergic responses to poison ivy and poison oak, as well as to mosquito bites, which used to generate tremendous welts. Consequently, she was able to decrease her antihistamine use, which in turn eliminated the need for drops to soothe her antihistamine-induced dry eyes.

A transformation (some days it seemed like a miracle) was unfolding before our eyes. The good news: Keri was increasing her participation in normal activities. The bad news: There were still times when fatigue and migraines slowed her down, causing her to lose days of her life.

Mitochondria

Mitochondria—little powerhouses contained inside every cell of the body—have their own separate DNA, mitochondrial DNA, or mtDNA for short. Mitochondria have been implicated in problems ranging from encephalopathies (brain dysfunctions), including autism, to muscle weakness, seizures, migraines, strokes, and vision impairments. They can affect a single organ, such as the brain, but more often they affect multiple organs or body systems, including muscles.

Mitochondrial dysfunction is frequently observed in the aged and/or in people diagnosed with Parkinson's, Alzheimer's, or severe psychiatric illness, although many doctors do not address this issue. Since the brain accounts for about 20 percent of the body's energy requirement, it has many mitochondria. Numerous factors can influence the function of mitochondria and mitochondrial DNA, including nutrition, medications, environmental toxins, and hormones such as thyroid.

Mitochondrial dysfunction also can be caused by mutations in mtDNA or in a part of a cell's regular (nuclear) DNA that influences the functioning of mtDNA. Or it can be due to what are termed epigenetic factors—problems with the proteins and processes controlling the functioning of DNA.

As mentioned earlier, mtDNA mutations can affect a single organ, one or more organ systems, or the entire body. They can range from subtle to severe, in the worst cases causing premature death. They can cause extreme disability, migraine-like symptoms, seizures, and strokes, even in children. The more subtle dysfunctions with oxidative stress (difficulty mopping up byproducts of metabolic energy production and having an excess of free radicals, which can damage cells) can cause fatigue, migraines, or cognitive decline, and they can mimic symptoms of aging.

I found more information about the necessity of nutritional support for mitochondrial function in children with autism than for those with other biological disorders affecting brain function. In literature on anti-aging and life extension, however, I found much about the effects of nutrition on the mitochondria. Only in retrospect did Greg and I understand how biomedical treatments for young children with autism, and integrative treatment for the elderly—processes perhaps better termed "functional medicine" or healing/treating the function of bodily systems responsible for a person's symptoms—had relevance for Keri. After all, her diagnosis was *mental illness*.

In 2007, when Keri was 19, we consulted Dr. Michael Hall, an anti-aging, integrative medicine specialist at the Life Extension Foundation. This consultation, which took place at my parents' urging, proved to be life-changing.

Keri sat facing Dr. Hall, her service dog nestled at her feet, while he looked over years of lab results carefully tabulated by Dr. Marwil. After some enlightening discussion, during which the doctor drew diagrams and graphs to illustrate his points, he suggested some nutritional supplements and referred us to another specialist in a city near our home, Dr. James Roach.

Keri was already taking a low dosage of melatonin to help her sleep soundly, but her sleep was still disturbed and she woke during the night. Dr. Hall suggested a slightly higher dosage of melatonin in extended-release form, along with a sleep-aid supplement, Nutrasleep, containing GABA, inositol, taurine, valerian, and other ingredients. We dutifully informed her psychiatrist of the changes being made to her regimen.

Amazingly, these small changes significantly reduced her need for Seroquel, her neuroleptic medication. By reducing the dosage of this psychopharmaceutical drug, she gained energy, felt more alert, and was more socially engaged.

Next came an even bigger miracle. Dr. Hall also suggested Keri take a specific, highly absorbable formulation of a supplement called co-enzyme Q10 (also called ubiquinone, CoQ10, and NADH dehydrogenase). CoQ10 is a powerful antioxidant that helps mitochondrial function by relieving the oxidative stress on these powerhouses of the cells. I had read previously about oxidative stress and mitochondrial dysfunction in illnesses that get diagnosed as schizophrenia,[80] but I didn't know how to apply this information to Keri specifically. What I hadn't read was that mitochondrial dysfunction also can be the cause of some children's severe, disabling migraines involving, as Keri's did, blood vessel dilatation—a condition referred to as encephalopathy.

> In addition to evidence that CoQ10 supplementation may help prevent some migraines in some people (a large testing of pediatric patients with migraines showed many of them to be deficient in ubiquinone[a]), melatonin may help as well. Three mg of melatonin has been shown to help prevent migraines in some sufferers, possibly because of its anti-inflammatory and free-radical scavenging effects.[b]
>
> [a] Hershey, et al., 2007.
> [b] Peres, et al., 2004.

Considering all the medications Keri had taken over the years, increasing her dosage of melatonin and adding CoQ10 seemed like minor adjustments. Little did we realize what a difference these "little" changes would make until several months had passed without her having a *single* migraine. By this time, she was leaving her teens behind. She'd had migraines since infancy.

Keri considered migraines to be her most disabling problem—more so, even, than the symptoms of schizoaffective disorder. And I was alarmed by reports appearing in scientific literature and newspapers associating migraines with an increased risk of stroke. So you can

---

[80] Prabakaran, Swatton, Ryan, and Huffaker, et al., 2004.

imagine our relief and gratitude—once her hormone levels were adjusted and nutritional supplements added to assist mitochondrial function and reduce oxidative stress—that her migraines stopped entirely. (As of this writing, researchers are working on even more powerful antioxidants directly targeting mitochondria. The options for those suffering from mitochondrial dysfunction are growing.)[81]

A few months later, Keri's neurologist decided she could slowly and carefully start lowering her Topamax dosage. Once she was taking less of this antiseizure (migraine) medication, her cognition improved. She became more talkative. She found she could do the crossword puzzle in the newspaper. Best of all, her migraines did not return. And at this point, with so many other issues also being addressed, neither did her seizure-like episodes of staring or catatonia, nor even her rare, psychotic-like episodes of fear.

Unraveling the mystery of Keri's sleep disorder was the last remaining challenge in understanding her complex medical history. Its profound impact on her life left us to ponder the thin line between a psychiatric problem and a medical problem causing psychiatric symptoms.

---

[81] Beil, L. 2009.

Chapter 39
Sleep

Addressing Keri's sleep problems proved critical in solving the puzzle of her schizoaffective disorder. Some of her symptoms—nighttime hallucinations, agitation, lethargy, insomnia, hypersomnia, fluctuating cognition, depression, and apparent psychosis—were, at least in part, *a direct result of her sleep disorders*. Sleep problems also had an *indirect* negative effect on her immune and endocrine systems, her emotional well-being, and her stress level. In combination, this plethora of sleep-related issues drastically lowered the quality of her life.

Her periodic hypersomnia episodes, which met the criteria for Kleine-Levin syndrome, had no depression associated with them, although at one time these episodes had been misdiagnosed as a symptom of depression. When reading about possible triggers for Kleine-Levin, I discovered infections, including chicken pox, were frequently mentioned,[82] along with a possible genetic susceptibility.

Sleep, or the lack of it, is inextricably intertwined with health and well-being. Many hormones are made primarily while we sleep. Lack of proper sleep and sleep architecture, including disturbed stages of sleep such as those seen in narcolepsy, can alter hormone production, including growth hormone. Some severe sleep disorders also can affect the immune system, increasing allergies and susceptibility to infections, which could explain why Keri had these issues.

As Keri's other symptoms became resolved, she continued to slowly lower the dosage of Topamax. She also lowered the dosage of Seroquel, her neuroleptic (antipsychotic) medication. By the time she was down to 150 mg of Seroquel per day, she realized her only

---

[82] Arnulf, et al., 2005.

remaining reason for taking it was to treat the non-psychotic symptoms she'd experienced since early childhood—problems with her sleep.

Sleep deprivation leads to an increased secretion of pro-inflammatory cytokines. These substances are elevated in disorders associated with excessive daytime sleepiness, such as sleep apnea, narcolepsy, and idiopathic hypersomnia. An elevation in body-wide inflammation may precede some cases diagnosed as psychiatric.[83]

In addition to impairing immune control, profound sleep disturbances can affect emotional control and frustration tolerance; they also can cause irritability and lead to meltdowns. Studies show that lack of sleep can cause people to have an amplified limbic response involving the amygdala (the part of the brain responsible for the fight or flight response), which causes them to greatly overreact to negative emotional stimuli. Such findings contribute to the idea that some cases of illnesses involving emotional dysregulation, such as bipolar and schizoaffective disorders, rather than having a comorbid sleep problem, may be, in fact, *caused* by sleep dysfunction.[84]

I thought back to Keri's earliest symptoms—sleep issues, pain, allergies, and ear infections. How much did her sleep disorders contribute to her immune and endocrine problems? Did the biological stress on her body trigger negative epigenetic changes that would otherwise have been left dormant?

I will never shake the idea that if Keri's sleep had been addressed *first*—when she was an infant or in early childhood—the entire course of her life might have been changed. Disturbed sleep is an early indicator of a neurological or other problem. It often precedes symptoms of mental illness and may indeed cause the mental illness.[85] It affects growth and immune function. Would Keri have had allergies resulting in intestinal malabsorption, nutritional problems, and

---

[83] Padmos, et al., 2008.
[84] Yoo, S., et al., 2007.
[85] Young, 2009.

osteoporosis, as well as chronic pain, fatigue, and symptoms of aging, if her sleep architecture had been improved as a young child?

> Some non-pharmacological methods to aid sleep and wakefulness (and help with symptoms of depression) are regular exercise and strict sleep/wake schedules. Others, such as broad-spectrum (sun) lights, dawn simulation, and/or high-density negative air ionization (said to simulate fresh country air), can be used seasonally or as needed. Dawn simulation and negative air ionization are considered to act as active antidepressants, without side effects.[a]
>
> Passive, non-pharmacological treatments used to augment pharmacological treatments may be especially useful when a child is unstable. These can include controlling the child's exposure to both light in the daytime and darkness at night. Research is being conducted into the effectiveness of specially tinted, amber-colored lenses to reduce exposure to light in the evening.[b]
>
> [a] Terman, et al., 2006.
> [b] Phelps, 2008.

Keri's profound tiredness was also reflected in her cortisol levels. Cortisol is supposed to be at its lowest in the middle of the night and peak just before we wake to jump-start our bodies into wakefulness. But Keri's levels were lowest first thing in the morning. No wonder she had trouble getting out of bed!

Resolving Keri's sleep issues was complex, involving hormonal interventions and the use of stimulating pharmaceuticals, Wellbutrin and Provigil, in the daytime and nutritional supplements at night.

Wellbutrin, considered an atypical antidepressant, had always made Keri feel more alert, less depressed, less anxious, and less prone to meltdowns. It also made her better able to concentrate and more easily tolerate frustration. For depression, most people use her type of Wellbutrin every 12 hours—morning and night. Keri uses it only in the daytime—one dose at dawn, a second dose after lunch. (The 24-hour extended-release form of this drug didn't work for her.)

We were later surprised to find, while Keri was under the care of Dr. Roach, that safe nutritional supplements could work for her in lieu of Wellbutrin. Fortunately, stopping Wellbutrin was easily accomplished without the horrendous withdrawal effects other psychotropic medications had caused.

Provigil/Nuvigil has been documented as reversing the atypical depression, sleepiness, and REM-sleep propensity attendant in some instances of narcolepsy.[86] In Keri's case, the drug has dramatically improved her daytime wakefulness as well as her mood.

After taking early-morning doses of these stimulating medications, along with her thyroid medications, she sometimes sleeps for another hour, giving them time to kick in.

The addition of supplements—specifically, melatonin and the additional sleep-aid supplement recommended by Dr. Hall, the anti-aging, integrative medicine specialist—helps her to remain asleep at night.

The last of Keri's sleep problems, her disturbed sleep with thrashing, moaning, crying, and horrific dreams, was resolved with the addition of one more nutritional supplement, the amino acid tryptophan. Interestingly, as far back as the early 1960s, studies have shown some gluten-intolerant individuals have diminished metabolism of tryptophan (and some other nutrients), even when on a gluten-free diet.[87]

With the addition of tryptophan, Keri was able to stop taking Seroquel. She'd been on this atypical neuroleptic, however, for more than eight years, and getting off it proved excruciatingly difficult. Beginning a day or so after each minute dosage lowering, she had severe withdrawal symptoms—nausea, vomiting, dizziness, anxiety, mood swings, head pain, and shakiness—that could last for several days. She took amino acids and sometimes a benzodiazepine to help alleviate these symptoms, and eventually the day came when she was able to eliminate the drug entirely and the withdrawal symptoms

---

[86] Rye, et al., 1998.
[87] Kowlessar, et al., 1994.

stopped. Months passed, and then years, with no return of her schizoaffective symptoms.

But if Keri no longer has any symptoms, and she is no longer taking any antipsychotic drugs, then where *is* her psychotic illness? In her psychiatrist's view, after so many years of active symptoms, her schizoaffective disorder is puzzlingly "in remission." Some of her other doctors feel she simply does not have it. One thing on which they all agree is that her illness has always been biological—that is, *medical*—even when it was identified by a psychiatric diagnosis.

Without the sedative, cognition-dulling effects of neuroleptic and antiseizure medications for conditions more effectively treated medically, biomedically, nutritionally, and functionally, Keri is feeling more alive than ever. She is open to the idea that she may need to return to a small amount of either type of these medications in the future. We cannot fix everything. After all, "in remission" does not mean cured. But at least for now, she can revel in the feeling of better health. Not excellent health. But better. *A lot better* than she has ever felt before.

Chapter 40
A Life Restored

Keri walked into the restaurant with her boyfriend and slid gracefully into the booth facing Greg and me. It was strange for us to see her without Kira by her side. It felt equally strange, she said, to *go* somewhere without Kira, and it was going to feel odder still to start classes without the dog. But Kira just didn't have enough work to do to remain a service dog. She lacked focus, because she no longer had to focus on Keri. Having done her job, she is now retired and a much-beloved family pet.

Keri was filled with news. Without the Topamax in her system, she was more verbal—more eloquently talkative—the way she'd been as a youngster. She relished the feeling of "getting my brain back," as she described it, even if not to the level it was before her acute, prolonged psychosis at the age of 12.

The conversation turned to age. Keri used to feel so old, yet now that she was chronologically older—turning 21—she said she felt almost *too* young for that age. She had missed so much. Only now did she feel ready to start taking on the life challenges of a teen facing independence and adult responsibilities.

I thought back to all the problems she had as an infant and a young child, to all the conversations when psychiatrists told us it was biology, not psychology, affecting her brain. Her second psychiatrist had given us information to read about autism, but he hadn't been quite able to put his finger on why. At the time, there wasn't nearly the wealth of research available today, but even then, parents and some scientists had the idea autism was not a mental problem. Instead, autistic kids had a neurodevelopmental, metabolic, immunological, or biological "something" going on. They also had associated behaviors resulting from their frustration, along with various symptoms, some of which were much like Keri's. Now I know Keri shared other traits commonly associated with autism—sensitivities to environmental allergens, food sensitivities, and intestinal malabsorption issues. Maybe her psychiatrist had noticed something subtle yet profound, but science had not yet caught up with his observation. It was only many years later that research began emerging that discussed genetic overlaps between autism and schizophrenia, and the prenatal factors that can contribute to both.

As a young child, Keri had no trait diagnosable as autism, yet her behavior was similar to children with autism spectrum disorder in areas such as a need for consistency, a need for guidance in learning to live with her own biology, hypersensitivity to both internal and external stimuli, allergies, lowered immune function, and even, we know now, particular dietary needs.

After she turned 16, two doctors said her problems were probably on a cellular level—body-wide. Even when she was much younger, pediatricians suspected endocrine problems, yet pediatric endocrinologists did not. Some doctors recognized she needed nutritional supplements and encouraged their use, but they couldn't tell us why. Tests detected she had intestinal malabsorption problems, yet again, nobody suggested how to correct them. In a nutshell, there was no source of comprehensive care.

In many ways, we worked backwards in our efforts to get Keri better. We just hadn't had enough information. We did a lot of things right in attempting to provide her with the nurture she needed to cope with her nature. And we were right to trust in her, respecting her chronic complaints of abdominal pain, fatigue, back pain, shoulder pain, eyesight problems, and so on, in spite of advice from doctors who ignored her symptoms and told us it was in her head. But I shake my head in amazement at how things unfolded. Sleep issues and diet were the *last* things we fixed; they should have been the *first*. We missed her hormone-deficiency problems for years. We tried and expanded upon food supplements only after trying psychological therapy and psychotropic medications—not before.

Unlike many teens and young adults who rebel against the idea they cannot live completely like a Chronically Normal[88]—someone who doesn't need to take medications or nutritional supplements, worry about food choices, or pay attention to sleep cycles—Keri has always accepted these aspects of her particular physiology. Of course, she wishes things were otherwise, but she accepts her biology and tries to work *with* it instead of against it. Is this because she was born the way she is? Is it "better" to be ill as a child than to become ill later in life?

I have pondered this question a lot. On the one hand, Keri grew up with tremendous challenges, challenges that influenced the woman she is today. On the other, she lost much of her childhood. Personality can have a huge impact on how we deal with adversity. Keri's self-motivation, deep thinking, and maturity—even her OCD-ishness—helped a great deal. But ultimately, I believe her ability to understand her brain and her illness has been the most significant contributor to the outcome of her ordeal. If she had not recognized and understood that her brain was affected (i.e., if she hadn't had insight), her life would have been completely different.

Based on old statistics about childhood-onset schizophrenia (COS) or schizoaffective disorder, Keri was destined to suffer permanent deterioration of cognition, emotion, maturity, motivation, and social skills, with ongoing psychosis rendering her mentally impaired for life. Thanks to a combination of modern medicine, modern knowledge, modern tests, modern medications, and modern pharmaceutical-grade food supplements, along with diet modifications based on her specific needs, she has escaped this dire prognosis. Various terms are used for the type of integrated care that helped my daughter, but the approach to such care is the same: individualized medical attention with the goal of treating (and preventing) the underlying causes of a serious, chronic disease, rather than just managing a patient's outermost symptoms.

---

[88] Chronically Normal is a euphemism applied to an individual who does not have a mental illness. Neurotypical, or NT, is another term sometimes used to describe a person with a brain and thought patterns the medical community would dub completely normal.

Even though the psychiatrists in Keri's early life recognized her depression as biological, they felt they had no recourse but to treat it psychiatrically. Since her illness was both severe, and not something psychological that could be helped by therapy, psychiatric medication seemed the only option. At the time, neither Greg nor I were aware of alternative tests or treatments. Yet depression can be a symptom of numerous testable and treatable conditions, including heart disease, hypothyroidism, Cushing's syndrome, vitamin deficiency, inflammatory and autoimmune processes, etc. (see Appendix B: Medical Tests), or it can be a reaction to prolonged pain, immune stress, cancer treatment . . . you get the idea. Treating only the outermost symptom—depression, may alleviate stress from that symptom, but it will not address the underlying cause(s). Few doctors look to see if there are other clues indicating a larger picture. My daughter calls such treatment the Band-Aid approach. Yet sometimes this is all we have. Sometimes it may be good enough. Other times it is not.

> Nonprofit organizations, including the Institute for Functional Medicine, the Life Extension Foundation, and Defeat Autism Now! along with pockets of scientists around the globe, are leading the way in scientific, nutritional, and integrative biomedical and functional medicine research. The emphasis of these groups is on wellness using pharmaceutical, nutritional, hormonal, exercise, and lifestyle approaches scientifically shown to benefit people.
>
> This is not "alternative medicine."

Testing is often required to uncover biological clues. In some instances, knowing what tests are needed, putting together a total picture, and determining appropriate treatments can be simple. At other times it can be a monumental task. Parents need more guidance than what is available in books. We need knowledgeable doctors to comprehensively test, analyze, and guide treatments. We hear about them here and there—those who get extra training; those who are willing to collaborate with other doctors—but they seem few and far between.

As Keri's schizoaffective symptoms dissipated with an *integrative* and *integrated*, functional, medical/biomedical approach to her treatment, we had to question the meaning of her schizoaffective order diagnosis. This label did not describe a cause, only a set of symptoms. Ultimately, it did guide us to the most effective treatment for her, but it did not indicate which precise set of biological problems comprised *her* set of symptoms, all of which were lumped under the broad category of schizoaffective disorder.

The *Diagnostic and Statistical Manual of Mental Disorders* (*DSM*) includes the instruction that psychiatric labels of major depressive disorder, schizophrenia, bipolar disorder, and schizoaffective disorder should not be given if the symptoms are caused by known medical conditions. To me, this means such diagnoses are to be given only after everything else that can cause a patient's symptoms has been considered and eliminated. There are so many conditions to look for, yet often only minimal testing is done. Sometimes, no testing is done at all!

In Keri's case, her schizoaffective disorder diagnosis resulted from many contributing problems. The earliest was profoundly disturbed sleep, although the underlying causes of this condition—possibly inflammation, and even lack of proper intestinal flora—may have preceded it. Even at the age of 20, with her schizoaffective disorder in remission, she found that reducing her sleep medication, i.e., the nutritional supplements that help to regulate her sleep patterns, led to her quickly becoming irritable, hypersensitive, and tearful, just as she had been when young. Looking back, she marveled she'd managed to stay as sane as she had, given the chronic, untreated sleep disturbances of her childhood.

We had long suspected that Keri's migraines, fatigue, sleep problems, dizziness, hallucinations, nightmares, sensitivity to pain and sound, falling down, muscle and joint pain, abdominal pain, lethargy, fatigue, and depression were all somehow connected. But the medical machine seemed to work well only when the answer was simple: one symptom, one diagnosis, one treatment.

338   It's Not *Mental*

Perhaps Keri's underlying issue was the mitochondrial dysfunction affecting her hypothalamus and causing body pain, allergies, immune dysfunction, sleep disorders, endocrine problems, and other escalating symptoms. Maybe it was her sleep disorder or celiac/gluten sensitivity that caused oxidative stress and mitochondrial dysfunction. We cannot know for sure. We do know that inappropriate treatment (the initial SSRI antidepressant and ADHD treatment instead of treatment for sleep, immune system, and hormonal issues) added to her sleep deprivation, escalated her anxiety, and precipitated her acute major psychotic break.

In her book *Probability Moon*, about a group of people who lived far in the future, author Nancy Kress creates a fascinating character. Other characters in the book consider this fellow a bit odd because he checks his hormone and body chemistry levels several times a day and is constantly adjusting them. To those who don't feel a need to have their chemical levels just right, his behavior seems obsessive. When the character is forced into a situation in which he can no longer check and adjust his chemicals, his brain function deteriorates. It turns out he has what today would be called schizophrenia, but in a future where everyone responsibly regulates his own chemistry, no one knows about his problem until he can not longer adjust his levels.

Some people view the anti-aging component of integrative medicine as having a goal similar to Nancy Kress's depiction of a futuristic, self-regulated neuropharmacology, except with a more holistic approach to wellness. Of course this would not work for every illness we currently label as schizophrenia. After all, some cases of schizophrenia may be due to parasitic infections; others are associated with a distinct loss of brain tissue, as visible on an MRI. Nevertheless, I found intriguing the author's contemplation of a future where at least one type of schizophrenia is so well-regulated.

In the world of the present, even more intriguing is a functional approach that seeks to help the body heal and regulate itself. This biopsycho-social treatment model is extremely important for long-term, chronic conditions, including diabetes, bipolar disorder, cancer, schizophrenia, epilepsy, autism, hypopituitarism, multiple sclerosis, and more. In fact, this is the model parents use for raising *all* children—we just don't usually have a need to label it "treatment."

Early on, before we had a method to help Keri's biology, Greg and I used the "psycho" (psychological/cognitive) portion of this model. This involved helping our daughter learn to cope with her sensitivities, pain, sleep disturbances, hallucinations, nightmares, feelings of irritability, and fatigue. We taught her words for feelings most children have no need to describe. We guided her to appropriate outlets for expression of feelings young children should not have to endure. We helped her to accept her condition and limitations without anger, to continue her education (which can help maintain cognition), and to foster her mental health, self-confidence, and self-esteem.

The "social" aspect of the model involved reliance on the strong family and social supports she already had, though many of the actions we took—choosing low-stress school environments with accommodations, giving her space, acceptance, and understanding—we did intuitively, without knowing they were part of any specific treatment. Keri appreciated that we separated the wonderful child she was from the horrific condition she had.

The social part of the model also included helping her foster friendships, even though she was often unable to participate in life. She was allowed to ease into adulthood without pressure, slowly learning the skills she missed during her earlier teens. Her dog was also an aide in this realm, assisting her cognitively, psychologically, and socially as well as physically.

The "bio" portion of the model was by far the most complex and puzzling. As our knowledge grew, the biological treatments changed and we found ourselves re-examining puzzle pieces from long ago.

Integrative, functional, biomedical (or anti-aging) medicine's approach is to do an initial assessment very much like the one the endocrinologist Dr. Fredericks did for Keri, and which an increasing number of treatment centers and doctors now perform for fibromyalgia, chronic fatigue syndrome, the non-behavioral aspects of autistic spectrum disorder, and other chronic neuroendocrinological, autoimmune, and neuroimmune disorders. First they run a set of blood and urine tests that look at a broad spectrum of hormonal, nutritional, and metabolic panels. They then try to move the person toward a more optimal balance through exercise, diet, bio-identical hormone replacements, pharmaceutical medications, and nutritional supplements. In other words, they do whatever is needed to get the body back to normal based on function. In this mode, the focus is not on age or arbitrary, non-testable diagnoses based on a list of symptoms. In the bio-psycho-social model, the focus is on wellness.

When we started down the path of medical (as opposed to psychiatric) treatments for Keri, our aim was simply to help her feel better physically. It was not to use "alternative medicine" or to get her off psychotropic medication. It was not to cure her schizoaffective disorder. We were searching for answers to puzzling problems. We wanted everything that could be treated to be treated so our daughter could have the best life possible. We knew she always would have limitations, but we felt her life deserved to be as good as it could be within those limitations.

We were thrilled for her when she began feeling better physically. We never expected that by addressing all of the biological problems within our power to address, her psychotic disorder would, as the psychiatrist put it, go into remission.

Keri herself made the necessary dietary changes—with support from the entire family. She exercises daily, takes hormones, supplements, and medications. Her bones are strengthening. Her muscles are getting stronger. Aches, pains, abdominal distress, and a general feeling of malaise are no longer a chronic part of her life. She looks healthy, and she feels better than she has ever felt. As her body continues to heal, she is looking forward to feeling even better.

Everything, of course, is not fixable. Conditions can be treated, but never perfectly. Sleep disorders fluctuate in intensity, and even with the most scrupulous of treatments, it is unrealistic—all other things being equal—to expect that someone with a sleep disorder will have the same amount of energy as a person without this condition. The same holds true for endocrine problems. We cannot mimic Mother Nature. Keri still has some minor tics, and she has her slow writing disability, for which she compensates by working harder, smarter, and more than someone without it, and for which she still has an accommodation at college.

She works at staying healthy, taking many pills each day, at many times during the day. One of them must be taken on an empty stomach. Others must be taken with food, some when she wakes up, some when she goes to sleep. She schedules exercise time religiously to maintain her strength and bone density and to keep her weight down, since weight gain is often a side effect of the very hormones she takes artificially to replace the ones she lacks. She has extra grocery shopping to do for fresh food, and extra food preparation time since she eats very little already-prepared or processed foods.

The idea of never being able to have children, which caused her much grief in the past, is now an open question as opposed to a certainty. Endocrinologically, the answer we were given as to whether she could someday become pregnant and deliver a healthy baby was "Yes, but maybe with assistance." But there are other areas of consideration beside hormones. Her thin bones need to be overcome before she can safely carry a baby. And she would want to be off the last remaining prescription medication she takes for her sleep disorder. Is this possible? The doctors believe it may be, though she could spend a large portion of her pregnancy sleeping. There are many unknowns. But there *is* hope.

Keri still has fragile health and limited energy, but she is living a fairly typical, semi-independent, college-student life. With her hallucinations and seizure-like episodes long gone, she is even learning to drive. She is also assuming ever-increasing responsibility for her life and health. Now, instead of me researching everything for her, she researches doctors' recommendations herself and informs me about the pros, cons, and wisdom of pursuing a course of action. She participates in NAMI, feeling well enough to give back and help others. She still needs assistance in dealing with medical details, medical bills, medical insurance, and the insurance appeals process.

But then, these issues are often extremely stressful for anyone with a chronic medical condition.

She has completed two associates degrees—one in the sciences, that other in the arts. At the age of 21, she is working toward a bachelor of science in dietetics, hoping to turn her strong interest into a career.

She has a renewed interest and personal enjoyment in playing a musical instrument, something I thought was gone forever. She is looking forward to marriage and being a mother, something on which she had given up. In other words, she has a life, a life filled with love, family and friends, school, hobbies, goals, motivation, and, above all, hope.

There are no guarantees in life. But Keri is grabbing all the fullness and joy she can. She is her own woman.

As it should be.

Epilogue

By the time Keri was 18 years old, she had received more than 15 diagnoses to explain her plethora of symptoms, including the diagnosis of schizoaffective disorder, a *mental illness*. Even though her GP has opined that when someone receives this many diagnoses, it tends to mean doctors don't really know what is going on, once she was transported from the realm of the *medical health system* to the much murkier world of the *mental health system*, several things changed:

- Keri (and to some degree, our entire family) was subject to the view of much of society, including some members of the medical profession, that her ills were psychological, the result of some character flaw, poor parenting, or abuse.
- Potential causes for her legitimate physical symptoms were not investigated, or not investigated thoroughly, or, in the worst cases, dismissed as being "just in her head."
- With no system of comprehensive care to identify biological sources of her mental issues, she was prescribed multiple drugs, many of which had side effects sometimes worse than the symptoms they were intended to alleviate.

Don't get me wrong. I am forever grateful to the pharmaceutical companies and scientists who develop psychotropic medications, and to the many conscientious doctors who helped Keri within the confines of their particular specialties. However, the structure of our medical system, coupled with diagnoses such as bipolar and schizoaffective disorder that describe a list of symptoms rather than defining an underlying cause, make it almost impossible to deal with the patient as a whole person or to design a treatment plan based on that individual's particular physiology. In short, the system is broken.

If we are to properly care for children like Keri in the future, we must look beyond relying solely on traditional psychiatric and behavioral treatment and move toward a truly collaborative approach that integrates all the research knowledge and medical/biomedical testing and treatment at our disposal. And we need to tailor such treatment to each patient's specific biological and emotional needs. In many cases, such an approach will still include cognitive therapies, behavioral therapies, and/or emotional therapies, which may be needed to deal with comorbid problems, damage done to a person's brain or psyche, or dysfunctional coping strategies an individual may have developed while sick. Under such a system, each patient should receive the best care available—not the best care available for a predefined set of symptoms, not the best care available from a particular medical specialty, but the best comprehensive care the profession can offer for that particular individual.

For years, my husband and I focused on helping our daughter live with her mental illness. Once we shifted our focus to her physiology and biological processes, we had no idea how (relatively) rapidly and profoundly her life was going to change, and how much better she was going to get. In healing her body, her "broken brain" mended as well. And as she got better, Keri badly wanted to know the answer to two questions: "What?" and "Why?" *What* actually went wrong with her biology, and *why* did it happen? The state of medical knowledge is not yet deep or broad enough to answer these questions, though the "what," her GP suggested, might ultimately turn out to be something inside her particular cellular structures, possibly resulting from a confluence of multiple DNA loci. Sadly, until more is known, definitive answers to both "what" and "why" will have to wait.

In the meantime, medical science cannot fix all of Keri's ills. She is not cured, but effective treatments based on research and tests have improved her health, her quality of life, her ability to go to school, and, ultimately, her contribution to society as a tax-paying, fully participating citizen. Perhaps, if the right things had been addressed—immunologically and nutritionally (dietary changes, probiotics, supplements for gluten intolerance/food sensitivities and sleep)—at infancy or during toddlerhood, many of the problems she developed down the road never would have happened. We may never know.

Comprehensive, integrated treatment comes at a price, and some people may argue it would not be cost-effective, that doctors do not have enough time to spend on these children, that testing costs too much. In the long run, I would counter, it is far cheaper for insurance companies and society at large to pay for testing and individualized care up front than to pay—perhaps over a lifetime—for repeated hospitalizations, residential treatment centers, the side effects of inappropriate medications, and disability support, not to mention the loss of tax revenue from the patient who is unable to earn a living due to illness, and the loss of productivity and income from a family taking care of an incapacitated child who grows up to become an incapacitated adult.

One cause for the financial burden many families must bear when trying to find treatment for their child is the current distinction between *medical* and *mental* health coverage. As the system stands today, it is worse than absurd. For example, one pediatric endocrinologist in Keri's life insisted all necessary endocrinological testing be done by the "prescribing physician," which in this case was the psychiatrist. Yet psychiatric appointments and related hospitalizations do not have to be covered by some health insurance policies because these services are not considered medical. It doesn't matter that some illnesses we call mental *are* medical. Treatment is not covered, even if the psychiatrist is performing the combined functions of endocrinologist, sleep disorder specialist, and neurologist—monitoring the patient for diabetes, hypothyroidism, sleep disorders, and more.

If such a division were made between *emotional* health and *medical* health, perhaps it would be more logical. Under emotional health would be treatments like talk therapy for dealing with traumas in one's life, marital counseling, etc. Therapy to help patients and their families learn to live with medical disorders such as diabetes, lupus, or cases of bipolar disorder or schizophrenia would fall under *medical* health and should be treated no differently than seeing a nutritionist for help in dealing with a metabolic disorder. Even talk therapy, if needed to rehabilitate, restructure, and strengthen parts of the brain, as in some cases of traumatic brain injury, depression, bipolar disorder, schizophrenia, autism spectrum disorder, or stroke, should be considered medical, rather than emotional, intervention.

I also do not want the type of treatment to be dictated by pharmaceutical or insurance companies, but, instead, by sane, integrative medical practices that treat each person as a functional human organism with unique physical properties. I want doctors to be as knowledgeable about environmental and food allergies, sensitivities, and nutritional support as they are about the medicines coming out of the pharmaceutical companies. And I want medical doctors to have the freedom to use anything in their arsenal, even if it is "off-label." The doctor is the one with intimate knowledge of the patient's problems—not the FDA or the insurance company.

Testing

As parents, we must recognize that prognoses for *all* diagnoses are based on past statistical data—data that may already be obsolete because of medical, functional, integrative, pharmaceutical, herbal, nutritional, dietary, hormonal, cognitive, and other therapeutic advances. More important, statistical data cannot be applied to any single individual. Parents need to acknowledge these realities and take control of their children's care in a way my husband, Greg, and I did not until it was almost too late.

The types of issues we struggled to understand for so many years are not unique to our daughter. For example, when reviewing recent research into gluten elimination and "remission" of symptoms of schizophrenia in a subset of patients, I was astonished to find that research in this area dates back almost 30 years. Yet no doctor ever mentioned gluten to us, let alone the possibility of a gluten intolerance/schizophrenia connection. This same lack of communication was repeated in relation to hormonal deficiencies and sleep disorders. No wonder the endocrinologists didn't concern themselves with our daughter's hormonal issues. If most members of the medical community aren't paying attention to the potential connection between physiology and psychiatric symptoms, it is easy to blame all physical symptoms on a psychiatric diagnosis, which leaves the psychiatrist to handle everything.

Medical science is far from being able to monitor and adjust all of the body's hormones, neurohormones, and necessary metabolic components to the same degree, for example, that insulin is monitored and adjusted for diabetics. Even pituitary and adrenal hormones are not available in a fashion that exactly matches Mother Nature.

Even so, a deeper understanding of the phrase *it's not mental* can change perspective. We can grasp more fully that a person's symptoms are the result of real medical problems—even if we don't know the exact nature of these problems or how to cure them. We can attempt to understand a child's (or an adult's, for that matter) unique biology and bring it into balance. We are no longer limited to a specific set of medications designated for mental illness.

I want children to be treated by a team of specialists, because it is only by combining our knowledge and treating patients collaboratively that we will make headway. (Note: Just because a clinic or medical center has many doctors and specialists on staff, it is not a given that they work *together* to investigate and solve cases.)

In addition to a GP or pediatrician, specialists, including nutritionists, endocrinologists, neurologists, immunologists, geneticists, therapists, psychiatrists (well-versed in these other fields), and integrative medical doctors need to be intimately involved in the diagnosis and treatment of children displaying brain symptoms that have no psychological cause. If doctors are not comfortable with this paradigm, or if they work in a facility that doesn't offer and support a collaborative approach, then they should not waste patients' time. Tell them up front and refer them to a facility that offers care for the entire person.

I want endocrinologists, especially, to step up to their responsibilities. If a child is under the care of a psychiatrist, there is no reason why the endocrinologist and psychiatrist should not work together to handle hormonal aspects of the patient's illness. In some cases, it may even turn out these "hormonal aspects" *are* the patient's illness, or, at the very least, may be exacerbating it.

The same goes for neurologists and sleep-disorder specialists. These physicians need to keep abreast of the latest research; it is not enough to rely solely on the scant information presented in medical schools that may gloss over nutrition in psychiatric presentations. Nor can such doctors depend exclusively for their knowledge on information from pharmaceutical representatives. Many aspects of illness—and wellness—are *not* addressed by prescription medications.

I want extensive biological testing to become routine. After all, when we don't know the real cause of an illness, we are treating blindly. I also want a comprehensive protocol established for testing children who exhibit sleep problems, excessive crying, or even subtle brain dysfunction. The focus of this protocol should begin in infancy and should list *all* known possible biological problems to be considered, along with appropriate tests to be performed for each. (A prime example: Testing for possible thyroid involvement should include more than just tests for TSH before ruling out thyroid hormone problems!)

Some children have a genetic makeup that makes them sensitive to a lack of nutrients in food (a problem perhaps more prevalent now than in the past). Some may seem to be getting sufficient nutrition, yet some metabolic difference may be preventing sufficient absorption or cellular utilization of the nutrition (micronutrients). Some are sensitive to heavy metals, chemicals in plastics, and God-only-knows what else. Some react to our lit-up homes at night, or to a lack of sunshine. Some of us have ancestors from cold climates, but we now live in warmer areas. Others came from desert environments, and we now live in humid ones. Any number of these factors, or all of them, may play a role, but we'll never know unless we look at the whole picture—not just genetics, and not just epigenetics.[89] We need to get out of the mode of limiting research to "populations" and start to treat each person as an individual, not just a set of symptoms with a label. It's terrific that 60 percent of people respond positively to medication "X," but this statistic is completely irrelevant to my child if she is made ill by medication "X" and really needs medications "Q" and "R," along with nutrients "W" and "Z."

Because of the fluctuating nature of their illnesses, once children like Keri are on medications, they should continue to receive periodic, comprehensive testing. Psychotropic medications affect hormones, neurohormones, neurotransmitters, histamines, etc. Hormones are responsible for growth, bone development, sexual development, and metabolism. Since a child's health can be compromised by the same medications he or she must take to maintain health, we are doing our children a grave disservice by not monitoring their health on a regular basis. Furthermore, because it is nearly impossible to take a child in for blood testing when he/she is most symptomatic, mobile units should come to the child's home to draw blood or to transport the child for blood draws.

Last but not least, since these tests are intended to determine, evaluate, or monitor *medical* problems, *medical* insurance should pay for them. In Appendix B: Medical Tests, I've included some of the tests Keri had, as well as tests recommended by others.

All of this may sound like I'm asking for a lot, but if we want to effectively diagnose, treat, and, someday, potentially prevent the complex issues presented by these children, a lot is required.

In the future, I am hopeful many people now being diagnosed with schizophrenia, bipolar disorder, or schizoaffective disorder will receive completely different medical diagnoses based on the underlying

---

[89] Epigenetics are elements influencing genetic expression that are not due directly to genes coded within chromosomal DNA. Such elements include mitochondrial DNA, histones, and DNA-methylation, all of which can be affected by environmental factors such as toxins, nutrition, and stress.

metabolic, endocrinological, and neurological physiology of their specific illness, determined, in part, by comprehensive testing administered in an integrated medical environment.

Comprehensive, Collaborative, Integrated Treatment

Even those individuals with a "legitimate" psychiatric diagnosis may have other things wrong with them. For example, a friend of mine with PTSD was taken to the emergency room three times. On the first two occasions, her PTSD and anxiety were blamed for what she kept saying was a problem with her heart. On her last trip to the emergency room, she nearly died before doctors found she had a congenital heart defect requiring emergency surgery. This woman *did* have a legitimate mental (psychiatric) diagnosis, but she also had something wrong with her heart!

Keri's medical care ultimately required a team of doctors that included neurologists, endocrinologists, allergists, psychiatrists, a bone metabolism specialist, her GP, and M.D.s who are integrative (anti-aging) specialists. Also involved were a chiropractor, gynecologist, and an expressive arts therapist, along with advice from an occupational therapist and education specialists. Fortunately, the majority of these professionals were not averse to conducting teleconferences with each other, but it took many years to find the right mix of individuals with both specialized knowledge and a collaborative philosophy.

Some people with schizophrenia spectrum illnesses show decreased brain tissue on an MRI. Some don't. Some have elevated indicators of infectious agents. Some don't. Some have genetic or biological markers for the schizophrenia spectrum illness. Some don't. Researchers around the globe are working to isolate these factors. In the meantime, I want the medical community to quit passing the buck whenever the brain is involved.

When she was a young girl, Keri used to play flute and violin to entertain patients at a nearby Shriners Hospital for Children. Spacious and airy, with friendly faces, diverse entertainment, and many recreational facilities, the hospital is a long-term-care setting for children undergoing extensive orthopedic or burn rehabilitation. At the time, I admired it a lot, but on my next visit—accompanying a school group after Keri had been a patient in a local behavioral hospital—I viewed it with sorrow, confusion, and envy. *This* is the type of place needed for children recovering from a brain illness, I thought. They, too, require long-term treatment and recovery. They, too, are emotionally fragile, traumatized, and prone to discouragement, confusion, and depression.

Children with disorders affecting brain function need access to safe and supportive hospital facilities where they can undergo comprehensive testing and/or stabilize and recover from major depressive and psychotic episodes. They deserve more than traditional behavioral hospitals and psychiatric wards. And the length of stay or type of testing must not be governed by an insurance company that decides, for example, that three days is enough when it might take three *months* to make a meaningful recovery.

Research and "Alternative" Medicine

In my quest to solve my daughter's puzzle I explored many different avenues. Some trails were called "alternative"; others, with seemingly no more convincing evidence, were considered "mainstream." As an example, one condition I read about is called pyroluria.[90] I was intrigued because the symptoms of this disorder matched many of the symptoms Keri experienced, and there were no symptoms listed she didn't have. As I read more about pyroluria, it seemed to fit with the inexplicable fact that Keri needed nutritional supplements to stave off her symptoms and that she suffered a

---

[90] Pyroluria (also called malvaria or mauve factor) is a controversial medical diagnosis alleged to be caused by the presence of excess pyrroles in the body, especially when under stress.

recurrence of those symptoms after several weeks of no longer taking the supplements (see Appendix C: Charting Symptoms). In my investigation, I uncovered credible research that found pyroluria is a fairly common condition in certain populations, including some diagnosed with schizophrenia,[91] just as metabolic syndrome is also more common in that population. Some doctors treat pyroluria; others don't.

Is this a real diagnosis? If it *is* real, then it would affect which supplements a person with the condition should and should not take. If it's real, testing for it should be routine and research should be done to learn more about it. Since such research is often propelled by pharmaceutical companies, however, it may be unfortunate no pharmaceutical medication is needed to correct this condition.

Pyroluria is listed under alternative medicine. But it's a diagnosis, not a treatment. How can a *diagnosis* be alternative medicine? I decided to have Keri tested; the results were negative. Later I met other parents whose children, diagnosed with symptoms of bipolar and other psychiatric disorders, had tested positive for pyroluria. These parents reported excellent results from treating the condition.

While the medical community dismisses many treatments (and, apparently, sometimes entire diagnoses) as alternative, many people may benefit from research to discover *why* these particular treatments work in the subgroup for which they do work. We need to learn more in order to develop diagnostic criteria for determining who falls into these subgroups. Individual nutritional needs must be taken out of the realm of "alternative" medicine. Medicine should be *medicine*.

There is no end to the number of paths a desperate parent can wander getting his/her child tested and trying different medications and supplements. People will argue they want to stick with medications that have been proven to help, but the truth is, no pharmaceutical for a psychotic disorder has been proven to help a specific child until tested on that child. We do not yet routinely implement genetic,

---

[91] McGinnis, 2004, and Bibus, 2000.

metabolic, and nutritional tests, coupled with the latest science-based biomedical research to help determine in advance which medication or supplement, and at what dosage, may help a specific individual. Because we don't know enough, many of our kids feel like guinea pigs. Each experiment begins anew, with a survey sample of one.

Diagnostic Software

I find it incredible that computer databases and software are not widely used to *help* doctors determine what illnesses a person might have and what additional tests might aid in diagnosis. Almost 30 years ago, when I was still in graduate school in computer science, we already had expert systems (also known as artificial intelligence [AI], because the software could "learn") that were capable of helping with diagnoses. Even having access to a simple relational database, one that keeps track of all illnesses in connection with each other and to all possible symptoms of those illnesses, could be useful in controlling medical costs as well as reducing the years wasted while patients' illnesses go undiagnosed or misdiagnosed.

Expert systems *are* in use today. Small versions learn individual shopping preferences so advertisers can target defined audiences. I played "Twenty Questions" with an amazing expert system online that was learning from people around the world. Think how powerful a major medical expert system could be today if it had been implemented years ago and doctors had been adding information ever since. If this technology is to be made as useful as it could be, it needs to be used not just within individual hospitals, but by *all* doctors. As a start, numerous people could simply "train" the system by adding existing case studies. (Yes, there is a learning curve for the software, but we have to start sometime.)

One reason these databases are so urgently needed is that a doctor cannot make a diagnosis unless he or she consciously *thinks* of that diagnosis. And no matter how excellent the doctor is, he/she cannot think of everything.

Sophisticated computer software (such as expert systems) could actually lead doctors through a thought process that asks about symptoms and test results. Such a review could allow them to consider symptoms they might not have even looked for and to order whatever tests are necessary to resolve unanswered questions. Of course, not every illness would be built in, but the greatest thing about expert systems is that they *learn*. With a centralized system, available on the Internet, each time a doctor discovered something new and added it, every doctor using the expert system could access the new information immediately.

If expert systems were augmented with a growing database of both pharmaceutical and non-pharmaceutical treatments that ameliorated conditions based on testing profiles—not just on diagnoses—what a wealth of information could be garnered for the benefit of humanity!

This technology would not be a substitute for diagnostic testing. It would not take the place of a doctor's keen observations and ultimate judgment. But it would help make sense of testing, symptoms, and treatments, and it would keep each doctor (and each parent) from having to reinvent the wheel.

Such a system would be especially helpful in cases now thought to be rare. (Right now, any child with chronic pain of an unknown cause, hallucinations, sleep disturbances, and/or incessant crying has a good chance of being put into the rare category.)

For complex symptoms, even a simple relational database would be useful if it were large enough. For instance, suppose I asked the system to find illnesses matching the word "fatigue"? No doubt I'd get back a long list of possible illnesses, which wouldn't be very useful. But if I added other symptoms to my query, the list generated would be further refined. It might still be large, but it would at least offer potentially relevant avenues for a doctor (and patient) to investigate. Although, in my opinion, a database this basic should be considered archaic by now, we don't have access to even this simple entity.

The potential downside of expert systems and relational databases is this: Lack of a particular symptom or symptoms doesn't mean someone doesn't have a particular illness. Take Wilson's disease, which on rare occasions gets misdiagnosed as schizophrenia. *Until other testing is done, hallucinations can be the only noticeable symptom of Wilson's.* On the other hand, a person can have Wilson's and never have a hallucination.

I cannot know my child might have central hypothyroidism, Kleine-Levin syndrome, gluten-sensitivity, narcolepsy, or a functional nutritional deficiency if I don't already know these terms and/or associate them with obscure symptoms. I can look up symptoms on Internet search engines and read for days without ever coming across the correct term. Instead, I am most likely to encounter the most obvious diagnosis for the most salient feature—schizophrenia for hallucinations, for example—regardless of accuracy.

On the other hand, once I know the name of a disease or disorder I have a diagnostic possibility, which then allows me to learn more about symptoms, testing, and treatment options.

Most of the medical diagnostic "expert systems" available for sale on the Internet are not representative of the software I am advocating. These systems are "wizards," which, while efficient at collecting and categorizing data, are *not* capable of learning. Such systems have their benefits, but they are of limited help for complex cases.

Advocacy

Less than 100 years ago, many children with hallucinations or other symptoms of brain dysfunction were locked in attics or upstairs bedrooms, out of sight while, in many cases, they truly went "out of their minds." Compared to these conditions, both the medical profession and society have come a long way. But there is so much farther to go. This is why I remain an advocate for children. This is why I volunteered at the Child and Adolescent Bipolar Foundation (CABF), and on various Internet discussion boards on childhood mental health and mental illness. It is why I trained as a National Alliance on Mental Illness (NAMI) volunteer support group leader and educator. I do it to give back. I do it to lend support to others, as others once gave support to me. I am only one tiny pebble, but I am hoping that my miniscule ripples will help someone, somewhere, in some small way. The care and nurturing of a child like Keri can be exhausting for individual parents, but the collective power generated by all who are interested in the well-being of such children is *awesome*.

The Stigma of Mental Illness

There are those who do not understand why some of us reject the euphemism *mental illness* in favor of terms like *neurobiological disorder* (a biological, non-psychological problem affecting the brain) to identify the type of depression, bipolar disorder, and schizophrenia with which Keri and others like her are diagnosed. Calling it something different, they say, doesn't change what it is—it's still *mental*.

But is it?

When a child's problems are non-psychological, modifying the term *illness* with the word *mental* is both unnecessary and often detrimental to the child's physical and emotional health and well-being. Children can sometimes accept they have an *illness*, even when they do not perceive it as mental. They know their sleep is messed up, that they see things other people don't, that their tummy hurts, their head hurts. They may be more likely to be compliant with treatment if they know they have an illness like any other, rather than stressing that their illness is a mental one.

Emotional and psycho-social therapies can help a child (or adult) cope with illness during treatment and when there is no cure. Rehabilitative and cognitive therapies can help patients regain brain function and improve their quality of life. They also can improve the mental health of a child who would otherwise be deteriorating under the strain of his or her illness. In fact, when coping with horrific symptoms, *above-average* mental health may be needed.

People with illnesses for which we have no cure—whether such illnesses are deemed psychiatric or medical—live with a level of uncertainty and pain most people can't fathom. I continue to be impressed by the astonishing strength of spirit in Keri and others battling illnesses affecting their brains—mental illnesses—who have managed to come out of the bowels of hell with spirit and mind intact. In fact, survivors of these disorders are some of the most mentally healthy people I know. They were mentally healthy when they became ill. That they remain as functional as they are is a testament to their mental strength.

It's *Medical*

As a teenager, my older daughter Candace also was diagnosed with a mental illness, first depression, then with bipolar disorder. After 13 years of psychotropic medications, repeated hospitalizations, and still no stability, the psychiatrist ran out of options. As he was about to start randomly prescribing previously tried drugs, Candace decided it was time to start down the same road her little sister had—biomedical testing and treatment. She switched GPs and eventually left her psychiatrist. She was found to have—not exactly the same issues, but the same *suite* of issues as her sibling. She was treated for a sleep disorder, received increased thyroid hormone, took food supplements, changed her diet according to the results of a food allergy test, and switched from synthetic to desiccated thyroid hormone. Stability at last!

Both my daughters' journeys raise the issue of the inherent danger of treating according to a set of diagnostic codes, which are based solely on symptoms rather than causes. Most medical insurances pay only for medications approved for specific diagnoses. Yet many mental illnesses, such as schizophrenia, bipolar disorder, and depression, should be considered placeholder diagnoses—merely temporary—while trying to find the underlying cause, whether it be a rare genetic duplication or deletion only a few people with that diagnosis have, or a metabolic disorder that may occur in more people.

Hopefully, such physical illnesses affecting brain function, currently labeled based on symptoms, will, someday, have their medical cause(s) determined in each individual. Someday.

In the meantime, it is incumbent upon us as individuals to become better educated and to seek the medical care our children deserve.

For my daughters, life is finally good. But I want it to be *better*, and not just for them. We always want improvement. It is a human failing, and a human greatness.

Appendix A: The Thyroid Connection

A few years after we learned that Keri's brain, along with the rest of her body, was suffering from a thyroid hormone deficiency, I came across a series of medical articles addressing the potential relationship between thyroid imbalances and psychiatric symptoms. The first, titled "Identifying Hyperthyroidism's Psychiatric Presentations,"[92] discussed the possible pituitary/thyroid involvement in a variety of psychiatric symptoms and suggested a thorough pituitary/thyroid workup be done on psychiatric patients.

The author, Thomas Geracioti Jr., M.D., is a psychiatrist and specialist in neuroendocrinology. Symptoms of *hyperthyroidism*, he wrote, can mimic those of schizophrenia and bipolar disorder, including psychosis, paranoia, anxiety, social withdrawal, intrusive thoughts of violence or bizarre sexual ideation, cognitive impairment, apathy, depression, mania, irritability, and emotional lability (instability). Patients with these psychiatric conditions can have a low (subclinical) level of hyperthyroidism; or, of course, someone with high thyroid hormone can have a psychiatric condition. Even after effectively treating a hyperthyroid condition, the author warned, residual psychiatric symptoms can persist for years.

The article concludes with a list of blood tests necessary to determine if hyperthyroidism might be causing, or contributing to, psychiatric symptoms.

When I read another article by the same author, "Identifying Hypothyroidism's Psychiatric Presentations,"[93] I felt he'd hit the nail on the head as far as Keri's case was concerned. Finally, I was seeing in writing what Keri and so many others had experienced. I dearly wished this information had been mandatory reading for every

---

[92] Geracioti, Dec. 2006.
[93] Geracioti, Nov. 2006.

pediatrician, endocrinologist, neurologist, and psychiatrist involved in my daughter's care.

In this second article, Dr. Geracioti explained that symptoms of *hypothyroidism* also can mimic, or be intertwined with, schizophrenia, bipolar disorder, anxiety, and depression. Moreover, patients diagnosed with mental illnesses (especially those with a mood component) are more likely to have a thyroid hormone imbalance than members of the general population. He also wrote that patients with thyroid disturbance and psychiatric symptoms are most often diagnosed with one of the following:

- Atypical depression (which may present as dysthymia).
- Bipolar spectrum syndrome (including manic depresssion, mixed mania, bipolar depression, rapid-cycling bipolar disorder, cyclothymia, and premenstrual syndrome).
- Borderline personality disorder.
- Psychotic disorder (typically paranoid psychosis).

Psychiatric symptoms of hypothyroidism, such as psychosis, depression, mood instability, mania, anxiety, hypersomnia, apathy, anergia (low energy level), impaired memory, psychomotor slowing, and attentional problems can be mistaken for mental illness. And symptoms such as hypersomnia, lethargy, hypercholesterolemia, galactorrhea, hyperprolactinemia, menstrual irregularities, and sexual dysfunction can be misconstrued as side effects of psychotropic medications being taken to alleviate psychiatric symptoms.

Treating an underlying thyroid hormone problem is critical to alleviating the psychiatric symptoms associated with it, and I completely agreed with Dr. Geracioti's statement that the first hurdle in treating underlying hypothyroidism is its diagnosis. In practice, tests to assess thyroid malfunction are usually limited to those measuring levels of the thyroid-stimulating hormone (TSH) . For patients exhibiting psychiatric symptoms, the article called for more extensive testing.

Because thyroid hormone levels have a circadian rhythm that peaks at night, Dr. Geracioti suggested blood tests for hypothyroidism be done before 9 a.m. in order not to miss subclinical (below the surface of clinical detection) hypothyroidism. Such tests may need to be repeated serially and should include measurements of the following:

- Thyroid-stimulating hormone (TSH).
- Free triiodothyronine (T3).
- Free levothyroxine (T4).
- Total T3.
- Total T4.
- Antithyroid antibodies.
- Serum cholesterol.
- Prolactin.

The author explained that hypothyroidism, because of its complex endocrinology, can stem from a problem in the hypothalamus, the pituitary gland, the thyroid, or the body's resistance to thyroid hormone, with varying levels of thyroid sensitivity in different organs of the body. When thyroid imbalances occur in pediatric patients, additional symptoms can include:

- Short stature.
- Learning problems.
- Attention-deficit/hyperactivity disorder (ADHD).

To my delight, the article outlined the hypothalamic-pituitary-thyroid endocrinology involved. It also discussed treatment. When augmenting psychiatric treatment with thyroid hormone, Dr. Geracioti asserted:

> *Psychiatric patients with subclinical hypothyroidism—especially those with incomplete responses to psychotropic therapy—should usually be treated with thyroid hormone. Free T3 levels in the lower 20% of the laboratory's normal range are cause for pause in a patient with a mood or psychotic disorder and any of hypothyroidism's clinical stigmata, even if thyroxine and TSH concentrations are normal.*

In regard to depressive symptoms, he proposed:

> *In some patients with no clear evidence of a biochemical or clinical thyroid disorder, mood symptoms nevertheless respond to thyroid hormone augmentation of antidepressants.* [94]

When hypothalamic function is believed to be involved in low thyroid levels, some doctors also recommend tests to measure hormones such as cortisol, growth hormone, and the sex hormones, which are influenced by the hypothalamus.

The "TRH stimulation of TSH" test is sometimes used to distinguish between secondary (pituitary) and tertiary (hypothalamic) hypothyroidism.

Since hypothyroidism also can affect lipid levels, cholesterol and triglycerides should be measured in these patients[95] and in *all* patients taking antipsychotic medications. (High cholesterol and triglycerides can lead to cardiovascular disease.)

I had wondered why a person with low-normal or perhaps even solidly normal thyroid hormone levels might respond well to thyroid augmentation. Peter C. Whybrow, M.D., and colleagues researched the connection between thyroid hormones and mood disorders for well over a decade. In a 2005 Expert Interview conducted by Randall F. White, M.D., on behalf of Medscape, Dr. Whybrow discussed gender differences in the development of ultra-rapid cycling (frequent cycling of moods that alternate between mania or hypomania, and depression or dysthymia). This type of cycling is much more common in females than males. Low thyroid levels, along with fluctuations in the levels of other hormones, such as progesterone, affect the severity and cycling of the mood symptoms.[96] Keri, it turned out, not only had

---

[94] Excerpts used with permission from "Identifying Hypothyroidism's Psychiatric Presentations" by Thomas D. Geracioti Jr., *Current Psychiatry Online*, Vol. 5, No. 11, Nov. 2006.
[95] "Mild Thyroid Failure and High Cholesterol May Go Hand in Hand: Changing Treatment Protocol," American Thyroid Association, Sept. 17, 2003.
[96] White, 2005.

low levels of thyroid hormones but also of other mood-affecting hormones, including progesterone, cortisol, and testosterone.

Exploring why low-normal levels of thyroid hormones might be insufficient in people with psychiatric symptoms, I read about the concept of thyroid resistance, which can affect the brain. Some patients with thyroid resistance may have high levels of TSH and normal levels of T3 and T4, but their bodies cannot effectively use the hormones available.

Another study investigated difficulties with transporting thyroid hormone to the brain, a problem manifested by many people with symptoms of paranoid schizophrenia.[97] The authors of this study noted that thyroid hormone dysfunction is relatively common in patients with schizophrenia and other psychiatric disorders and may even be genetically linked to such disorders.

In addition to cases in which a thyroid T4 hormone is administered to augment treatment of psychosis with a mood component, thyroid T3 hormone is sometimes used to augment treatment of depression, even while the patient is on an antidepressant. At a continuing medical education (CME) seminar, Keri's GP learned that augmenting treatment with T3 was associated with a better outcome, especially in patients with lower T3 levels to begin with—not necessarily levels *below* normal, mind you, just in the low-normal range.[98] Keri's T3 level, when tested at age 16-1/2, was *below* normal.

The results of my investigations convinced me that some people are being diagnosed with mental illness when what they actually have is a highly complex disorder affecting the endocrine system and, by extension, the entire body. Sadly, most endocrinologists are woefully unprepared to treat these patients. In fact, many refuse to even acknowledge they have a job to do.

---

[97] Huang, J. T., Leweke, F. M., Oxley, D., Wang, L., Harris, N., et al., 2006.
[98] Barclay, Laurie, and Lie, 2007.

Appendix B: Medical Tests

Before doctors give a neuropsychiatric diagnosis such as schizophrenia, schizoaffective disorder, or even depression or OCD, *they need to run the necessary tests* to rule out other illnesses! Sometimes test results will point to a biomedical condition that may be causing the patient's psychiatric symptoms. Sometimes they will not. Regardless of outcome, however, the tests are valuable. After all, a person with a legitimate diagnosis of schizophrenia, etc., can *also* have exacerbating medical conditions that need to be addressed.

Some illnesses and tests are still being researched, such as tests for the Borna virus. Other illnesses can manifest neuropsychiatric symptoms but are more likely to be noticed because of other symptoms. For example, acute intermittent porphyria can cause symptoms of psychosis, anxiety, depression, agitation, and altered mental status, but its predominant physical symptom is severe stomach pain.

If a child is already on medication for psychiatric symptoms, and new or worsening symptoms occur, the medications themselves should be considered suspect. As ironic as it seems, not only can medications for depression, anxiety, or psychosis actually *cause* or *worsen* depression, anxiety, or psychosis, other seemingly unrelated or benign medications can cause psychiatric symptoms. Withdrawal from medications also can cause or worsen psychiatric symptoms. Although such symptoms are often of a temporary nature, there are times when they can persist for a prolonged period.

The chart below lists a few of the illnesses that can cause symptoms similar to those of neuropsychiatric disorders, along with common tests to detect these illnesses. Keri turned out to have several of these medical problems, though in some cases this took years to determine because the proper tests were not administered.

Table 27: Tests: Diagnoses with Neuropsychiatric Symptoms

Illness	Test(s) to Be Performed
Sleep disorders Excessive REM Narcolepsy Sleep apnea	Sleep study, genetic testing, CSF (cerebrospinal fluid) (Note: Insurance will usually pay for only one night of a sleep study. However, it may take two nights for a patient to relax enough for an accurate study.)
Sprue (celiac/coeliac) disease, gluten sensitivity, and other intestinal autoimmune, food sensitivity, and malabsorption issues	• Antibody blood tests, skin scratch tests, fecal tests, absorption tests • Possible DNA test • Possibly endoscopy and biopsy
Seizure disorder, including temporal lobe seizures	Can be complex, including brief EEG If negative: 24-hour sleep-deprived EEG If negative: 3-day EEG Possible video EEG
Autoimmune disorders (lupus, multiple sclerosis, rheumatoid arthritis, AIDS)	Varied, including MRI with contrast and blood tests
Hypothyroidism, hyperthyroidism	Test for: • Thyroid-stimulating hormone (TSH) • Free triiodothyronine (T3) • Free thyroxine (T4) • Total T3 • Total T4 • Antithyroglobulin & antithyroid peroxidase antibodies • Serum cholesterol • Prolactin
Cushing's (hypercortisolism) & Addison's (hypocortisolism)	• Blood tests • Urine testing of cortisol over 24-hour period
Turner syndrome/mosaic	DNA test
Lyme disease	Testing is complex

Illness	Test(s) to Be Performed
Hypothalamic-pituitary dysfunction, including pituitary or brain tumor	• MRI of brain & pituitary • Test of hormone levels: blood, urine, saliva
Hemochromatosis	Blood tests (see Centers for Disease Control Web site for "Iron Overload and Hemochromatosis: Detection and Diagnosis")[99]
Wilson's disease	• Urine test • Ophthalmologic exam (99% of patients with neurological or psychiatric symptoms due to Wilson's disease have Kayser-Fleischer rings—dark rings around the cornea)[100] • Blood tests
Mitochondrial dysfunction (mitochondrial encephalopathy)[101]	• Family history • Urine, blood, and CSF tests • Nuclear DNA testing (nDNA) • Mitochondrial DNA testing (mtDNA)
Vitamin/mineral toxicity, vitamin/mineral deficiency, or a vitamin utilization problem	• Blood tests, including tests for the levels of B vitamins, zinc, copper, iron, CoQ10, cellular micronutrients, etc. • DNA tests • Blood tests to measure methylmalonic acid and homocysteine levels (levels increase during early vitamin B_{12} deficiency) • (controversially) Urine tests, including: — Test for excessive pyrroles/mauve factor (indicating vitamin B_3, vitamin B_6, zinc, manganese, and antioxidant supplements may be necessary)[102]

---

[99] "Iron Overload and Hemochromatosis: Detection and Diagnosis," http://www.cdc.gov/ncbddd/hemochromatosis/detection.htm, accessed July 20, 2007.
[100] Brewer, 2000.
[101] Mancuso, et al., 2007.
[102] Testing for pyroluria or mauve factor—elevated pyrroles in the urine—as an indicator of vitamin B_6 and zinc deficiency is *not* accepted as a mainstream medical diagnostic test.

There are other illnesses to consider, such as PANDAS (pediatric autoimmune neuropsychiatric disorders associated with streptococcal infections), hormonal problems not listed in the table above, PTSD (Keri's PTSD was actually *caused* by her hallucinations), and even reactions to medications a child is currently taking.

Functional magnetic resonance imaging (fMRI) is sometimes used to garner more information about the brain and its hallucinatory, manic, and depressive symptoms, as well as about ADHD.

Because each person has unique sensitivities and biological quirks, effects of excess vitamins and minerals or, conversely, vitamin/mineral deficiencies cause symptoms that vary by individual.

- **Manganese:** Excess manganese can cause apathy, irritability, headaches, insomnia, weakness of the legs, impulsivity, absentmindedness, hallucinations, aggressiveness, and uncontrollable laughter at inappropriate times.[103]
- **Mercury:** Symptoms of mercury poisoning include loss of appetite, weakness, insomnia, indigestion, diarrhea, gingivitis, irritability, hallucinations, manic-depressive psychosis, loss of memory, irritability, and tremors. It can also cause irreversible brain damage.[104]
- **Iron (hemochromatosis, a hereditary illness):** Excessive buildup of iron in the body can cause endocrine abnormalities. Low reproductive hormones levels would indicate the hypothalamic-pituitary-adrenal axis is affected (see figure 1 and table 10). The condition can result in hypogonadism; dysmenorrhea; amenorrhea; low levels of thyroid hormones, luteinizing hormone (LH), and follicle-stimulating hormone (FSH);[105] fatigue; lethargy; sensory processing problems; hypothyroidism; muscle and joint pain; diabetes; cognitive impairment; depression; and psychiatric illnesses.[106]

---

[103] Haman and Bottcher, 1986.
[104] Haman and Bottcher, 1986.
[105] O'Neil and Powell, 2005.
[106] Cutler, 1994.

Periodic Tests

Most of the following tests (table 28) were part of the structural ecology workup performed by Dr. Robert Fredericks, the endocrinologist who identified several of Keri's medical issues. Other endocrinologists, along with her GP, Dr. David Marwil, now perform some of these tests yearly. While her medications were being adjusted, some tests were performed more frequently to continue to monitor her health. Hormone levels can be affected by medications, so repeating certain tests periodically may be warranted. Since hormone levels can fluctuate from day to day, or even within a day, some tests may need to be performed more than once over a multi-day period.

As medical knowledge and technology advances, more tests should be added to the list.

Table 28: Tests for an Endocrine Workup

- Aldosterone
- Angiotensin II
- Cholesterol
- Comprehensive metabolic panel
- Cortisol
- Dehydroepiandrosterone (DHEA)
- Estradiol
- Ferritin
- Folate (Vitamin B_9)
- Follicle-stimulating hormone (FSH)
- Free fatty acids
- Free T3
- Free T4
- Hemoglobin A1c
- Homocysteine
- Insulin
- Insulin-like growth factor-1 (IGF-1)
- Leptin
- Lipid panel
- Luteinizing hormone (LH)
- Intact parathyroid hormone (PTH)
- Parathyroid hormone-related protein (PTHrP)
- Prolactin
- Progesterone
- Testosterone
- Thyroid-stimulating hormone (TSH)
- Urine calcium
- Urine cAMP
- Urine creatinine
- Urine microalbumin
- Urine phosphorus
- Vitamin B_{12}
- Vitamin D (1,25-D)
- Bone density
- Growth hormone stimulation test (GHST) – done once

Monitoring Adrenal Function/General Health and Well-Being

Children with chronic conditions—especially those affecting brain function—are under a great deal of stress. Their innate biology may render them exquisitely vulnerable to stressors. Their symptoms create additional stressors. The combination of chronic symptoms and severe illness can deplete the body's resources, making it more difficult for the adrenals glands to protect the body from stress. Adrenal-gland malfunctions also can impact the proper functioning of body and brain, leading to further stress and a spiral of deterioration. That's why it's so important to monitor these children's general health and well-being.

It may be advisable to test periodically for adrenal function—and to test with increased frequency if a problem is found for which the patient is receiving treatment. Many of the tests listed below were included in Keri's structural ecology workup. Samples for some of them can be obtained via blood, urine, and/or saliva.

Table 29: Tests: Adrenal Function

- ACTH (ACTH stimulation/challenge test if other adrenal hormones are low)
- Cortisol
- Aldosterone
- Progesterone
- DHEA-S
- Testosterone
- Pregnenolone
- Estradiol
- Androstenedione
- Thyroid levels: free T3, free T4, and rT3

Keri was given other tests by a bone metabolism specialist, tests he recommended be repeated annually for patients taking medications that can affect bone metabolism, such as some medications for anxiety and depression, neuroleptics, antiseizure medications, and lithium.

Table 30: Tests: Bone Metabolism

- Bone density scans
- Blood tests
  - PTH (parathyroid hormone), PTH-CAP, PTH-CIP, CAP/CIP ratio
  - N-telopeptide
  - BCE (bone collagen equivalents)
  - Osteocalcin
  - Vitamin D_3
  - Bone-specific alkaline phosphatase
  - Plasma total homocysteine
  - Blood urea nitrogen
  - Creatine
  - Electrolytes: sodium, potassium, chloride CO_2, calcium, phosphorus, albumin, magnesium, and serum aldosterone
- 24-hour urine tests
  - Creatinine
  - Calcium, sodium, and magnesium
  - Phosphorus/protein
  - Creatinine clearance
  - Urinary calcium/creatinine ratio
  - Excretion of phosphorus and sodium
  - UPEP (urine protein electrophoresis)
  - UIFE (urine immunofixation electrophoresis to test for Bence Jones proteins)
  - Urine aldosterone
  - Urinary free cortisol

Glucose Tests

Many medications have adverse metabolic side effects. Therefore, if a person is taking medication that can cause dyslipidemia, metabolic syndrome, glucose intolerance, insulin resistance, or diabetes, or that lists any of these conditions as a side effect, it is reasonable for him/her to be tested periodically for pre-diabetes.

In addition, there is evidence that a subgroup of patients diagnosed with mood and psychotic disorders are simply more prone to problems with insulin resistance[107] and therefore should be tested for it. Undiagnosed insulin resistance can have far-reaching consequences, including a higher risk of cardiovascular disease; thus, the blood lipids profile and blood pressure of such patients should also be monitored.

Table 31: Tests for Medication Side Effects: Glucose

Two tests for impaired glucose tolerance or impaired fasting glucose (both known as pre-diabetic conditions) are:

- **Oral Glucose Tolerance Test (OGTT).** This very sensitive test for diabetes and pre-diabetes is considered the gold standard. However, many doctors do not think it is practical, because it takes several morning hours to complete.

- **Fasting Plasma Glucose Test** (FPG). This test requires a blood draw after at least eight hours of fasting.

A study on the most cost-effective method of testing for diabetes and glucose metabolism impairment in this high-risk group found the FPG missed more than half the cases![108] However, because of the expense of running the more accurate OGTT on everybody, the World Health Organization suggests a two-step screening process: If the results of an FPG indicate any sign of impairment, then an OGTT

---

[107] Cohen, et al., 2006.
[108] Van Winkel, Ruud, et al., Oct. 2006.

should be performed. This two-step method has been found to have a 96-percent success rate.

The random plasma glucose test, another glucose-measurement tool, is a good diagnostic aid for a patient who already has symptoms of full-blown diabetes, including increased thirst, increased urination, fatigue, and unexplained, sudden weight loss. However, it is even less reliable than the FPG as an indicator of a pre-diabetic condition.

A urine test is not useful when trying to determine impaired glucose tolerance. A urine test that is positive for glucose can indicate the kidneys are damaged or that the person has very high plasma glucose, as in the case of uncontrolled diabetes. The presence of ketones in the urine can also indicate uncontrolled diabetes, but it can just as easily indicate that the patient is fasting or simply on a low-carbohydrate diet.

Fatty Acids, Vitamin B, Homocysteine, and Mitochondrial Function

Because some medications can adversely affect vitamin, fatty acid, and homocysteine levels, periodic testing of these levels is a reasonable precaution, especially for patients who do not take nutritional supplements. There also is evidence that a subgroup of patients diagnosed with schizophrenia is prone to problems in this area.[109] Elevated levels of homocysteine can increase the risk of cardiovascular disease, and pregnant women with high levels of this amino acid may be at increased risk for having children who later develop symptoms of bipolar disorder or schizophrenia.

---

[109] Kemperman, et al., Feb. 2006.

Table 32: Tests of Metabolic & Mitochondrial Health

Specifically, levels of the following should be tested:

- Cholesterol (LDL/HDL)
- Triglycerides
- Homocysteine
- Vitamins B_{12}, B_9 (folate) and B_6
- Glucose and electrolytes
- CBC (check for neutropenia, thrombocytopenia, and anemia)
- BUN
- Lactate, pyruvate
- Ammonia
- Creatine kinase (CK); often mildly elevated with muscle involvement
- Amino acids (blood and urine)
- Organic acids
- Acetyl-carnitines (blood and urine)

Nutritional support (under advice from a physician) might consist of a combination of foods and/or supplements high in pyridoxal (B_6 or P-5-P), methylated cobalamin (B_{12}) and folate (B_9), glycine, trimethylglycine (TMG) or betaine (DMG), carnitine, choline or S-adenosylmethionine (SAM-e), omega-3 fatty acids, ubiquinone (CoQ10) and antioxidants. Since people diagnosed with autism spectrum and bipolar/schizophrenia spectrum disorders can have a higher-than-normal incidence of genetic variants affecting the metabolism of folate and vitamin B_{12}; for these people, supplements containing the methylated forms of folate and vitamin B_{12} (methylcobalamin) may be more suitable.

Appendix C: Charting Symptoms

Over the years, we used many kinds of charts, some given to us by sleep specialists and psychiatrists, some we created or modified ourselves. We'd remove irrelevant items such as "alcohol abuse" while adding items like "spaciness at school." Keri refused to chart her moods, even when doctors requested it. Just the act of charting, she said, made her feel worse. Not wanting to ask her what she was thinking, we modified thought items to be behavior items. For example "thoughts of death or suicide" can be modified to "hitting oneself."

We also kept notes about symptoms during treatment changes so we could know if, and how, things changed. When we charted and kept notes, patterns emerged from the overwhelming sea of details.

The example included here (see table 33) represents a period when Keri resumed taking a specific type of nutritional multivitamin/mineral/herbal ("micronutrient") supplement called EMPowerPlus. She had previously taken this supplement for approximately one year but had stopped a month prior to the charting, during which time her condition deteriorated. At the time she also was taking several other medications, including antihistamines, the antidepressant Wellbutrin (bupropion), and the atypical neuroleptic Seroquel (quetiapine), but neither the doses nor the frequency of these medications had changed.

Since stopping the supplement had been the only significant change in Keri's routine, we wanted to determine if resuming it would really help or not. Table 33 shows two weeks of charting, one for the week *prior to* restarting the supplement, the other for the fourth week *after* restarting it.

Because some symptoms, such as hallucinations, can be minor and not visible to a parent, there are days when the entry was "0," meaning *not at all*. This turned out to be inaccurate. We chart what we observe, which means that sometimes the *internal* experience of a "1" or "2" (*just a little* or *somewhat*) can manifest itself *externally* as a "0." Even so, by the sixth week, we had no doubt the supplement was helping. By the eighth week, Keri begged never to be removed from it again.

Table 33: Charting Key Symptoms

Week Before Restarting Supplement EMPowerPlus

Week of: dd mm yyyy to dd mm yyyy
0= Not at all   1= Just a Little   2= Somewhat   3=Very Much

Symptoms	Sun	Mon	Tues	Wed	Thur	Fri	Sat
Hallucinations or delusions	1	1	0	0	0	2	2
Extremely disorganized thoughts	1	1	0	0	0	2	2
Inappropriate emotional responses	2	1	1	1	1	2	2
Social withdrawal	1	1	0	0	0	2	2
Intense depression	2	2	1	1	1	3	3
Inability to concentrate	2	2	0	0	0	2	2
Avoiding activities and hobbies	0	0	0	0	0	3	3
Forgetfulness	1	1	1	1	1	1	1
Unusual sensitivity to stimuli	3	3	2	2	2	3	3
Emotional rigidity or stubbornness	1	1	0	0	0	0	0
Motor tics	2	2	2	2	2	2	2
Vocal tics	1	1	1	1	1	1	1
Headaches/migraines	3	2	1	1	3	3	3
Excessive sleeping	0	3	0	0	0	0	0
Disturbed sleep/terrors	3	3	3	3	3	3	3
Extreme anxiety	3	3	2	2	2	3	3
Extreme frustration intolerance	3	3	2	2	2	3	3

Week Four on Supplement EMPowerPlus

Week of: dd mm yyyy to dd mm yyyy
0= Not at all   1= Just a Little   2= Somewhat   3=Very Much

Symptoms	Sun	Mon	Tues	Wed	Thur	Fri	Sat
Hallucinations or delusions	1	0	0	0	0	0	0
Extremely disorganized thoughts	0	0	0	2	0	0	0
Inappropriate emotional responses	0	0	0	2	0	0	0
Social withdrawal	0	0	0	3	0	0	0
Intense depression	1	1	1	3	1	1	1
Inability to concentrate	0	0	0	0	0	0	0
Avoiding activities and hobbies	0	0	0	3	0	0	0
Forgetfulness	0	0	0	0	0	0	0
Unusual sensitivity to stimuli	1	2	0	3	0	0	0
Emotional rigidity or stubbornness	0	0	0	3	0	0	0
Motor tics	1	1	1	1	1	1	1
Vocal tics	0	0	0	0	0	0	0
Headaches/migraines	0	3	0	0	0	0	0
Excessive sleeping	0	1	0	0	0	0	0
Disturbed sleep/terrors	0	0	0	0	0	0	0
Extreme anxiety	0	0	0	2	0	0	0
Extreme frustration intolerance	1	1	1	0	0	1	1

Appendix D: Preparing for Doctor Visits

For some doctors, all that is necessary is a list of all medications (both prescription and over-the-counter [OTC], food supplements, and dosages). Since some food supplements are composed of many ingredients, having separate sheets with those ingredients may be necessary to include in the child's chart. For example, for doctors who care about it, I provide a list of ingredients in my daughter's EMPowerPlus and Nutrasleep supplements.

We always carry a one-page sheet with the names of all medications, a list of current doctors and their phone numbers, and insurance information. This makes filling out paperwork in doctors' offices simpler, and it is good emergency information to have on hand. I include a list of current diagnoses, but I've found it is sometimes (depending on the circumstances) better not to share a list of previous diagnoses.

When I was journaling (or charting) my daughter's sleep and moods, I brought this raw data with me to appointments for my own reference, along with a short summary to give to the doctor (see figures 4 and 5 and table 33).

As shown in table 18, I also created a table of medication history (including food supplements). From this I created a table of current medications, which I continue to keep current. One important detail in each of these tables is *why* the child is taking the medication.

Initially, I kept a year-by-year list of symptoms, which I took to consultations with new specialists. However, I realized that many symptoms were the same each year; some disappeared from one year to the next, and new ones emerged. I also realized we needed to know which medications had been tried and the outcome of each. Sometimes much can be gleaned from what helped in the past and what made things worse.

I replaced the year-by-year symptom list with a symptom history chart, beginning from infancy. For each symptom, I asked myself, "What happened to that symptom? When did it start? What helped? When did it end?"

Here is an excerpt from Keri's symptom history spreadsheet. I actually started with perinatal symptoms, but for illustration I have just included the segment from birth through age two.

Table 34: Symptom History Chart

Age Began or Diagnosed	Problem or Diagnosis	Age Addressed	Treatment or What Ameliorated Condition	Result or Reason for Treatment Discontinuation
Infancy	Severely disturbed sleep, insomnia. **See age 3**. Throughout infancy, slept in 5–90 minute intervals day and night. Would bizarrely fall asleep in the daytime (for example, at 6 months of age, each time she was turned on her back to float in swimming pool). **See Insomnia & parasomnias** at age 3.	N/A	See age 3	N/A
Infancy	Excessive Startle Reaction, Sensory hypersensitivity (touch, sound)	7	Therapy	Helped with coping and expression
		9.5	SSRI antidepressant (Zoloft)	Wonderful while it lasted, but eventually resulted in mania/psychosis
		12.5	Seroquel	Still happened frequently but not chronically
		16.5 – 20	Hormones and diet changes	Symptoms became rare, then ended
Infancy	Fits of prolonged screaming for no apparent reason. Diagnosed as "colic." Possibly migraines? Terror? Panic?	N/A	Colic medication did nothing.	Later, screaming fits became rare with multimodal treatment of dietary changes, hormones, psychotropic medications (phased out), and nutritional supplements.

Age Began or Diagnosed	Problem or Diagnosis	Age Addressed	Treatment or What Ameliorated Condition	Result or Reason for Treatment Discontinuation
Infancy	Below-average flexibility (muscle tear in leg at ~18 months)	2.5	Tots gymnastics & play	Immense improvement over the years
		~7	Yoga	
Infancy-2	Infantile seborrheic dermatitis	N/A	Resolved on its own	
Infancy	Migraines (diagnosed at age 2). Developed prodromes & auras, with duration, frequency, and severity increasing over the years. Prodromes included, at various times, ataxia, confusion, aphasia, mood change (severe but brief depression), vision changes similar to hallucinatory phenomena. Cluster headaches as a young teen.	2	Rx Pediatric Liquid Advil	Insufficient control
		4	Chiropractic therapy	Only relieved some headache pain from neck - did nothing for migraines
		8	Ibuprofen + caffeine	Insufficient control
		~13	Cranio-facial osteopathic manipulation	Consistently triggered Kleine-Levin sleep episodes, so was discontinued after about 4 sessions
		~14	Imitrex at start of migraine	Not much help
		14	Topamax	Partial control
		~15	Zomig at start of migraine	Worse.
		~15	Axert at start of migraine	Shortened duration and severity *if* taken very early in prodrome
		16	Service dog could detect prodromes (same as seizures)	Began to be able to take medication more effectively—early in prodrome stage
		19	Added LEF super-absorbable CoQ10 to Topamax	Complete control (Was able to eliminate Topamax by 21)

Age Began or Diagnosed	Problem or Diagnosis	Age Addressed	Treatment or What Ameliorated Condition	Result or Reason for Treatment Discontinuation
1	Intermittent growth / delayed growth. Size (but not weight) fell from 50th percentile to below 5th. Pediatrician suspected endocrine system problems.	1.5	GH checked during period of growth and found normal.	
		16.5	Human Growth Hormone (was also put on other hormones over the next few years)	Many accumulated problems improved: (growth, bone density, pain, lethargy, etc.)
1	Environmental allergies	2	Long-term antibiotics, antihistamines, eye drops, hypoallergenic bedroom, allergy shots	Partial control.
		14	Singulair added to 2 other antihistamines	Great relief except when exposed to specific antigens (such as tobacco smoke).
		17	Quercetin & Boswelia seasonally	Better control seasonally
		19.5	Gluten, dairy, soy, egg-free diet	Eventually, maybe diet and shots combined (?) improved allergies to the point where Singulair was needed only periodically.
		20.5	Allergy shots again	
1	Frequent ear and sinus infections with gunky eyes	age 1–12	Antibiotics, saltwater, antihistamines	Partial relief. Adding additional antihistamines resolved this
1 or 2	Intermittent pain in knees, ankles, back and neck	16, 19	T3/T4 and growth hormone	Increasingly infrequent

Appendix D: Preparing for Doctor Visits 383

Age Began or Diagnosed	Problem or Diagnosis	Age Addressed	Treatment or What Ameliorated Condition	Result or Reason for Treatment Discontinuation
2	Chronic low-level depression and Intermittent, more severe depression at age 10	N/A	Fluctuated with psychotropics, nutritional supplements, & hormonal therapies, but ultimately remains today. Not psychological	
2	Huge hard balls of stool, too large to flush (family called it mini-megacolon) Frequent abdominal pain. Bloated (distended) belly.	19.5	Elimination of gluten, dairy, soy, peanuts, egg whites. Addition of food supplements. Hormones.	Controlled. Not as frequent
2.5	Screaming, wailing meltdowns (non-aggressive, nonviolent) from sensory overload and frustration (increased in autumn and spring). One-quarter-hour-long screaming/crying/wailing fits, sometimes with urination followed by sleep (*not* behavioral). Tapered off as a preteen but replaced by psychotic- and PTSD-like fits.	3	Antihistamine change for allergies	Slightly decreased frequency, esp. seasonally
		7	Therapy	Helped with articulation of feelings and needs, but did not treat cause
		9.5	SSRI antidepressant	Resolved sensory issues, but created anxiety and OCD. Increased until mania & psychosis (see age 12)
		12	Seroquel plus vitamin supplement (EMPowerPlus)	Back to intermittent status. Slowly getting better.
		16.5	Hormones and more nutritional supplements added	*Much* relieved. No longer as sensitive. Was able to reduce Seroquel dosage
		21	Tryptophan added to NutraSleep (has GABA) and extended-release melatonin	Was able to get off the rest of Seroquel. No return of symptoms

Photos

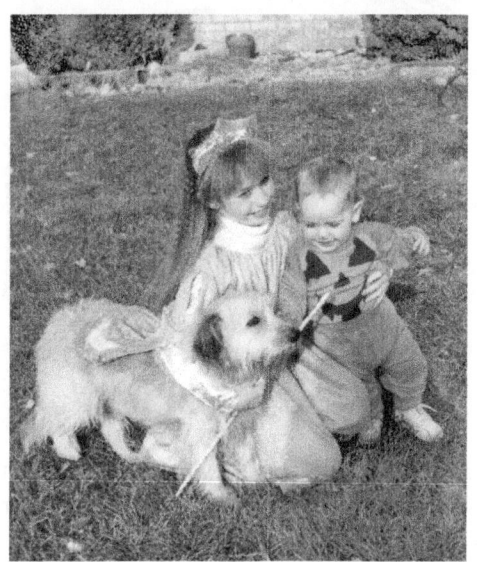

Big sister Candace (9) and dog Napkin on Halloween with Keri (12 months) with a "boo-boo" on the tip of her nose.

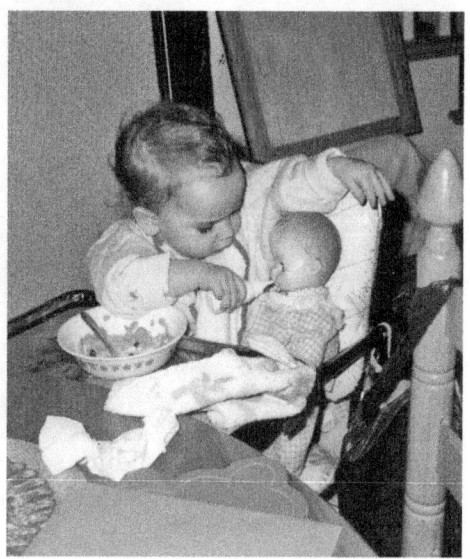

After feeding herself breakfast, the nurturing Keri (16 months) gives her doll a bottle.

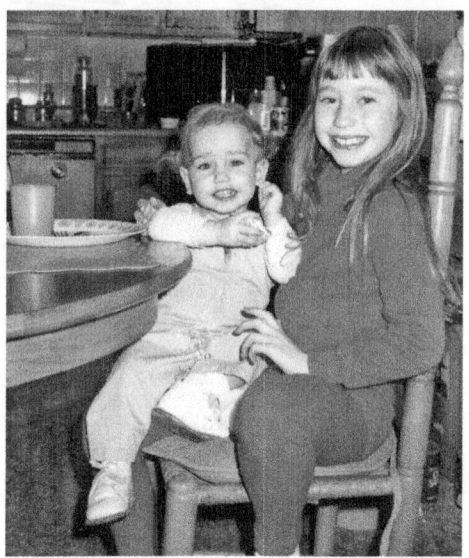

Keri (17 months) and Candace (9) playing a game of "dinging" each other's ears. Candace loved the way it made her baby sister LAUGH!

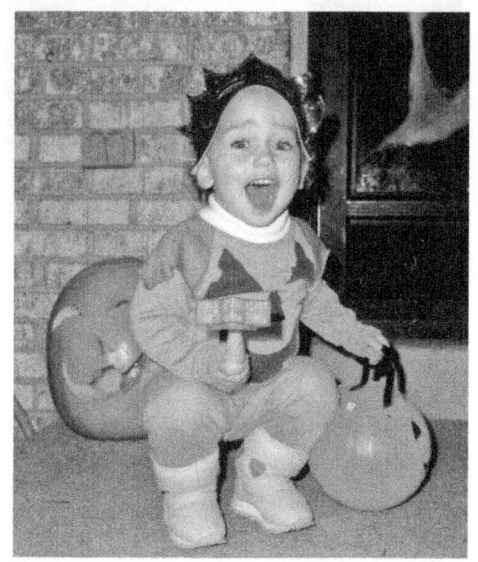

Keri, just turned 2, enjoying Halloween.

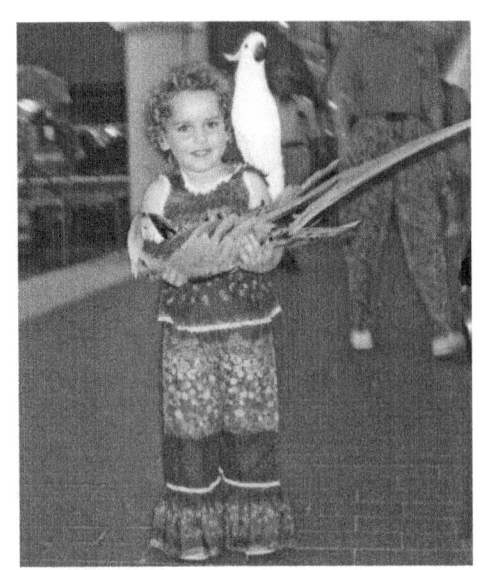

Keri (3) thrilled to be holding some large birds while on vacation in Florida.

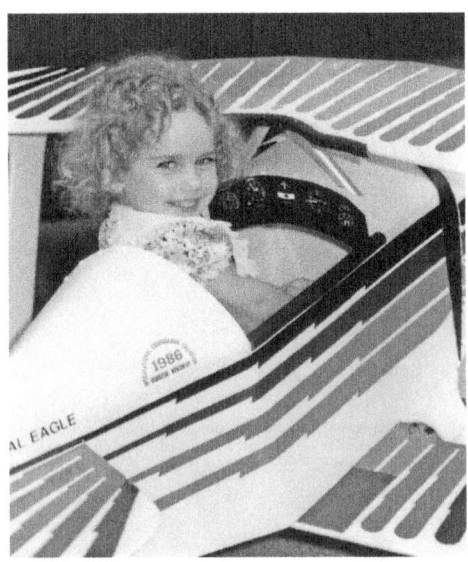

Keri (3½) being the little aviator in the Christen Eagle pedal biplane her father built for her.

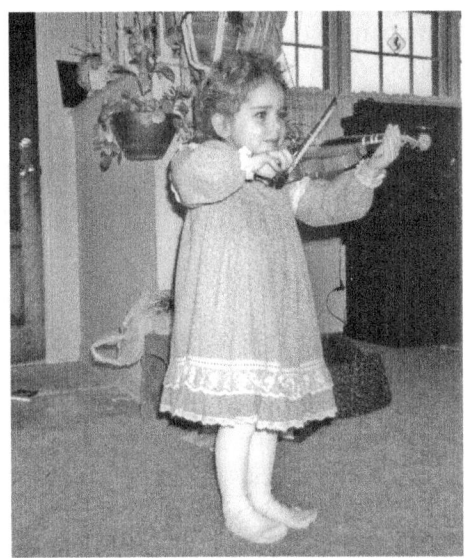

Keri (4) playing violin shortly before quitting the first time.

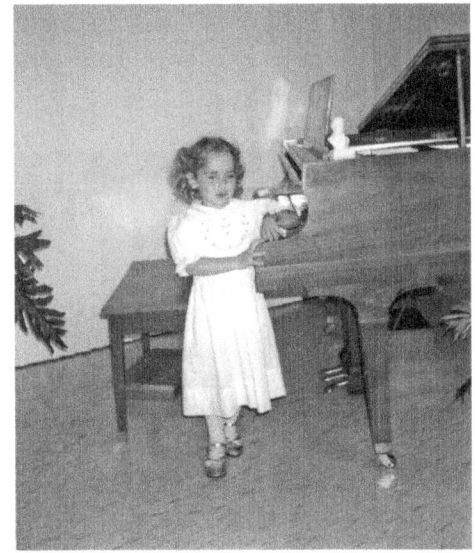

Proud Keri (5) at a piano recital. In addition to her assigned music, she played a cute little piece she wrote herself.

Photos 387

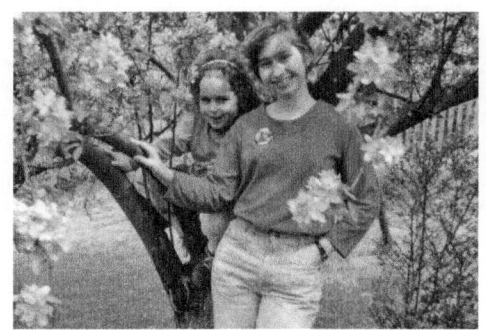

Keri (5) & Candace (13) in the backyard, with the crabapple tree in full bloom.

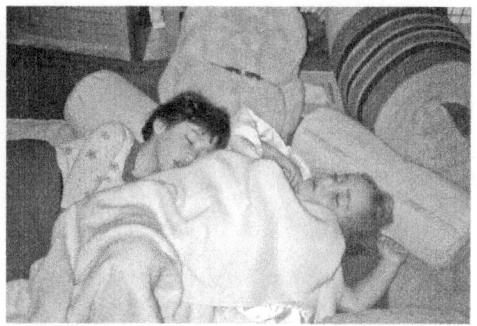

Keri (right) and her cousin Roberta (both age 5) sleeping after a hard day of playing.

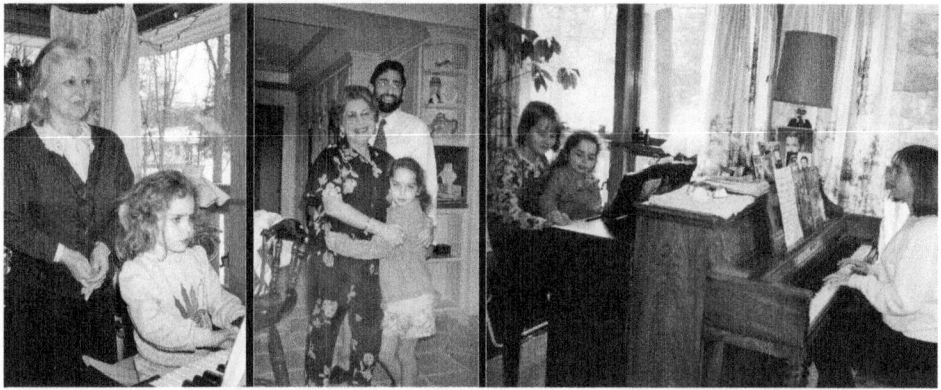

Keri (6) playing on her Grandma Edie's organ; at 8, with her Grandma Sylvia and her Uncle Sam; at 8, on the organ with cousin Nichole (12) and sister Candace (16).

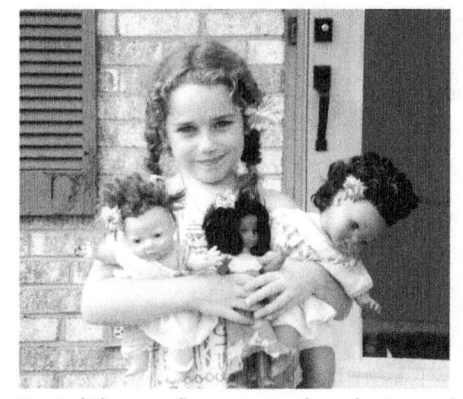

Keri (8) put flowers in her hair and her dolls' hair, too.

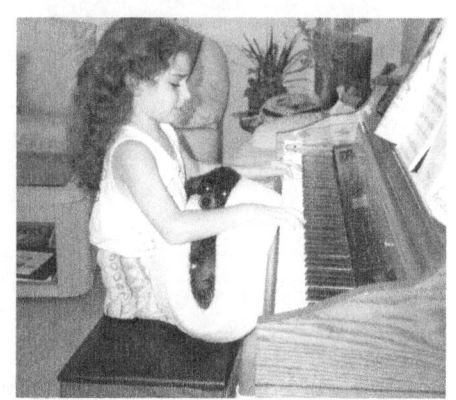

Keri (9½) smiling down at Mugsy while playing piano with him on her lap. That summer she was overcome by symptoms of depression.

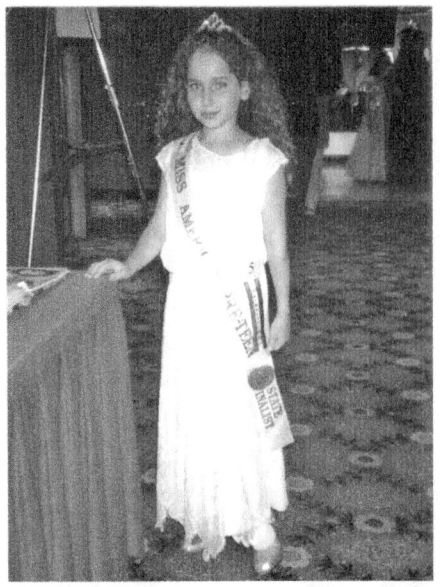

Keri (10) in a pre-teen pageant. She played piano and sang her own music and lyrics. A classmate of hers won.

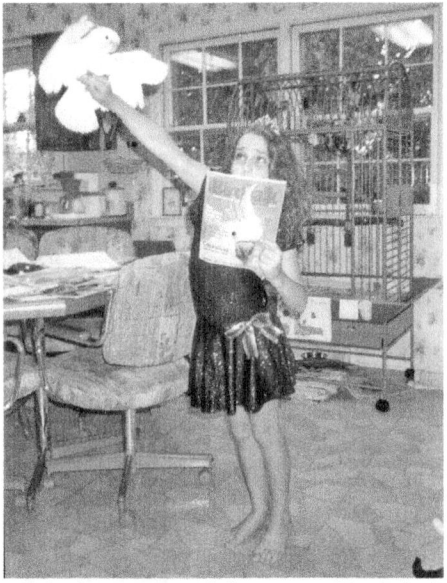

With her typical humor, Keri (10) poses as "The Statue of Birdety" while holding Chieena, her Goffin's cockatoo.

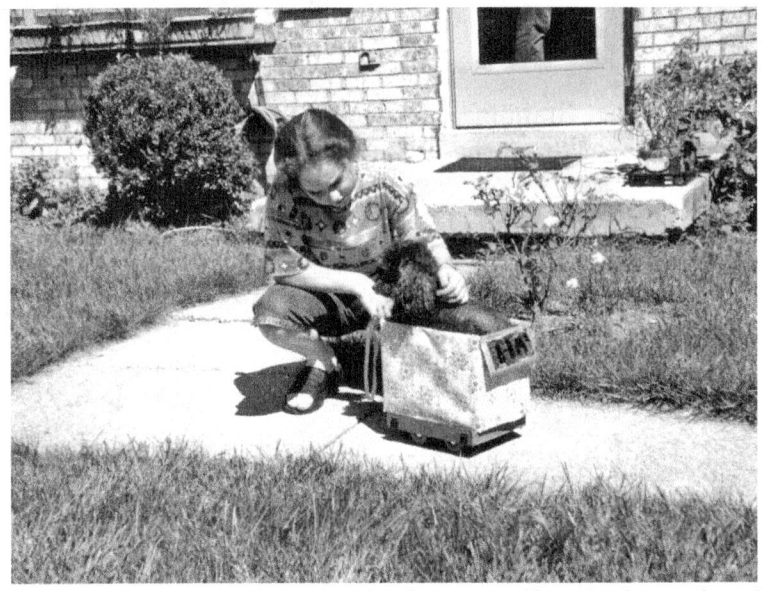

Mugsy in his Boo-Boo Mobile, made from Waffle Blocks and a decorated cardboard box. Keri (12) wheeled him around the neighborhood when his hind legs became temporarily paralyzed.

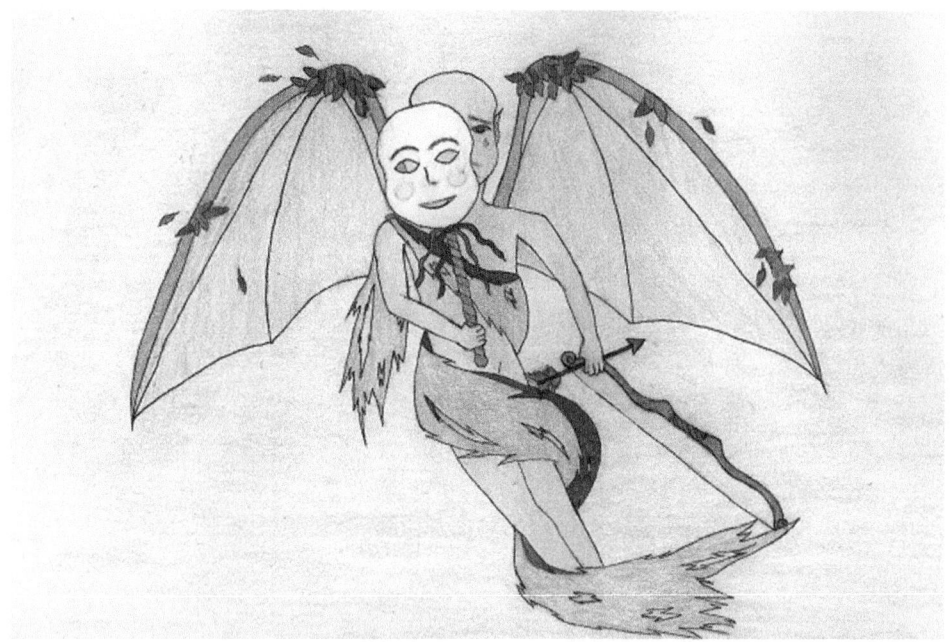

Keri (13) created this drawing during one of her sleepless nights. She titled it Masked. A picture truly can speak a thousand words.

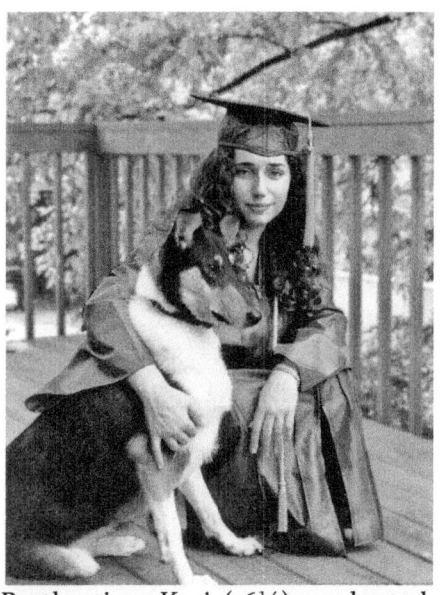

By the time Keri (16½) graduated high school, she had her service dog, Kira, a smooth-coat, tricolor collie.

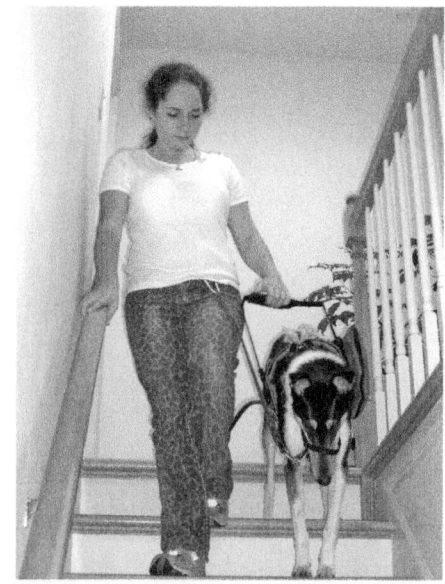

Kira helped Keri (17) with stability issues on sleep days and at other times of dizziness and severe fatigue.

References

Books

Alcott, Louisa May. *Little Women*. New York: Signet Classics, 2004.
Amador, Xavier. *I Am Not Sick, I Don't Need Help*. 2nd ed., Peconic, NY: Vida Publishers, 2007.
Brooks, Robert and Sam Goldstein. *Raising Resilient Children*. New York: McGraw-Hill, 2002.
Carlson, Trudy. *The Life of a Bipolar Child*. Duluth, MN: Benline Press, 2000.
Comings, David E. *Tourette Syndrome and Human Behavior*. Duarte, CA: Hope Press, 1990.
Dornbush, Marilyn Pierce and Sheryl K. Pruitt. *Teaching the Tiger: A Handbook for Individuals Involved in the Education of Students with Attention Deficit Disorders, Tourette Syndrome or Obsessive-Compulsive Disorder*. Duarte, CA: Hope Press, 1995.
Earley, Pete. *Crazy: A Father's Search Through America's Mental Health Madness*. New York: Penguin Group, 2006.
Greenberg, Joanne. *I Never Promised You a Rose Garden*. New York: Signet, 1964.
Greene, Ross W. *The Explosive Child: A New Approach for Understanding and Parenting Easily Frustrated, Chronically Inflexible Children*. New York: Harper Paperbacks, 2005.
Hoffman, Martha. *Lend Me an Ear: The Temperament, Selection and Training of the Hearing Ear Dog*. Irvine, CA: Doral Publishing, 1999.
Kay, Kiesa, ed. *Uniquely Gifted: Identifying and Meeting the Needs of the Twice-Exceptional Student*. Gilsum, NH: Avocus Publishing, 2000.
Keyes, Daniel. *Flowers for Algernon*. Orlando, FL: Harcourt, 2004.
Kress, Nancy. *Beggars and Choosers*. New York: Tom Doherty Associates, 1996.
—. *Beggars in Spain*. New York: HarperCollins Publishers, 2004.
—. *Beggars Ride*. New York: Tor Books, 1997.
—. *Probability Moon*. New York: Tor Books, 2002.
Loiselle, Beth, RD. *The Healing Power of Whole Foods*, Healthways Nutrition,1999.
Marsh, Tracy Lynne, ed. *Children with Tourette Syndrome: A Parents' Guide*. 2nd ed., Baltimore, MD: Woodbine House, 2006.
Montgomery, Lucy Maud. *Anne of Green Gables*. New York: Sterling Publishing Company, 2004.
Munsch, Robert N. and Sheila McGraw. *Love You Forever*. Richmond Hill, Ontario: Firefly Books, 1995.
Neufeld, John. *Lisa, Bright and Dark*. New York: Penguin Young Readers Group, 1999.
Papolos, Demitri and Janice Papolos. *The Bipolar Child*. New York: Broadway Books, 1999.

Poe, Edgar Allan. *The Works of Edgar Allan Poe*. New York: Avenel Books, 1985.
Salinger, J. D. *Catcher in the Rye*. New York: Little, Brown & Company, 1951.
Steel, Danielle. *His Bright Light: The Story of Nick Traina*. New York: Delacorte Press, 1998.
Taylor, Sydney. *All-of-a-Kind Family*. New York: Random House Children's Books, 1984 (part of a series).
Torrey, E. Fuller. *Surviving Schizophrenia*. 4th ed., New York: HarperCollins Publishers, 2001.
Waltz, Mitzi. *Obsessive-Compulsive Disorder: Help for Children and Adolescents*. Sebastopol, CA: O'Reilly Media, 2000.
Wilder, Laura Ingalls. *Little House on the Prairie*. New York: HarperCollins Children's Books, 1953 (part of a series).

Articles

Agarwal, R. "Nonhematological Benefits of Iron." *American Journal of Nephrology*, Vol. 26, No. 7, 2007, pp. 565–571.
Anderson, Kristina A. "Low Cortisol Caused by Quetiapine: Presented at APA." *Doctor's Guide*, May 23, 2007, http://www.docguide.com (accessed July 6, 2008).
Aneja, A. and E. Tierney. "Autism: the role of cholesterol in treatment." *International Review of Psychiatry*, Vol. 20, No. 2, Apr. 2008, pp. 165–170.
Arnulf, I., et al. "Kleine-Levin syndrome: a systematic review of 186 cases in the Literature." *Brain*, Vol. 128, No. 12, Dec. 1, 2005, pp. 2763–2776.
Barclay, Laurie and Désirée Lie. "Liothyronine Plus Sertraline May Be Helpful for Major Depression." Medscape Medical News, June 8, 2007, http://www.medscape.com/viewarticle/557949 (accessed June 8, 2007).
Bauer M., A. Heinz, and P. C. Whybrow. "Review Article: Thyroid Hormones, Serotonin and Mood: Of synergy and significance in the adult brain." *Molecular Psychiatry*, Vol. 7, 2002, pp. 140–156.
Bauer M., et al. "Original Research Article: Suraphysiological doses of levothyroxine alter regional cerebral metabolism and improve mood in bipolar depression." *Molecular Psychiatry*, Vol. 10, No. 5, May 2005, pp. 456–469.
Beil, L. "Mitochondria Gone Bad." *Science News*, Feb. 28, 2009, pp. 20–23.
Bhat, Shyam K. and Redentor Galang. "Narcolepsy Presenting as Schizophrenia." *American Journal of Psychiatry*, Vol. 159, July 2002.
Bibus, Douglas M., et al. "Fatty Acid Profiles of Schizophrenic Phenotypes," abstract. San Diego, CA: 91st AOCS Annual Meeting and Expo, April 25–28, 2000, http://www.hriptc.org/fatty_acids.html (accessed Sep. 21, 2008).
Bierkowska, B. and I. Rybakowski. "Rapid cycling bipolar affective illness." *Psychiatria Polska*, Vol. 28, No. 4, July–Aug. 1994, pp. 443–454.
Brewer, George J. "Recognition, Diagnosis, and Management of Wilson's Disease." *Proceedings of the Society for Experimental Biology and Medicine*,

Vol. 223, 2000, pp. 39–46, http://www.ebmonline.org/cgi/content/full/223/1/39#SEC3 (accessed May 17, 2006).

Brown, Colin H. and David R. Grattan. "Does Maternal Oxytocin Protect the Fetal Brain?" *Trends in Endocrinology & Metabolism*, Vol. 18, Issue 6, Aug. 2007, pp. 225–226.

Busko, Marlene. "Oxytocin Affects Brain Function and Behavior in Autism in Preliminary Study." Medscape Medical News, May 10, 2007, http://www.medscape.com/viewarticle/556321 (accessed Feb. 28, 2008).

Busko, Marlene and Désirée Lie. "Estrogen Relieves Psychotic Symptoms in Women with Schizophrenia CME." Medscape Medical News, Aug. 7, 2008, http://www.medscape.com/viewarticle/578772 (accessed Aug. 11, 2008).

Cascella, N. G. et al. "Prevalence of Celiac Disease and Gluten Sensitivity in the United States Clinical Antipsychotic Trials of Intervention Effectiveness Study Population." *Schizophrenia Bulletin*, June 2009.

Clark, Susan F. "Iron Deficiency Anemia." *Nutrition in Clinical Practice*, Vol. 23, No. 2, Apr–May 2008, pp. 128–141.

Cochen, V., et al. "Vivid dreams, hallucinations, psychosis and REM sleep in Guillain-Barré Syndrome." *Brain*, Vol. 128, Issue 11, Nov. 2005, pp. 2535–45.

Cohen, Dan, et al. "Hyperglycemia and Diabetes in Patients with Schizophrenia or Schizoaffective Disorders." *Diabetes Care*, Vol. 29, 2006, pp. 786–791, http://care.diabetesjournals.org/cgi/content/abstract/29/4/786 (accessed May 21, 2006).

Cohrs, S., et al. "The atypical antipsychotics olanzapine and quetiapine, but not haloperidol, reduce ACTH and cortisol secretion in healthy subjects." *Psychopharmacology*, Vol. 185, No. 1, Mar. 2006, pp. 11–18.

Conklin, L. S. and Oliva-Hemker, M. "Nutritional Considerations in Pediatric Inflammatory Bowel Disease." *Expert Review of Gastroenterology and Hepatology*, Vol. 4, No. 3, June 2010, pp. 305–317.

Corcoran, Cheryl and Dolores Malaspina. "The Relevance of the Stress Cascade to Schizophrenia." Psychiatry: Schizophrenia and Stress Cyberounds Web site, Mar. 5, 2001, http://www.cyberounds.com/conferences/psychiatry/conferences/0301/conference.htm (accessed May 7, 2001).

Correl, Christoph U. "Atypical Antipsychotics in Child and Adolescent Psychiatry: A Comparison of Adverse Events." Continuing Medical Education (CME), Apr. 25, 2006, http://www.docguide.com (accessed May 10, 2006).

Cutler, Paul. "Iron overload and psychiatric illness." *Canadian Journal of Psychiatry*, Vol. 39, No. 1, Feb. 1994, pp. 8–11.

"Daily Dose of Fish Oil May Keep Schizophrenia at Bay." *eBiology News*, Nov. 29, 2007, http://www.ebiologynews.com/4001.html (accessed Dec. 11, 2007).

Dohan, F. C. "Coeliac disease and schizophrenia." *British Medical Journal*, Vol. 3, No. 5870, July 7, 1973, pp. 51–52, http://www.pubmedcentral.nih.gov/articlerender.fcgi?tool=pmcentrez&artid=1587927 (accessed Nov. 13, 2008).

Emory University Press Release. "Study Focuses on Teens at Risk for Psychosis." Nov. 10, 2008, http://www.emory.edu/home/news/releases/2008/11/teens-at-risk-for-psychosis.html (accessed Nov. 13, 2008).

"Evidence of genetic overlap of schizophrenia and bipolar disorder." *American Journal of Medical Genetics Part B: Neuropsychiatry Genetics*, Sept. 8, 2005, pp. 54–60.

Froling, Joan. "Service Dog Tasks for Psychiatric Disabilities." http://www.iaadp.org/psd_tasks.html (accessed Sep. 10, 2001–Nov. 13, 2007).

Geoffroy, G. M., et al. "Daycare attendance, stress, and mental health." *Canadian Journal of Psychiatry*, Vol. 51, No. 9, Oct. 2006, pp. 607–615.

Geracioti Jr., Thomas D. "Identifying Hypothyroidism's Psychiatric Presentations." *Current Psychiatry Online*, Vol. 5, No. 11, Nov. 2006, http://www.currentpsychiatry.com/article_pages.asp?AID=4545 (accessed Jan. 15, 2007).

—. "Identifying Hyperthyroidism's Psychiatric Presentations." *Current Psychiatry Online*, Vol. 5, No. 12, Dec. 2006, http://www.currentpsychiatry.com/article_pages.asp?AID=4580 (accessed Jan. 15, 2007).

Goldberg, J. F. and C. L. Ernst. "Features associated with the delayed initiation of mood stabilizers at illness onset in bipolar disorder." The *Journal of Clinical Psychiatry*, Vol. 63, No. 11, Nov. 2002, pp. 985–991.

Gupta, B. K., et al. "Nasopharyngeal EEG recording in psychiatric patients." *Journal of Clinical Psychiatry*, Vol. 50, No. 7, July 1989, pp. 262–264.

Haman, Dorota Z. and Del B. Bottcher. "Home Water Quality and Safety." University of Florida, Florida Cooperative Extension Service, Circular 703, May 1986, http://edis.ifas.ufl.edu/pdffiles/AE/AE00900.pdf (accessed May 17, 2006).

Hellander, Martha. "Girls with Bipolar Disorder: Special Concerns." Child and Adolescent Bipolar Foundation e-bulletin, Sept. 29, 2004, http://healthyplace.com/communities/bipolar/children_girls.asp (accessed Oct. 1, 2004).

Hershey, A. D., et al. "Coenzyme Q10 deficiency and response to supplementation in pediatric and adolescent migraine." *Headache*, Vol. 47, No. 1, Jan. 2007, pp. 73–80.

Horrobin, D. F. "What should be done about schizophrenia?" *Journal of the Royal Society of Medicine (JRSM)*, Vol. 74, No. 3, March 1981, pp. 180–182, http://www.pubmedcentral.nih.gov/articlerender.fcgi?tool=pmcentrez&artid=1438286 (accessed Nov. 13, 2008).

"Iron Overload and Hemochromatosis: Detection and Diagnosis." http://www.cdc.gov/ncbddd/hemochromatosis/detection.htm (accessed July 20, 2007).

Johns Hopkins University Bloomberg School of Public Health News Center. "Celiac Disease Is a Risk Factor for Schizophrenia." Feb. 19, 2004, http://www.jhsph.edu/PublicHealthNews/Press_Releases/PR_2004/celiac_schizophrenia.html (accessed June 25, 2006).

Kalaydjian, A. E., et al. "The gluten connection: the association between schizophrenia and celiac disease." *Acta Psychiatrica Scandinavica*, Vol. 113, No. 2, Feb. 2006, pp. 82–90, abstract http://www.ncbi.nlm.nih.gov/pubmed/16423158?dopt=abstractplus (accessed Oct. 12, 2008).

Kemperman, R. F., et al. "Low essential fatty acid and B-vitamin status in a subgroup of patients with schizophrenia and its response to dietary supplementation." *Prostaglandins, Leukotrienes, and Essential Fatty Acids*, Vol. 74, No. 2, Feb. 2006, pp. 75–85. http://www.ncbi.nlm.nih.gov/ (accessed May 23, 2006).

Kowlessar, O. D., et al. "Abnormal Tryptophan Metabolism in Patients with Adult Celiac Disease, with Evidence for Deficiency of Vitamin B_6" *Journal of Clinical Investigation*, Vol. 43, No. 5, 1964, http://www.pubmedcentral.nih.gov/articlerender.fcgi?tool=pmcentrez&artid=2 89568 (accessed Nov. 13, 2008).

Kuitunen, M., M.D., et al. "Probiotics prevent IgE-associated allergy until age 5 years in cesarean-delivered children but not in the total cohort." *Journal of Allergy and Clinical Immunology*, Vol. 123, No. 2, Feb 2009, pp 335–341.

Layton, Lyndsey. "Chemical in Plastic Is Connected to Health Problems in Monkeys." *Washington Post*, Sept. 4, 2008, p. A02.

Lee, P. R., et al. "Prenatal Stress Generates Deficits in Rat Social Behavior: Reversal by Oxytocin." *Brain Research*, Vol. 1156, July 2, 2007, pp. 152–167.

Ludvigsson, J. F., et al. "Coeliac disease and risk of schizophrenia and other psychosis: a general population cohort study." *Scandinavian Journal of Gastroenterology*, Vol. 42, Issue 2, Feb. 2007, pp. 179–185.

Mancuso, Michelangelo, et al. "Autosomal dominant psychiatric disorders and mitochondrial DNA multiple deletions: Report of a family." *Journal of Affective Disorders*, Vol. 106, Issues 1–2, Feb. 2008, pp. 173–177.

McGinnis, Woody. "Pyroluria: Hidden Cause of Schizophrenia, Bipolar, Depression, and Anxiety Symptoms." May 21, 2004, http://www.alternativementalhealth.com/articles/pyroluria.htm (accessed Sep. 21, 2008).

NARSAD. "Scientists Find Genetic Factor in Stress Response Variability." Apr. 8, 2008, http://www.narsad.org/news/press/rg_2008/res2008-04-08.html (accessed May 12, 2008).

Nasrallah, Henry A. "Is Schizophrenia a Psychotic Disorder?" *Current Psychiatry Online*, Vol. 6, No. 12, Dec. 2007, http://www.currentpsychiatry.com (accessed Jan. 12, 2008).

Obreitan, et al. "Excitatory actions of GABA increase BDNF expression via a MAPK-CREB-dependent mechanism—a positive feedback circuit in developing neurons." *Journal of Neurophysiology*, Vol. 88, No. 2, Aug. 2002, pp. 1005–1015.

O'Neil, Jillian and Lawrie Powell. "Clinical Aspects of Hemochromatosis." *Seminars in Liver Disease*, Vol. 25, No. 4, Nov. 2005, pp. 381–391.

Overeem, S., et al. "Somatotropic axis in hypocretin-deficient narcoleptic humans: altered circadian distribution of GH-secretory events." *American Journal of Physiology: Endocrinology and Metabolism*, Vol. 284, No. 3, 2003, pp. 641–647.

Padmos, R. C., et al. "Discriminating Messenger RNA Signature for Bipolar Disorder Formed by an Aberrant Expression of Inflammatory Genes in

Monocytes." *Archives of General Psychiatry*, Vol. 65, No. 4, Apr. 2008, pp. 395–407.

Papadimitriou, George D., et al. "Rapid cycling bipolar disorder: biology and pathogenesis." *The International Journal of Neuropsychopharmacology*, Vol. 8, No. 2, June 2005, pp. 281–292.

Peres, M. F., et al. "Melatonin, 3 mg, is effective for migraine prevention." *Neurology*, Vol. 63, No. 4, Aug. 24, 2004, p. 757.

Perrin, M. A., et al. "Growth trajectory during life and risk of adult schizophrenia." *British Journal of Psychiatry*, Vol. 191, Dec. 2007, pp. 512–520.

Phelps, J. "Dark therapy for bipolar disorder using amber lenses for blue light blockade." *Medical Hypotheses*, Vol. 70, No. 2, 2008, pp. 224–229.

Prabakaran, S., et al. "Mitochondrial dysfunction in schizophrenia: evidence for compromised brain metabolism and oxidative stress." *Molecular Psychiatry*, Vol. 9, No. 7, July 2004, pp. 684–697.

Sapolsky, Robert and Yvette Sheline. "Depression and the Brain." *The Infinite Mind*, Apr. 23, 2006, Lichtenstein Creative Media, http://www.lcmedia.com (accessed Apr. 23, 2006).

Silverman, Linda Kreger (of the Gifted Development Center). "The Two-Edged Sword of Compensation: How the Gifted Cope with Learning Disabilities." *Uniquely Gifted: Identifying and Meeting the Needs of the Twice-Exceptional Student* (Ed. Kiesa Kay).

Smith, Stephen E. P., et al. "Maternal Immune Activation Alters Fetal Brain Development through Interleukin-6." *Journal of Neuroscience*, Vol. 27, No. 40, Oct. 3, 2007, pp. 10695–10702.

Swerdlow, N. R., et al. "Startle gating deficits in a large cohort of patients with schizophrenia: relationship to medications, symptoms, neurocognition, and level of function." *Archives of General Psychiatry*, Vol. 63, No. 12, Dec. 2006, pp. 1325–1335.

Terman, Michael and Jiuan Su Terman. "Controlled Trial of Naturalistic Dawn Simulation and Negative Air Ionization for Seasonal Affective Disorder." *The American Journal of Psychiatry*, Vol. 163, Dec. 2006, pp. 2126–2133.

Tierney, E., et al. "Abnormalities of cholesterol metabolism in autism spectrum disorders." *The American Journal of Medical Genetics, Part B: Neuropsychiatric Genetics*, Vol. 141B, No. 6, Sept. 5, 2006, pp. 666–668.

Tyzio, R., et al. "Maternal Oxytocin Triggers a Transient Inhibitory Switch in GABA Signaling in the Fetal Brain During Delivery." *Science*, Vol. 314, No. 5806, Dec. 15, 2006, pp. 1788–1792.

University of Guelph news release. "BPA Impairs Synapses Formation in Brain, New Study Finds." Sept. 3, 2008, http://www.uoguelph.ca/news/2008/09/bpa_impairs_syn.html (accessed Sep. 6, 2008).

Vaillancourt, C. and P. Boksa. "Birth insult alters dopamine-mediated behavior in a precocial species, the guinea pig. Implications for schizophrenia." *Neuropsychopharmacology*, Vol. 23, No. 6, Dec. 2000, pp. 654–666.

Van Winkel, Ruud, et al. "Screening for Diabetes and Other Metabolic Abnormalities in Patients with Schizophrenia and Schizoaffective Disorder:

Evaluation of Incidence and Screening Methods." *Journal of Clinical Psychiatry*, Vol. 67, No. 10, Oct. 2006, pp. 1493–1500.

Vliagoftis, H., et al. "Probiotics for the treatment of allergic rhinitis and asthma: systematic review of randomized controlled trials." *Annals of Allergy, Asthma, and Immunology*, Vol. 101, No. 6, Dec. 2008, pp. 570–579.

White, Randall F. "Mood Disorders at the Turn of the Century: An Expert Interview with Peter C. Whybrow, M.D." *Medscape Psychiatry & Mental Health*, May 19, 2005, http://www.medscape.com/viewarticle/503013 (accessed May 10, 2007).

Witmans, M. B. and V. G. Kirk. "Infancy Onset of Symptoms of Narcolepsy in a Child." *Clinical Pediatrics*, Vol. 41, No. 8, Oct. 2002, pp. 609–612.

Wolfson, Jeanie. "How a Psychiatric Service Dog Changed Our Lives." *International Association of Assistance Dog Partners* newsletter, Vol. 9, No. 4, 2004.

Yel, L., et al. "Thimerosal induces neuronal cell apoptosis by causing cytochrome c and apoptosis-inducing factor release from mitochondria." *International Journal of Molecular Medicine*, Vol. 16, No. 6, Dec. 2005, pp. 971–977.

Yoo, S., et al. "The Human Emotional Brain Without Sleep—A Prefrontal Amygdala Disconnect." *Current Biology*, Vol. 17, Oct. 23, 2007, pp. R877–R878.

Young, Emma. "Are bad sleeping habits driving us mad?" *New Scientist*, Feb 18, 2009, http://www.newscientist.com/article/mg20126962.100-are-bad-sleeping-habits-driving-us-mad.html (accessed Feb. 27, 2009).

Music, Poems

Cross, Keri, composer. "The Bells." Sept. 1, 1997.
—. "Running Through Time." Lyrics and music by Keri Cross, 1998.
Poe, Edgar Allan. "Annabel Lee." 1847.
—. "The Bells." 1849.

Index

9
911 call, 195

A
abdominal pain, 71
absence seizures. See seizures
acetylcholine, 306
acidosis, 245
ADHD, 78, 113, 145, 146, 163, 287, 338, 361
adrenal function, 371
adrenals, 283, 309, 315
adrenocorticotropic hormone (ACTH), 124, 291
Advair, 298
advance directive, 299
advocate, 121
agoraphobia, 193
akathisia, 203
alienation, 57, 157
allergies, 41, 46, 65, 83, 107, 245, 264
    metal, 47, 252
    propylene glycol, 104
alternative medicine, 352
amblyopia, 161
amenorrhea, 258, 283, 368
American with Disabilities Act (ADA), 280
amygdala, 124
Angiotensin II, 291
anosognosia, 298
anovulation, 258
anti-aging, 306, 323, 350
antibiotics, 26, 28, 36, 41
antihistamines, 36, 46, 160, 245, 264, 377
antileukotriene, 264
antioxidants, 115, 315, 324, 367, 375
anxiety, 187, 276, 279, 296, 350
anxiolytic, 151
aphasia, 183
assistance dogs. See service dogs
ataxia, 160, 183
attention surplus, 145
autism, 322
Autistic Spectrum Disorders (ASD), 123
autoimmune, 19, 27

B
bad days, 142, 157
bat mitzvah, 207
Benadryl (diphenhydramine HCl), 160, 187
benzodiazepine, 151
bioidentical hormone replacement, 340
bio-psycho-social model of treatment, 338
bipolar disorder, 163, 167
blood draws, 181
    phobia, 168
bone metabolism, 291, 372
Borna virus, 365
BPA. See plastics
braces, 252

C
calcium, 291, 320
car locks, 176
carnitine, 290, 375
catatonia, 206, 251
celiac disease, 318, 366
Cesarean section, 26, 27, 36
charting moods, sleep, symptoms, 30, 162, 211, 377
chicken pox, 27, 36, 327
Child and Adolescent Bipolar Foundation (CABF), 159, 257, 355
cholesterol, 291, 317
choline, 221, 290, 375
cholinergic urticaria, 264, 294
chronic fatigue syndrome, 305
Chronically Normal, 335
clonazepam, 187, 193
Clozapine, 191
co-enzyme Q10, 304, 324, 375
cognition, 251
cognitive behavior therapy (CBT), 233
cognitive impairment, 193, 203, 205, 251, 285, 294, 359, 368
cold
    abnormal feeling of, 157, 190
colic, 17, 28, 29, 31, 380
College
    Disability Support Services (DSS), 273
    Test accommodations, 273

Comprehensive Test of Basic Skills
    (CTBS), 207
constipation, 70
coping strategies, 232, 281
copper, 367
cortisol, 291, 313, 314, 315, 363, 366, 372
creativity, 117, 118, 140, 150
cross titration, 161
crying, 45, 86, 108, 111, 131, 144, 153
    wailing, 218
Cushing's syndrome, 366
cussing, 192, 194
cytokines, 328

D

dairy, 319
delayed menarche, 258, 261, 283
delirium, 65
delusions, 144
dessicated thyroid, 310
DHEA (dehydroepiandrosterone), 306, 315
Diagnostic and Statistical Manual of
    Mental Disorders (DSM IV), 19
diet, 304
Dispense As Written (DAW), 308
dopamine, 306
drug use, 231
dysmenorrhea, 262, 368
dysthymia, 163
dystonia, 160

E

ear infections, 41, 245
EEG, 207
electroencephalogram (EEG)
    Nasopharyngeal, 144
emotional
    meltdowns, 79, 84, 105, 111, 122, 163, 203, 270, 313, 328, 329
    regression, 190
    resilience. See resilience
EMPowerPlus. See micronutrients
encephalopathy, 322
endocrine
    dysfunction, 126
    symptoms, 259, 283, 359, 360
    tests, 359
epigenetics, 322, 328, 349
epilepsy, 144
essential fatty acids (EFAs), 115, 163, 239, 290

deficiency, 164
estrogen, 47, 48, 305, 306
extrapyramidal symptoms (EPS), 155, 241
    acute dystonia, 160

F

family psychoeducation, 74, 222, 339
Fasting Plasma Glucose Test (FPG), 373
fibromyalgia, 305
folate, 221, 317, 375
Follicle Stimulating Hormone (FSH), 124
food supplements, 304, 309
Fredericks, Robert, 287
Froling, Joan, 275, 276
functional medicine, 323
functional nutritional deficiency, 290, 317

G

gamma-aminobutyric acid (GABA), 27, 306, 323
generic, 308
gifted-LD, 100
gingivitis
    causes, 253
gluten, 317, 318, 319, 338, 345, 366
glycine, 221, 290
growth hormone, 42, 43, 124
Growth Hormone Stimulation Test
    (GHST), 370
growth pattern, 42
Guillain–Barré syndrome, 185

H

Haldol (haloperidol), 164, 191
hallucinations, 13, 18, 144, 145, 150, 153, 164, 181, 185, 189, 192, 197, 199, 203, 206, 207, 224, 230, 231, 232, 233, 236, 239, 240, 243, 246, 259, 261, 265, 269, 276, 281, 282, 285, 296, 303, 304, 305, 313, 316, 327, 337, 339, 341, 354, 355, 368, 377, 393
    as a side-effect, 66
    auditory, 185, 233, 275, 279, 303
    dealing with, 190, 199, 232, 233
    dismemberment, 152
    maggots, 157
    migraines, 249
    pain, 152, 184, 194
    prodromal, 303
    residual, 303
    tactile, 157, 194

visual, 233, 303
voices, 72, 73, 74, 151, 152, 153, 155, 160, 185, 186, 211, 231, 232, 303
hemochromatosis, 315, 367, 368
hives, 264
homebound instruction, 115
homework, 133, 142, 149, 180, 233, 244
   math, 98
Homocysteine, 367
hormone
   replacement, 303
hormone replacement, 305, 310, 315
hormones, 19, 26, 27, 37, 48, 124, 126, 127, 264, 284, 291, 303, 304, 306, 308, 309, 310, 313, 314, 315, 318, 320, 321, 322, 327, 340, 341, 347, 349, 362, 363, 368, 371, 380, 382
hunger, 186
Hydroxyzine (Atarax), 294
hyperlexia, 122
hypersomnia, 114
hyperthyroid, 292, 311, 359
hyperthyroidism
   psychiatric symptoms, 359
hypervigilance, 279
hypnogogic and hypnopompic hallucinations, 185
hypoglycemia, 186
hypogonadism, 368
hypomania, 149
hypopituitarism
   idiopathic, 315
hypothalamic-pituitary axis, 126
hypothalamic-pituitary hypothyroidism, 355
hypothalamic-pituitary-axis hypothyroidism, 308
hypothalamic-pituitary-thyroid axis
   feedback mechanism, 311
hypothalamus, 124, 163, 264, 311, 315
hypothyroidism, 283, 291, 300, 308, 360, 361, 362, 368
   psychiatric symptoms, 360
   tests, 361

I

Imitrex (sumatriptan), 250, 251
immune system, 306, 327
impaired fasting glucose, 373
impaired glucose tolerance, 373
independence, 147

inflammation, 28, 37, 113, 239, 252, 306, 313, 319, 328, 337
inositol, 323
insight, 335
insomnia, 286
integrative medicine, 221, 339, 346, 350
International Association of Assistance Dog Partners (IAADP), 275
invisible disabilities, 276
Iron, 368

K

Keratosis Polaris, 210
kindling theory, 145
   bipolar disorder, 308
Kleine-Levin syndrome, 259, 263, 287, 293, 327
Klonopin, 187, 193

L

light therapy, 186
limbic system, 123
lithium, 210, 249
   suicide, 249
   withdrawal, 249
lorazepam, 168
Lorenzo's Oil, 304
Luteinizing Hormone (LH), 124

M

magnesium, 320
manganese, 368
mania, 167
marijuana, 231
markers, 318
medical databases, 353
medical diagnostic software
   AI Expert Systems, 353
Medical Power of Attorney, 299
medications while sick, 245
melatonin, 221, 323, 324
meltdowns. See emotional meltdowns
menstruation, 258, 261, 283, 284, 303, 360
mercury, 368
metabolic syndrome, 373
methylmalonic acid, 367
micronutrients, 240, 241, 242, 290, 317, 377, 379
   discontinuation, 241
microsleeps, 286
migraine, 322

migraines, 113, 144, 183, 230, 246, 285, 294, 296, 304, 323, 324, 337
    auras, 249
    cigarette smoke, 247
    cluster headaches, 250
mitochondria, 70, 123, 221, 253, 290, 291, 304, 314, 321, 322, 323, 324, 325, 338, 349, 367, 375, 395
mitochondrial dysfunction, 367
MRI, 161

N

NADH dehydrogenase, 324
narcolepsy, 19, 30, 34, 285, 286, 291
National Alliance on Mental Illness (NAMI)
    Family-To-Family class, 222
    Visions for Tomorrow class, 248
neurohormones, 124, 349
neurological evaluation, 144
neurologist, 145
neuropsychiatric diagnosis, 365
neurosarcoidosis, 290
neurotransmitters, 306
neurotypical, 335
night terrors, 163
nightmares, 45, 79, 126, 151, 154, 157, 163, 183, 184, 186, 195, 197, 203, 206, 265, 277, 285, 313, 337, 339
    that don't stop, 184
    while awake, 185
nutrigenomic, 318
nutritional supplements, 242, 340, 377
    discontinuation, 241

O

obsessive-compulsive disorder (OCD), 131, 133, 272
    CBT, 104
occupational therapy, 100
omega-3 fatty acids. See essential fatty acids (EFAs)
OmegaBrite, 163
osteo-cranial manipulation, 285
osteopenia, 291
overdosed, 245
oxytocin, 27

P

P-5-P. See vitamin B6

pain sensitivity, 157
PANDAS, 368
panic attacks, 187, 276, 279, 296
pantothenic acid. See vitamin B5
paradoxical reaction, 193
parathyroid, 290
petechiae, 259
Phinergan (promethazine), 65
phthalates, 48
pituitary, 283, 291, 315
plastics, 48
Pleurisy, 113, 245
Pneumonia, 141, 245
Porphyria, 365
post-traumatic stress disorder (PTSD), 157, 166, 184, 206, 350, 368
pregnenolone, 315
prepulse inhibition (PPI), 33
probiotics, 28, 107, 345
progesterone, 291, 303, 306, 313, 321, 362
Prolactin (PRL), 124
propylene glycol, 104
Provigil (modafinil), 287, 293, 329
psychosis, 207
psychotic disorder-NOS, 181
pycnogenol, 115
pyridoxal. See vitamin B6
Pyroluria, 351, 367

R

rages, 85, 122, 163, 185
Random Plasma Glucose Test, 374
Rapid Eye Movement (REM), 285
recovery (in mental illness), 19, 20, 304
REM while awake, 185
remission, 331, 340, 346
reproductive hormones, 368
residential treatment center (RTC), 194
resilience, 92, 146, 269
resveratrol, 115
risk vs. benefit, 156, 195
Risperdal (risperidone), 106, 155, 191
    side-effects, 157, 159, 160

S

SAM-e, 221, 375
schizoaffective disorder, 167
schizophrenia, 73, 167
Scholastic Aptitude/Achievement Test (SAT), 271, 273

school
   absences, 115, 186, 245, 246, 259
   accommodations, 264
   distractibilty, 143
   fluctuation in abilities, 83, 204
   lost assignments, 244
   organization, 244
   while hospitalized, 179, 180
   seizures, 91, 113, 144, 161, 205, 207, 249, 251, 322, 325, 366
      complex partial, 206, 251
      temporal lobe, 251
self-harm, 108, 143
sensitivity to
   sound, 33
sensory gating deficit, 123
sensory integration (processing) disorder (SID/SPD), 71, 123
Seroquel (quetiapine), 191, 309
   titration, 191
   withdrawal, 330
serotonin, 306
service dogs, 233, 275
   etiquette, 280
   tasks, 275, 296
   trainer, 276, 279, 280, 281
sibling relationship, 44
side effects, 112, 145, 155, 161
   dystonia, 160
   hormonal, 155
   movement, 145, 155
sleep, 41, 105, 183, 327
sleep days, 159, 250, 287, 292, 294
sleep deprivation, 30, 210
sleep disorders, 185, 325, 338, 340, 341, 345, 357, 366
sleep disturbances in infancy
   colic, 29
   emotional sensitivity, 34
sleep episodes, 115, 259, 263, 293
sleep study, 19, 285, 286, 366
somatotropin, 306
St. John's Wort, 220
staring spells, 113, 251
statistics, 13, 15, 43, 258, 287, 335
stimulants, 145
stress, 147, 247, 294, 307
stress cascade, 146, 294
stress intolerance
   compensatory strategies, 69, 146
stretch marks (striae), 259, 288
Structural Ecology Workup, 288, 369
suicidal, 195, 219

Sunday school, 56, 75, 159, 247

T

tardive dyskinesia, 191
taurine, 323
temperature
   sensitivity, 126
temperature dysregulation, 162
temperature fluctuation, 41, 189
testing for learning disabilities, 271
testing protocols, 348, 365
testosterone, 291, 306, 313, 315, 363
tests, 290, 292
therapy, 132
   cognitive behavior therapy (CBT), 233
   expressive arts, 87, 129
   group therapy, 180
   parental, 153, 191
   speech, 203
   talk, 87
thimerosal, 122, 253
thyroid, 161, 259, 283, 291, 292, 294, 303, 306, 307, 308, 309, 310, 311, 313, 315, 321, 322, 330, 336, 345, 348, 355, 357, 359, 360, 361, 362, 363, 368, 371
   hormones, 311
   tests, 312, 361
thyroid disorder, 70, 307
thyroid hormone, 291
thyroid stimulating hormone (TSH), 124, 308, 310, 311, 348, 360, 363, 370
tics, 39, 80, 94, 101, 103, 104, 105, 106, 110, 112, 119, 135, 140, 142, 145, 155, 203, 269, 285, 287, 341, 378
   CBT, 104
   fatigue, 104
   motor tics, 104
   mouth irritations, 104
   treatment, 106
   vocal, 103
   vocal tics, 159
titration, 156, 161
Topamax (topiramate), 250, 251, 325, 327, 333
   humor, 251
Tourette syndrome, 17, 101, 103, 105, 106, 121, 143, 146, 149, 156, 273, 287, 291
toxins, 36, 37, 322, 349
Truehope. See micronutrients
tryptophan, 221, 330
TSH Releasing Hormone (TRH), 311
Turner syndrome, 43, 161, 283

U

ultradian cycling, 158, 191, 192

V

vaccinations, 122, 253
Valerian, 323
verbal development, 44
viral infections, 27, 112
vision, 148, 322
    changes, 112, 210
    prism reading glasses, 148
    problems, 142
    testing, 148
vitamin B, 290
    MTHFR, 319
vitamin B12, 221, 290, 317, 367, 375
    deficiency, 290
vitamin B3, 367
vitamin B5, 314
vitamin B6, 221, 367, 375
vitamin C, 315
vitamin D, 291, 321
vitamin/mineral toxicity or deficiency, 367

voice changes, 73, 157, 190, 209, 211

W

wakeful dreams, 185
weight gain, 187
Wellbutrin
    seizures, 252
Wellbutrin (bupropion), 203, 204, 207, 220, 240, 309, 329, 377
white noise, 32
writing problems, 244, 272
    accommodations, 293
    compensation, 141
    overcoming, 75, 86, 244, 245
    stress, 264

Z

zinc, 367
Zoloft (sertraline), 110, 112
Zomig (zolmitriptan), 251
Zyprexa (olanzapine), 161
    hunger, 186
    itchiness, 187
    side effects, 161

A Note from Keri

When my mother first asked me if I would be okay with her writing this book, my response consisted of a shrug and an offhand "Umm... yeah, sure. That's cool." My only defense for this less-than-eloquent response is that I was 16, entirely more concerned with boys and starting college than what seemed no more than a random parental whim. It took several years for the ideas that were rattling around inside my mom's skull to come together into the manuscript you have, presumably, just read, which gave me ample time to think about just how important this book, and its creation, really is.

If I were to write a book it would be dedicated to my mother. I'm not writing a book though, just this note! Still, I'd like to say a little about her, a woman I've seen go above and beyond the norm my entire life, yet persist in saying she only did what any mother would have. I know better. Without such an incredible champion, I never would have made it to where I am today—going out with friends, enjoying hobbies, working, volunteering, and going to school full-time. In a year I'll graduate with a B.S. in dietetics to begin a career I'm really excited about. As a dietitian I may be able to help prevent situations like mine or to assist those already mired in such situations get out of them.

But, as I am so often wont to do, I digress!

People have asked how I feel about so much of my life story—the good times, the bad times, especially the painful and ugly times—being out there for anyone to read. It's as if they're shocked I don't want to keep it all quiet. Sure, I value my privacy, but if my story helps even one person or makes even one doctor take a second glance at how he or she does things, giving up some of that privacy will be worth it a hundred times over.

All doctors are familiar with the mantra of Primum non nocere—first, do no harm. Often, this directive seems to be interpreted as "Don't make things worse." But making things worse is subjective. For example, medicating away symptoms is an improvement, right? Maybe, maybe not... Taking away the warning flags doesn't make the problem go away; it only allows it to be ignored. When symptoms are masked by medication, the cause is allowed to run rampant. As a result, while no self-respecting doctor would admit to ignoring the problems of his or her patients, this is exactly what many of them are doing.

I don't blame the doctors for everything. And that's important. They are only human, full of flaws and as easily exhausted by the big picture as the rest of us. To expect them to do no harm—in other words, to be infallible—is perhaps unfair. A better mantra, for doctors and patients alike, would be this: "If it doesn't seem right, question it." My psychiatrist used to say, "When you hear hoofbeats, think horses, not zebras." In other words, look for the most straightforward answer first. But the human body is anything but straightforward. It's fine to be looking for horses, but it's also wise to keep an eye out for zebras. And if, out of the corner of your eye, you see something that looks like a unicorn, don't be too quick to dismiss the possibility.

About the Author

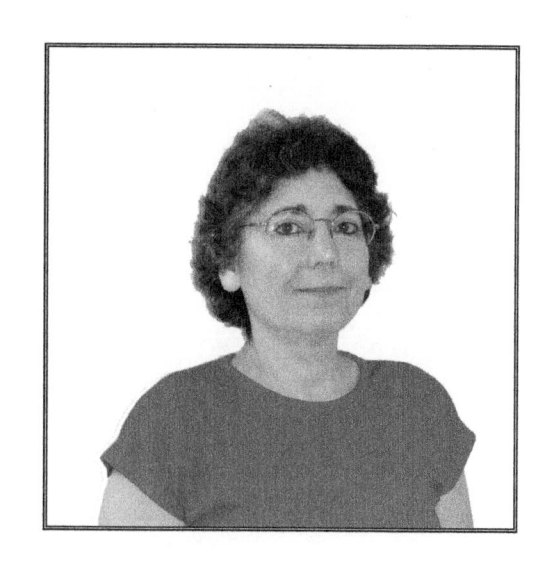

Jeanie Wolfson was raised in the U.S.A. and in Central America.

She received her Bachelor of Science in Zoology from the University of Florida followed by graduate studies in biology at the University of Kentucky before receiving her Master of Science from the college of engineering there. She worked for 22 years at IBM while teaching on the side.

In the last decade, she has been writing science-based news article summaries and blog entries, teaching, and volunteering for non-profit organizations such the Child and Adolescent Bipolar Foundation (CABF), a schizophrenia site, and in support group leadership and educator roles with the National Alliance on Mental Illness (NAMI). Since more knowledge is continually needed in today's world, she also has occasionally dabbled in extra post-graduate studies in education at the University of Kentucky and technical studies at Spencerian college.

But to her daughter Keri, she's just the smart mommy who never gave up on her, and helped her get better.